i

ii

The Great Cholesterol Con

Why Everything You've Been Told About Cholesterol, Diet and Heart Disease is Wrong!

Anthony Colpo

iv

Second edition, revised and updated.

© Anthony Colpo, 2006.

ISBN 978-1-4303-0933-8

To order additional copies of this book, please visit www.Lulu.com

Medical Disclaimer

The contents of this book are presented for information purposes only and are not intended as medical advice, nor to replace the advice of a physician or other health care professional. Anyone wishing to embark on any dietary, drug, exercise or lifestyle change for the purpose of preventing or treating a disease or health condition should first consult with, and seek clearance and guidance from, a competent health care professional.

The information in this book should not be construed as specific advice; it is a review of the available scientific and empirical evidence. It is presented for the sole purpose of stimulating awareness and further investigation of important information that has received woefully inadequate attention from mainstream providers of health and nutrition information.

Any individual wishing to apply the information in this book for the purposes of improving their own health should not do so without first reviewing the scientific references cited and consulting with a qualified medical practitioner. All patients need to be treated in an individual manner by their personal medical advisors.

The decision to utilize any information in this book is ultimately at the sole discretion of the reader, who assumes full responsibility for any and all consequences arising from such a decision. The author and publisher shall remain free of any fault, liability or responsibility for any loss or harm, whether real or perceived, resulting from use of information in this book.

If the above conditions are not acceptable to the reader, he/she should return this book immediately to the place of purchase for a refund.

Financial Disclosure

The author wishes to make it perfectly clear that he does not, and never has, received any form of financial assistance from industry groups that may stand to benefit from the information presented in this book. This includes those from the meat, egg, dairy, nutritional supplement, food, beverage, drug, and agriculture industries. The author does not hold, trade or speculate in the stock of companies whose financial status or share price could potentially be affected by the information presented in this book.

The author is a certified fitness professional who has worked in the capacity of both salaried fitness instructor and freelance personal fitness consultant. The author does not sell food products, nutritional supplements, medical apparatus or fitness equipment.

vi

Dedicated to my late father Peter Colpo, who might still be alive had the information in this book been available to him after his first heart attack in 1990.

Contents

Acknowledgements

The publication of this book would not have been possible without the valued insight, help and encouragement of a number of very special individuals. Foremost among these is Dr. Uffe Ravnskov, M.D., Ph.D., author of the groundbreaking *The Cholesterol Myths: Exposing the Fallacy that Saturated Fat and Cholesterol Cause Heart Disease*. Uffe's book was nothing short of a revelatory experience for me, one that ignited my own desire to conduct a thorough investigation into the cholesterol theory of heart disease. I am most grateful to Uffe for his valued advice and warm praise for my own writing and research efforts.

Helping me along my investigative path were the research and writings of numerous other individuals including, but not limited to, Duane Graveline, M.D., MPH, Mary Enig, Ph.D., Sally Fallon, George V. Mann, Sc.D., M.D., the late Russell L. Smith, Ph.D., and the late John Yudkin, M.D. All of these individuals have my utmost admiration and respect for their willingness to question and criticize faulty paradigms already accepted as gospel truth by their peers. By publishing their contrarian findings, these individuals risked the alienation, derision and financial disadvantages that can arise from speaking out against the status quo--a status quo propagated by extremely powerful vested interests. Thankfully, the risk of ruffling some very well connected feathers was of less concern to them than their allegiance to the truth and to public health.

A huge thank you is owed to Anna Dimasi, who did a terrific job of putting together the cover design for this book at short notice.

Last but definitely not least, I am deeply indebted to my wonderful, selfless mother Eleonora for her never-ending love and encouragement, and for adding to her already long list of known talents by proving to be a valuable research assistant. During the research for this book there were a number of key scientific papers that I could not find in the Melbourne libraries I frequented. Mum's readiness to hunt down and retrieve, at short notice, many of these papers from the well-stocked medical libraries of Adelaide was invaluable, and allowed the writing of this book to continue at a relatively smooth pace.

x

Foreword

The assertion that animal fat and high cholesterol cause atherosclerosis and coronary heart disease, known as the 'lipid hypothesis', is probably one of the greatest and most harmful misconceptions in the history of medicine. As a result of this hypothesis, millions of people around the world have made drastic changes to their eating habits and exposed themselves to the many well-documented side effects of cholesterol-lowering drugs. Their efforts have been almost entirely in vain.

An endless stream of studies, published in renowned medical journals, has shown that the anti-cholesterol campaign is not based on scientific evidence, yet it continues to flourish. It is exceedingly difficult to abandon a hypothesis when large numbers of supporting scientists are guaranteed generous financial support from the incredibly prosperous and powerful food and drug producers. Instead, there is great incentive to ignore contradictory studies or misquote them as if they were in fact supportive, which is just what many scientists in this area have done. Most doctors and members of the public, who rarely examine these studies for themselves, remain blissfully unaware of the true facts concerning cholesterol, diet and heart disease.

For decades, a steady procession of concerned, critical researchers has tried to inform the rest of the scientific community and the public about the many fallacies of the diet-heart idea, but with little success. In recent years, however, an increasing proportion of the public has embraced high-fat/low-carbohydrate diets, with their subsequent positive experiences on these diets stimulating an increased scepticism towards the low fat paradigm. Concern is also mounting with each passing day over the ill effects of widely prescribed cholesterol-lowering drugs, the aggressively promoted cash cows of the pharmaceutical industry. The time is ripe, therefore, for an able commentator to demonstrate to the public in no uncertain terms that the lipid hypothesis is scientifically invalid, and why it is so dangerous.

Anthony Colpo is just such a person.

In this timely and urgently needed book, Colpo starts by pointing out the many contradictions inherent in the lipid hypothesis. Meticulously, he dissects the numerous fallacies of the anti-cholesterol campaigners and highlights their blatant misuse of statistics. Colpo presents the reader with numerous examples of how these campaigners have misleadingly presented insignificant findings as 'strong evidence' and kept quiet or explained away any finding that runs counter to their pet hypothesis.

Colpo doesn't stop there. After having thoroughly demolished the cholesterol hypothesis, he tells the reader what really matters. One of the truly sad effects of the preoccupation with the reigning diet-heart idea is that progress in the search for the real causes of atherosclerosis and cardiovascular disease has been retarded. In his book, Colpo reviews the most important theories; the harmful effects of inactivity and stress, the dangers associated with high blood sugar, nutrient imbalances, homocysteine, trans fats and smoking, the intriguing question about the influence of too much iron and the fascinating research that points to infections as the initiator of arterial damage. Most important of all, Colpo has many suggestions as to how we can improve our chances of living to a ripe old age and maintaining good health without using expensive and dangerous drugs. He tells us about the benefits of vitamins, antioxidants, exercise, stress avoidance and good food. He explains in clear, easy-to-understand terms what exactly constitutes healthful eating and why.

If you are thinking that Colpo is just another guru peddling unsubstantiated claims about health and disease, you are wrong. The most amazing thing about this book's author is that, although he lacks a formal university education, his writing bears witness of an analytic and critical mind far superior to that of most doctors and medical researchers. And as a true scientist, Colpo gives you a chance to question his conclusions. All of them are based on thorough studies of the medical literature to which he refers. If you find something hard to believe, you can go to a medical library with the relevant references (there are over 1400!) and check for yourself.

Uffe Ravnskov, MD, PhD.
Independent researcher, spokesman for The International Network of Cholesterol Skeptics (www.thincs.org) and author of *The Cholesterol Myths: Exposing the Fallacy that Saturated Fat and Cholesterol Cause Heart Disease.*

Foreword

For over thirty years, the anti-fat, anti-cholesterol paradigm has formed the cornerstone of heart disease prevention policy the world over. I recall clearly, as a medical graduate in 1955, the first rumblings of the cholesterol juggernaut. I remember vividly the novelty and newness of this fledgling theory, and just how quickly it ascended to its present-day exalted status. As the cholesterol tsunami proceeded to sweep over America and subsequently the rest of the world, my colleagues and I rode happily along. We strove to keep our blood cholesterol levels under control by eating low-fat diets, and enthusiastically admonished our patients to do the same. When the first inklings of the Atkins diet surfaced in the media in the early seventies, we heartily laughed at the absurd concept of a liberal-fat, liberal-protein diet. When cholesterol-lowering medicines hit the market around the same time, we wasted no time in prescribing them to patients with elevated cholesterol levels. Like one giant collective sponge, we doctors readily soaked up the anti-cholesterol propaganda, so easily brainwashed by the powers that be.

Because of my unswerving belief in the cholesterol theory, I offered no protest in 1990 when my medical colleagues at NASA instructed me to begin taking the cholesterol-lowering drug Lipitor. After commencing this popular statin drug, I twice experienced an unsettling form of memory loss known as transient global amnesia (TGA). This rare phenomenon can last anywhere from fifteen minutes to twelve hours, in which time sufferers fail to recognize familiar surroundings and even their own families, often becoming disorientated and confused. In the worst of my two TGA episodes associated with Lipitor use, my memory loss extended for twelve terrible hours and transported me all the way back to my high school days. During that interval, my entire adult life had been eradicated and I had no awareness of my marriage and four children, my medical studies, nor my adventure-filled career with NASA.

Without exception, all the medical professionals I consulted with refused point blank to even consider the idea that Lipitor had anything to do with my memory loss. Unable to obtain any help from my doctors, and with no other feasible explanation for my TGA, I began my own search for the facts. I didn't know it then, but this search would turn into a remarkable journey, one which would see my story reported in media outlets around the world. I would eventually find out that TGA had befallen hundreds of other patients taking cholesterol-lowering statin drugs. During this time, I would also witness the seminal acknowledgement of statin-induced memory loss in the scientific literature. As a result of my extensive research into the relationship between cholesterol and cognition, I came to realize that cholesterol was in no way the heinous foe we had been led to believe it was. Instead, I realized that cholesterol was the most important substance within our bodies, a substance without which life as we know it would simply cease to exist. That billions of dollars have been spent in an all-out war on a substance that is so fundamentally important to our health is undoubtedly one of the great scientific travesties of our era.

The experiences that led Anthony Colpo to write the book you presently hold in your hands are remarkably similar to those of my own. Like myself, Colpo had fallen hopelessly for the low-cholesterol paradigm, with its golden promise of improved health and freedom from heart disease. Like myself, he was eventually jolted into reality when this baseless paradigm exerted unwelcome and harmful effects upon his health.

In *The Great Cholesterol Con: Why Everything You've Been Told About Cholesterol, Diet and Heart Disease is Wrong!*, Anthony Colpo presents a damning exposé of one of modern medicine's most deeply-held paradigms. With merciless logic and an unapologetic presentation of the cold, hard facts-- facts that the reigning health orthodoxy would rather you did not hear--he thoroughly destroys the claim that elevated blood cholesterol and dietary saturated fats cause coronary heart disease. Citing data from over fourteen hundred published studies, Colpo delivers blow after blow to the cholesterol theory, exposing it for the unscientific myth that it is.

Colpo does not just limit his efforts to destroying the cholesterol theory. He is well aware that medicine's overwhelming focus on cholesterol and saturated fats has given rise to a most regrettable consequence--the diversion of valuable scientific attention and precious research funds away from the factors that really do cause heart disease. One shudders to think how many lost lives could otherwise been saved had the medical establishment not been so obsessed with the mythical cholesterol bogeyman.

The greater part of Colpo's book is devoted to informing readers what really does cause coronary heart disease, and what can be done to halt the march of this insidious killer. Refreshingly, the preventive measures outlined by Colpo are not based on preconceived opinion, dogma, politics, or vested financial considerations---as is so much of popular health advice--but on data obtained from tightly controlled clinical research.

Colpo is a truly independent commentator who has pieced together the most thorough, extensive and up-to-date critique of the anti-cholesterol phenomenon I have ever read. I wholeheartedly urge you to read *The Great Cholesterol Con* from cover to cover--it could well be your life that is saved by the valuable information gracing the pages of this long overdue book.

Duane Graveline, M.D., MPH.
Former astronaut, NASA physician, author of *Lipitor: Thief of Memory* and *Statin Drugs, Side Effects and the Misguided War on Cholesterol.*

Introduction

"It seems to be a constant throughout history: In every period, people believed things that were just ridiculous, and believed them so strongly that you would have gotten in terrible trouble for saying otherwise. Is our time any different? To anyone who has read any amount of history, the answer is almost certainly no."
Paul Graham

The book that you hold in your hands contains information that could quite literally save your life. For it to achieve this goal, however, will depend on your willingness to consider an explanation for heart disease that is very different from the one promulgated by governmental and private health officials. These groups would have us believe that the primary cause of coronary heart disease (CHD) is elevated blood cholesterol. Furthermore, because saturated fat has demonstrated an ability in clinical studies to raise blood cholesterol concentrations, health authorities insist that saturated fat itself is a major cause of CHD. This overly simplistic paradigm has been used to cajole millions of people the world over into consuming low-fat diets and to commence therapy with cholesterol-lowering drugs.

What mainstream health officials have not been so quick to point out is that, despite this massive offensive against saturated fat and cholesterol, the incidence of coronary heart disease has not declined over the past forty years. In *The Great Cholesterol Con: Why Everything You've Been Told About Cholesterol, Diet and Heart Disease is Wrong!* you will learn that:

- A massive volume of scientific literature proves that heart disease is *not* caused by saturated fat *nor* by elevated blood cholesterol levels.
- Despite having no basis in scientific fact, the anti-cholesterol/anti-saturated fat paradigm continues to be promoted for reasons *other* than the welfare of the general public.
- Many of the dietary recommendations made by health and nutrition 'experts' to reduce heart disease have actually been shown in animal and human studies to *increase* heart disease, cancer, diabetes and obesity!

The above may be difficult for many readers to fathom initially, but after reading this book they will have no doubt the cholesterol-CHD paradigm is, as University of Vanderbilt Professor George Mann stated, *"the public health diversion of this century . . . the greatest scam in the history of medicine."*

Rude Awakening

The seeds of my own personal interest in the charade that constitutes modern CHD prevention policy were sewn back in 1989 at the tender age of twenty-one, when a blood work-up revealed my cholesterol level to be 213mg/dl. The physician who ordered these tests solemnly warned that such a blood cholesterol concentration placed me at 'moderate risk' of future heart disease, and made it clear that this 'elevated' reading had to be reduced.

Telling a healthy young man of twenty-one that he harbors an increased susceptibility to heart disease on the basis of a single test of an essential blood lipid is nothing short of absurd. Unfortunately, I didn't know this back then. Alarmed by this alleged threat to my health, I began religiously following a low-fat, high-carbohydrate diet. I ate only the leanest meats and fish and, in keeping with advice given to highly active athletes, I began consuming large amounts of 'healthy' complex carbohydrate foods. Almost without exception, mainstream 'experts' were adamant that such an eating pattern would greatly reduce the incidence of heart disease.

It was in 1996 that I began to realize these health authorities had gotten it seriously wrong. Despite my 'wholesome' diet and daily strenuous exercise, my blood pressure had risen from 110/65, a reading characteristic of highly conditioned athletes, to an elevated 130/90. Instead of the lean, athletic look to which I had become accustomed, my physique started to become increasingly smooth and bloated. My digestive function began to deteriorate dramatically, with my stomach often feeling heavy, gaseous and distended after meals. I developed a surprisingly long list of irreversible food sensitivities, and frequently felt tired and fatigued. My fasting blood glucose level was below the normal range, indicative of reactive hypoglycemia--a manifestation of low blood sugar caused by the consumption of too many carbohydrates.

Ironically, the elevated blood pressure and disturbed blood sugar metabolism precipitated by my low-fat, high-carbohydrate diet *increased* my risk of the very thing I had sought to avoid, the very ailment that had claimed my father's life at only fifty-five years of age: *heart disease!*

This extremely disheartening revelation was the catalyst for an extended period of self-experimentation, in which I anxiously tried a number of highly touted popular diets. It was only after settling into a high-fat, high-protein, low-carbohydrate eating plan--the exact opposite of that recommended by most health authorities--that I was able to attenuate the negative changes bought about by years of high-carbohydrate eating. My blood pressure and glycemic control finally returned to normal levels, while my digestive function, mental focus, energy levels and overall sense of well being improved dramatically.

This seemingly paradoxical experience caused me to question everything I had ever learnt about nutrition. I became adamant in wanting to know why the revered low-fat paradigm had failed me, while a diet in which the bulk of calories were obtained from supposedly 'dangerous' animal fats made me feel better than I had in a long, long time.

Rather than simply take for granted the existence of data showing saturated fat to be harmful--as does so much of the public, medical and research communities--I became insistent on viewing this data for myself. My burning desire for the unadulterated facts drove me head first into an intensive search of the medical literature.

What I subsequently discovered truly astounded me:

- Of the numerous controlled clinical trials examining dietary interventions for heart disease prevention, *none* had ever demonstrated a beneficial effect of saturated fat restriction!
- Of the twenty-six long-term studies monitoring selected populations for the occurrence of heart disease, only four were able to demonstrate even *desperately weak* associations between saturated fat and heart disease!
- Numerous populations consuming high amounts of saturated fat have been observed to enjoy extremely low rates of heart disease. These populations have been consistently ignored by promoters of the anti-fat/cholesterol theory.
- A staggering amount of evidence indicates that by lowering their cholesterol, many people will *worsen* their physical and mental health and *increase* their risk of dying prematurely!

Most people would be truly amazed at just how little evidence exists in support of the cholesterol paradigm--the same paradigm that has firmly entrenched itself as a central pillar of modern-day health policy.

How Can We Really Prevent Heart Disease?

The greatest tragedy emanating from the medical establishment's myopic obsession with saturated fat and cholesterol is that the dietary and lifestyle factors that do increase the risk of heart disease have remained neglected or even completely ignored. As a result, the massive amounts of money and scientific manpower that have been poured into the fight against heart disease have so far completely failed to yield any cure for this most common of killers. Despite almost half a century of intense research, the indisputable fact is that heart disease is still the industrialized world's number one killer and occurs with the same frequency as fifty years ago. Millions of precious lives that could have been saved have been lost.

This book, therefore, seeks not just to highlight the falsity of the cholesterol hypothesis, but to inform readers as to what really does contribute to heart disease and what they can do to prevent it. *The Great Cholesterol Con* reveals the factors that scientists have shown to directly contribute to heart disease, and discusses others that are rapidly emerging as potential culprits. *The Great Cholesterol Con* describes practical and easily implemented steps that can help neutralize each of these potentially deadly assailants of cardiovascular health.

This book, in short, has been written for those who wish to learn the true facts about heart disease. In Section One, readers will learn about the origins of the cholesterol myth and why it completely lacks any foundation in scientific reality. Section Two discusses the dietary and lifestyle factors that have either been strongly implicated or clearly shown to cause heart disease, while Section Three shows how we can all immediately set about to significantly lower our risk of ever experiencing a cardiovascular crisis.

Good health is the foundation upon which we build our entire lives. To this author, uncovering little known facts that facilitate major improvements in wellbeing is like unearthing hidden treasure; it is one of the most liberating and satisfying sensations he has ever known. It is my sincerest wish that readers gain as much from reading this book as I did researching and writing it.

Join me now, as I explain why modern-day heart disease prevention policy has been built around a big, fat lie!

Anthony Colpo,
Melbourne, Australia,
February, 2006.

SECTION ONE
Why Saturated Fat And Cholesterol Do Not Cause Heart Disease.

Chapter 1

"A lie told often enough becomes the truth"
Lenin

The Big Fat Lie

Why claims of a coronary heart disease 'epidemic' caused by saturated fat and cholesterol are completely false.

Over the last forty years, billions of dollars have been allocated to research examining the link between saturated fat, cholesterol and heart disease. Despite the staggering amounts of money and time that have been poured into this undertaking, no direct role for these substances in the causation of cardiovascular disease has ever been established. The saturated fat and cholesterol hypothesis remains just that--a hypothesis.

As you shall learn throughout this book, there exists a massive volume of scientific evidence that completely absolves dietary cholesterol, saturated fat, and elevated blood cholesterol of any harmful role in heart disease. This evidence does not stem from a small group of axe-grinding fringe lunatic researchers; some of the most damning evidence against the mainstream anti-cholesterol dogma comes from research that has actually been funded and conducted by the mainstream itself.

Despite the fact that this contradictory research has been published in prestigious, peer-reviewed medical journals, and despite the complete failure of the massive low-fat, anti-cholesterol campaign to lower the overall incidence of heart disease, the cholesterol/saturated fat theory of coronary disease enjoys almost unanimous acceptance among health authorities. These are the same 'experts' that most of us look to for credible, scientifically-sound advice on matters pertaining to diet and health; the same experts who design nutrition guidelines, who tell us whether a particular food is 'heart-healthy' or harmful, and who set the prescribing guidelines for cholesterol-lowering drugs.

The Decline in Heart Disease that Never Was

It is these same authorities who repeatedly tell us that the death rate from coronary heart disease (CHD) climbed rapidly during the twentieth century, reached a peak in the late 1960's, then began a gradual decline that continues to this day. The rise in CHD mortality, so the story goes, was primarily a result of America's predilection for fatty foods--especially those high in 'artery-clogging' saturated fats. While the increase in CHD has been attributed to the nation's gluttony, the subsequent fall in heart disease mortality was, allegedly, a direct result of public awareness campaigns that steered people away from saturated fats and towards 'healthy' low-fat foods. These promotional efforts lowered the population's blood cholesterol and blood pressure levels, reduced the rate of smoking, and provided a shining example of how both government and private health agencies could work together in harmony and save millions of lives in the process.

That is the official version of events. It is, quite frankly, a self-serving fantasy.

It is only natural that health authorities would like us to believe that they were the prime movers behind any drop in CHD, because they have spent astounding amounts of our money researching and promoting dietary measures purported to fight this ubiquitous killer. The National Institutes of Health, the government's foremost diet and medical research agency, is without question the world's biggest spender on diet-heart disease research. The NIH has fervently spent well in excess of a *billion* taxpayer dollars trying to implicate saturated fat and cholesterol in the causation of heart disease, so far without any success whatsoever.

The American Heart Association (AHA), the first prominent health organization to officially embrace the lipid hypothesis, is an incorporated entity with assets totaling over one *billion* dollars and revenue that exceeds 650 million dollars per year(1). Of this, 540 million dollars is derived from public support, while another 115 million dollars is earned through activities that include the sale of educational materials and the lucrative 'heart check' program. The latter is a licensing agreement in which food manufacturers can capitalize on the AHA's 'credibility' by paying a first-year fee of $7,500 per product, and a subsequent annual renewal fee of $4,500 per year. This permits them to display the Association's logo on their product labels and to market their wares as 'heart healthy'(2). Despite its 'non-profit' status, top-level executives at the AHA receive six-figure salaries that would be the envy of many CEOs heading for-profit firms; during the 2005 fiscal year, the AHA's CEO, M. Cass Wheeler, received a hefty $656,608 in compensation. Remuneration to the AHA's five Vice-Presidents ranged from $249,235 to $414,928(3).

Clearly, fighting CHD is big business. And there is nothing worse for business than the realization by customers that one's products and services are ineffective. Imagine the potential financial repercussions for an organization that has invested heavily in a product or service of questionable worth, that has unwisely promoted the new offering with unbridled enthusiasm, and has begun to draw criticism from some quarters that it acted prematurely. To compound this organization's woes, published scientific findings have emerged which strongly suggest these critics are correct. Imagine further that this entity has no foreseeable way of improving upon this product or service. Impending doom, in terms of prestige and financial loss, is a very real possibility--unless of course, the entity in question can prevent the paying public from ever discovering that there was anything wrong with its offering in the first instance.

This is the exact situation in which promoters of the saturated fat and cholesterol theory of CHD have found themselves for the last four decades. Despite massive propaganda efforts to convince the medical profession and public alike of the validity of their theory, numerous independent commentators over the years have questioned its scientific tenability. In order to counter such concerns, the reigning health orthodoxy has formulated several key arguments that have been repeated with such prolific frequency they are now deeply ingrained in the public psyche. As a result, they have come to be accepted by much of the population as self-evident facts.

The notion that increasing saturated fat consumption precipitated an 'epidemic' of CHD, and that the low-fat, anti-cholesterol campaign has played a major role in reversing this epidemic, is one such 'fact'. The ubiquity of this myth is sad testimony to the ease with which so many of us uncritically accept the information presented to us from authoritative-sounding figures. It can readily be disrobed using national vital statistics data freely available to anyone with an internet connection.

The Real Story Behind the Rise and Fall of CHD

Before we begin to dismantle the 'Big Fat Lie', it is important to define the difference between coronary and non-coronary heart disease. When we talk of CHD, also known as *ischemic heart disease*, we are referring to the blockage of a coronary artery that impairs or completely blocks blood flow to the heart. This blockage can be caused by the build-up of arterial plaque, the formation of blood clots, or arterial spasm, and if severe enough causes a heart attack, also referred to as a *myocardial infarction.*

Non-CHD heart stoppage is most commonly referred to as *heart failure,* and can occur from such conditions as *cardiac arrhythmia, cardiomyopathy, endocarditis, myocarditis* and *pericarditis*. It is CHD that is invariably the focus of diet-heart theories, for heart failure has long been attributed mostly to non-dietary causes such as viral infection, aging, and genetic defects of the heart.

Having made this vital distinction, let us now cast our eyes upon Figure 1a. It presents the death rate from CHD, non-coronary heart disease and all heart conditions combined, for the period 1900-1993. When we glance at the plotted line for CHD, we see that it does indeed travel an upward path throughout most

Figure 1a. Unadjusted CHD, all heart disease except CHD, and all heart disease mortality between 1900-1993.

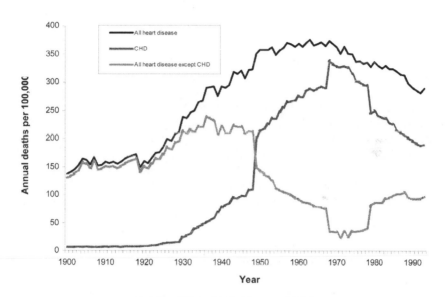

Adapted from: US National Vital Statistics, years 1900-1993. Available online:
Available online: http://www.cdc.gov/nchs/products/pubs/pubd/vsus/vsus.htm

of the twentieth century, sometimes swinging violently skyward, before reversing direction in 1968.

The death rates depicted in Figure 1a are derived from the National Center for Health Statistics, and are based on the International Classification of Diseases (ICD). The ICD provides a standardized system for classifying causes of death in an effort to ensure uniformity of reporting amongst different regions and nations. The first ICD came into effect in 1900, and has since been modified about once every ten years, the last revision occurring in 1999. These frequent revisions are necessary to keep the ICD current with rapidly growing scientific knowledge about life-threatening diseases.

At the beginning of the 1900's, doctors and scientists knew very little about CHD. It was not until 1912 that a Dr. James B. Herrick first described an unusual form of heart disease resulting from hardening of the arteries(4). The paucity of knowledge surrounding this 'new' condition was reflected in the ICD system, where deaths attributable to CHD were classified as *"Angina pectoris"*. Angina is actually a symptom of CHD and not the disease itself (angina pectoris literally means 'pain in the chest' and results from inadequate blood flow to the heart).

It was not until 1929 that the classification was changed to *"Diseases of the coronary arteries, Angina pectoris",* and it was at this point that the number of recorded CHD deaths, which had shown little change since 1900, underwent a sudden and sharp increase. This increase was accompanied by a leveling-off in the number of recorded non-coronary heart disease deaths, as can be seen in Figure 1a.

In 1948, the sixth ICD introduced a major new category, entitled *"Arteriosclerotic heart disease, including coronary disease".* This new classification included three subcategories; 1) *"Arteriosclerotic heart disease so described",* 2) *"Heart disease specified as involving coronary arteries",* and 3) *"Angina pectoris without mention of coronary disease".* As you can see in Figure 1a, this new addition was accompanied by a massive vertical leap in CHD death rates, and a similarly massive drop in non-coronary heart disease deaths.

In 1968, the eighth ICD came into effect. For the first time ever, heart attack was given an explicit listing, under the category *"Acute myocardial infarction".* This landmark change was immediately followed by yet another abrupt jump in the CHD mortality curve.

The ninth ICD update in 1979 introduced five new sub-categories to the *"All other forms of heart disease"* category. This is the umbrella classification into which all non-CHD categories of heart disease are placed. Among the new arrivals were heart failure and arrhythmia, which refers to a disturbance in the normal rhythm of heartbeat. Nowadays, both heart failure and arrhythmia are known to be major causes of cardiac death. The establishment of specific categories for these was accompanied by a sudden downturn in CHD mortality and an instantaneous upswing in non-CHD deaths.

There are two possible explanations for the CHD mortality pattern shown in Figure 1a. The first one is that, during the twentieth century, coronary and non-coronary heart disease victims were doing an outstanding job of timing their deaths to correspond precisely with the new ICD classification changes--a highly unlikely occurrence to say the least. The second and far more realistic explanation is simply that doctors were increasingly classifying victims into CHD- and non-CHD-related categories as the classifications became more specific, ECG machines became more widely used, and medical knowledge of heart disease increased. When the 1968 additions to the ICD criteria allowed doctors to assign the maximum possible percentage of heart disease deaths to the CHD category, CHD mortality hit its 'peak' then immediately began to decline in line with the overall heart disease trend(5,6).

Adjusted Versus Unadjusted Data

CHD fatalities occur most commonly in old age. In 1900, the average life expectancy in the US was only forty-nine years, due in no small part to a rate of infant mortality far higher than that seen today. As ninety-four percent of CHD deaths occur after the age of fifty-five, and because average life expectancy in the US had increased to seventy-seven years by the year 2000, one need not be a genius to identify a major reason why so many more people began dying of CHD throughout the last century. Quite simply, many more people were living long enough to die of CHD.

To gain insight into whether any increase in mortality from a specific disease is real or simply an artifact of increased life expectancy, researchers calculate what are known as 'age-adjusted' death rates. These are figures that have been arrived at only after making allowances for any increase in average life span. The heart disease trend lines seen in Figure 1a--the same figures cited by health authorities when commenting on the rise and decline of CHD--are not age-adjusted. Those in figure 1b are.

In Figure 1b, the plot for CHD mortality (for which age-adjusted data is only available from 1960 onwards) hits a peak in 1968 before turning around and heading southeast, similar to what we saw in Figure 1a. Take a closer look, though, at the trend line for overall heart disease mortality. It hits a peak, not in the late sixties, but in 1950. We know that the 1968 peak for CHD mortality is simply an artifact of changing diagnostic criteria; that when the maximum possible number of deaths were finally being placed into this category, its trajectory instantly fell into line with that of overall heart disease mortality. We therefore have every reason to believe that the historical age-adjusted peak for CHD occurred, not in 1968, but somewhere around 1950. As such, the true decline in CHD appears to have begun over a decade before the health establishment launched its campaign against saturated fat and cholesterol!

Postponing the Inevitable

It is an extremely interesting exercise to sit back and take in all the proffered explanations for the reduction in CHD mortality. While orthodoxy assures us its anti-fat, anti-cholesterol efforts have helped instigate the drop in CHD, others have tried to link the decline with the increased or decreased consumption of specific food items, or to food fortification with certain vitamins. There's just one problem with all these theories, and that's the little-publicized fact that while CHD deaths have been declining, numerous studies show that the overall age-adjusted incidence of CHD--which includes non-fatal disease--is remaining steady or even *increasing*(7-10). In other words, people are having just as many heart attacks as ever--if not more--but emergency medical care has become increasingly adept at saving their lives(11-14).

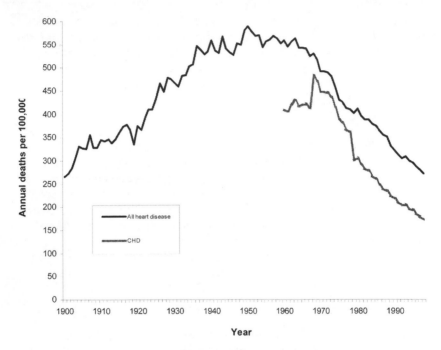

Figure 1b. Age-adjusted CHD and total heart disease mortality, 1900-1998.

Adapted from National Center for Health Statistics. HIST293: Age-Adjusted Death Rates for Selected Causes, Death Registration States, 1900-32, and United States, 1933-98; http://www.cdc.gov/nchs/dataw h/statab/unpubd/mortabs/hist293.htm

The authors of the famous Framingham study, frequently cited in support of the cholesterol hypothesis, wrote in a 1990 article; *"Our data indicate that the decline in mortality was primarily the result of improved survival among persons with new cases of cardiovascular disease, rather than the result of a substantial decrease in the incidence of the disease"*(9).

In 1996, a high-ranking member of the health orthodoxy revealed at an annual gathering of his colleagues that deaths from heart disease had not dropped nearly as much as officials had claimed and that the prevalence of the disease may actually be increasing. So why the erroneous assertions about an establishment-led drop in CHD?

"Our philosophy was that to get more money from politicians, we had to show that good things were happening". The individual responsible for these words,

quoted in a 1996 edition of the *Wall Street Journal*, was none other than Jan L. Breslow, the then newly-appointed president of the AHA(15).

Ambulance and paramedic networks, the development of CPR techniques and electrical defibrillators, anti-clotting drugs, coronary care units, and campaigns to raise awareness of heart attack symptoms are the true stars responsible for the decline in CHD deaths. If highly touted 'risk factor' changes were responsible for the decline in CHD mortality, they would surely reduce the incidence of CHD itself.

The Anti-Cholesterol Campaign Has Been Counter-Productive

Throughout the twentieth century, there has been a steady and substantial decline in the number of people smoking cigarettes(16). Because smoking unarguably contributes to heart disease, the incidence of CHD should, by all rights, have undergone a marked decline during this same period--but it hasn't! Clearly, some other factor(s) has acted to counter the beneficial impact of this reduction in cigarette smoking. As we will explore in later chapters, a number of the establishment's recommended dietary modifications actually encourage the onset of CHD (and various other lethal diseases).

The Increase in Saturated Fat that Never Was

Even after adjusting the mortality data for increased life expectancy, a substantial increase in coronary and overall heart disease mortality is still evident during the first half of the last century. Is this increase in any way due to increasing saturated fat consumption?

Absolutely not.

Take a good look at Figure 1c, which shows the consumption of various types of fats during the last century(17). Beginning in the 1920's, total fat consumption increased steadily, due entirely to the accelerating use of vegetable oils, shortenings, and margarines. The increasing popularity of these unsaturated fat-rich vegetable fats also explains the rise in polyunsaturated and monounsaturated fat intake. Saturated fat intake, on the other hand, has remained relatively stable in the face of increasing total fat intake. While vegetable fats do contain some saturates, the richest source of these in the American diet is animal fats, whose consumption slightly *declined* during the twentieth century(18). As can readily be seen from the graph, saturated fat is the only type of fat whose consumption did not rise during the twentieth century. Whether you choose to believe the historic peak in CHD mortality occurred in 1950 or in 1968, saturated fat intake during the decades prior to

Figure 1c. Average daily U.S. intake of various types of fat, 1909-2000.

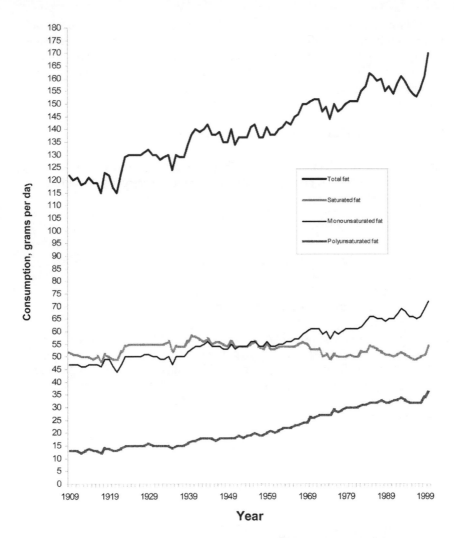

Source: USDA US Food Supply database: http://www.cnpp.usda.gov/nutrient_content.html

either of these dates shows no increase. Neither animal fats nor saturated fat can be logically blamed for any increase in CHD deaths.

Much Ado About Nothing

It seems that, during the last four decades, saturated fats from animal foods have been implicated in just about every health ailment to have ever befallen humankind. However, for the same reason that animal fats cannot possibly be associated with any increase in CHD, they cannot logically be implicated in any real or imagined increases in cancer, diabetes, obesity, teenage acne, falling sperm counts or global warming.

In the next chapter, we will examine the relationship between cholesterol and CHD, and find out why efforts to lower cholesterol via dietary means are more likely to cause harm than good.

Chapter 2

"To arrive at a contradiction is to confess an error in one's thinking; to maintain a contradiction is to abdicate one's mind and to evict oneself from the realm of reality."
Ayn Rand.

Cholesterol is Not a Killer

The true relationship between saturated fat, cholesterol, heart disease, and mortality.

One of the major reasons for the continual barrage of vitriol against saturated fats is that they possess the ability to raise blood cholesterol levels. These elevated cholesterol levels, in turn, are alleged to increase the risk of heart disease. According to health authorities, if we could all hammer our cholesterol levels down to 150 or lower then freedom from heart disease and a long, healthy life would be ours for the asking.

You are now about to find out why such a contention is little more than a deluded pipe dream, and how an abundance of published research has shown that lowering your blood cholesterol levels can actually *increase* your risk of dying prematurely!

What Is Cholesterol?

Before we examine the many problems with the 'saturated fat-raises-cholesterol-which-causes-heart-disease' theory, known in research circles as the 'lipid hypothesis', it is imperative that we take a quick look at cholesterol. What exactly is it, and what does it do?

Cholesterol is most accurately defined as a sterol or alcohol, but because it is a waxy substance that has little in common with the merchandise sold in liquor stores, it is typically referred to as a lipid. It is produced mainly in the liver, although smaller amounts are generated in the intestines and other organs. Far from being a poisonous substance that must be avoided at all costs, cholesterol is a critical substance that we simply cannot live without.

Because cholesterol's unique structure makes it impossible to dissolve in water, it forms a crucial component of cell membranes, which rely heavily on its waterproofing properties in order to function efficiently in a fluid environment. The ability of cells to resist saturation from external fluids is especially important for nerve cells and, not surprisingly, the highest concentrations of cholesterol are found in the brain and nervous system. Cholesterol also acts as an antioxidant, protecting cell membranes from free radical damage.

Because cholesterol is water-resistant, and because blood is a water-based medium, cholesterol must be carried through our bloodstream inside special water-soluble particles known as *lipoproteins*. There are different types of lipoproteins, the two most abundant being HDL (high density lipoprotein) and LDL (low density lipoprotein). The main function of LDL is to transport cholesterol from the liver to our organs and tissues, where it is incorporated into cell membranes. In contrast, HDL carries 'old' cholesterol that has been discarded by the body's cells back to the liver for recycling or excretion. The liver does a number of things with recycled cholesterol; it can be incorporated into bile (which is used to break down the fat we eat), or used to produce hormones that are essential for our continued wellbeing, such as testosterone, estrogen, dehydroepiandrosterone (DHEA), progesterone and cortisol. Cholesterol is also deployed to the nervous system, where it enables the facilitation of messages along our nerve pathways. The brain, in particular, is especially rich in cholesterol.

Cholesterol is, quite simply, one of the most important substances within our bodies.

The Association Between Cholesterol and CHD

Amongst free-living individuals in the real world, it is difficult to find a consistent, uniform correlation between saturated fat consumption and serum cholesterol levels. Individuals with similar saturated fat intakes can possess markedly different serum cholesterol concentrations, and individuals with high saturated fat intakes can have serum cholesterol readings far lower than individuals with low intakes. Serum cholesterol levels are influenced by a whole host of factors aside from fat intake, including stress, physical activity, obesity, illness, smoking, genetics, alcohol, and medicine usage. However, in clinical studies where all these other variables are controlled to the greatest possible extent, saturated fats do tend to raise total serum cholesterol in comparison to monounsaturated fats, which have a neutral effect. Polyunsaturated fats, on the other hand, exert a lowering effect(1).

Those of you adhering to Spartan low-fat diets in the hope of lowering your cholesterol levels should be aware that, when caloric intake is held constant, fat restriction itself is useless for lowering cholesterol. In a carefully controlled study, researchers fed a group of healthy men diets that were identical in every respect except that one contained twenty-two percent fat, the other thirty-nine percent. Unlike previous experiments, where researchers had modified the ratio of saturated and unsaturated fatty acids in the low-fat diet, both diets in this study featured an identical saturate/monounsaturated/polyunsaturate ratio. Only the overall amount of fat varied between the low- and high-fat diets. Each subject served as their own control by consuming both diets for fifty days each. The study was conducted with the utmost scientific rigor; the participants were housed in a research facility for the entire duration of the study, and had no opportunity to consume any food other than that supplied by the researchers. All food was monitored and weighed, and the participants were required to consume all the food provided. A spatula was even provided to ensure that all food was scraped from the plates and eaten! To avoid the confounding effects of weight loss, the participants were fed sufficient calories to maintain their weight throughout the study.

The particpants' cholesterol levels at the start of the study ranged from 133 to 240 mg/dl. During the study, the researchers observed that cholesterol levels barely changed from baseline. They also found *no* difference in mean serum cholesterol levels during the low- and high-fat diets (173 versus 177 mg/dl, respectively). When put through the wringer of tightly controlled clinical examination, the low-fat diet—so aggressively promoted for its alleged cholesterol-lowering capabilities—is promptly shown to be a fraud(2).

So while fat restriction itself has little effect on cholesterol levels, saturated fat restriction can affect blood cholesterol. Does the potential cholesterol-raising action of saturated fat have any actual impact upon CHD? According to the purveyors of the lipid hypothesis, the answer is an uncontestable *"yes!"*. The 'strong' association between serum cholesterol and CHD deaths, they say, leaves no doubt that the cholesterol-raising effects of saturated fat increase the risk of CHD.

Before we discuss the studies examining the cholesterol-CHD association, readers should carefully consider one of the most fundamental rules of science: *Association does not automatically equate to causation.* What this means is that even if a certain factor, like high cholesterol, is frequently observed in CHD patients, this does not mean it actually causes the disease. To illustrate the folly of equating association with causation, researcher John Yudkin published a study in 1957 showing that TV and radio ownership were far more closely associated with coronary mortality in England than any dietary factor(3). Despite the strength of Yudkin's correlation, we know that TV sets and radios do not cause heart disease; none of us seriously believe that throwing our television sets out in the trash will grant us immunity from CHD. The association between television and radio ownership and CHD demonstrated by Yudkin was secondary, meaning that some other causal factor--reduced physical activity, perhaps--was more prevalent among owners of these appliances than non-owners.

It never seems to have occurred to promoters of the lipid hypothesis that any rise in cholesterol associated with CHD may not necessarily be the cause of the aforementioned ailment, but may actually be part of the body's response to some other destructive process that was truly causing coronary deterioration. No-one in their right mind would suggest that the dramatic rise in white blood cell count that often accompanies infection is the 'cause' of infection; everyone knows that pathogenic microbes are the guilty party. Increased white blood cell activity is simply an important part of the body's effort to destroy the invading pathogens. No authority with even a micron of intelligence would recommend 'white-blood cell-lowering' diets for the prevention of infection, no sooner than they would recommend drink-driving to improve road safety. Millions around the world, however, have been coaxed and cajoled into following cholesterol-lowering diets and taking dangerous cholesterol-lowering drugs in an effort to reduce blood cholesterol levels.

Does cholesterol cause heart disease, or are cholesterol elevations part of the body's response to whatever else causes heart disease? Can lowering blood cholesterol levels improve one's survival prospects--or does it actually cause more harm than good?

Let's find out…

Framingham Follies

One of the studies most frequently mentioned by proponents of the lipid hypothesis is the famous Framingham study. This project commenced in 1948 and proceeded to monitor the occurrence of CHD in over 5,000 Framingham, Massachusetts, residents who were initially free of any outward signs of CHD. After following these folks for sixteen years, the Framingham researchers claimed to have found that the risk of CHD in those under 50--but not over-- was *"strikingly related to the serum total cholesterol level."*

Exactly how *"striking"* was this relationship? Take a look at Figure 2a, which shows the distribution of serum cholesterol levels among residents who developed CHD and those who remained free of the disease. Notice that the range of cholesterol amongst the majority of subjects in both groups was very similar. The *mean* serum cholesterol level of those with CHD was a mere eleven percent higher than those without. The majority of patients were in the normal range, with CHD afflicting those whose cholesterol levels were as low as 150(4). Despite what some claim, low cholesterol levels do not guarantee immunity against CHD, and high cholesterol levels are anything but a sure sign of impending coronary disaster.

In 1987, the Framingham researchers published a thirty-year follow-up paper, reporting on the incidence of all-cause mortality and cardiovascular disease mortality. The researchers again found that higher cholesterol levels were associated with increased mortality before the age of fifty, but after this age

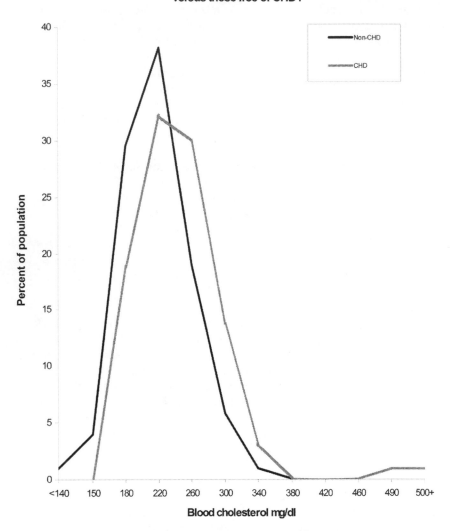

Figure 2a. Blood cholesterol levels in men aged 30-49 years with CHD versus those free of CHD .

Data from: Kannel WB, et al. Cholesterol in the prediction of atherosclerotic disease. New perspectives based on the Framingham Study. *Annals of Internal Medicine* , 1979; 90: 85-91 cholesterol levels in men and women showed *no* relationship with CVD or total mortality(5).

The Framingham study is hardly alone in demonstrating that cholesterol is not a risk factor for older folks. Study upon study has repeatedly shown that higher cholesterol levels do not increase the risk of CHD, nor stroke, nor overall mortality, in seniors(6-24). In fact, several studies have found that higher cholesterol levels are predictive of increased survival and greater longevity in older age groups!(20-24) As we learnt in chapter one, ninety-five percent of CHD deaths occur in those over fifty-five, which means that only a miniscule percentage of CHD deaths can claim to have even a statistical relationship with blood cholesterol!

If you are over fifty, and starting to become a little agitated by the idea that for years you have abstained from many of your favorite foods for no good reason, wait--it gets worse! The above-mentioned lack of association in older Framingham adults was for those whose cholesterol levels had remained constant. Those whose cholesterol levels had *decreased* during the study experienced an *increase* in both total and CVD mortality. That's right--an increase! Even the researchers had to admit; *"There is a direct association between falling cholesterol levels over the first 14 years and mortality over the following 18 years..."*

For every 1mg/dl per year drop in cholesterol levels during the first fourteen years of the Framingham study, there was a fourteen percent increase in cardiovascular death and an eleven percent increase in overall mortality during the subsequent eighteen years. The authors tried to dismiss this astounding revelation by claiming; *"After age 50 years the association of mortality with cholesterol values is confounded by people whose cholesterol levels are falling--perhaps due to diseases pre-disposing to death"*. This unconvincing piece of doublespeak inferred that people over 50 were dying of diseases that also happened to lower their cholesterol levels.

There are at least two factors that make such a proposition highly unlikely. Firstly, the considerable fourteen-year time lag employed by the researchers weighed heavily against the possibility of cholesterol reductions occurring due to the development of disease. Secondly, CVD mortality, which includes deaths from CHD and ischemic stroke--the very diseases that are supposedly caused by high cholesterol levels--increased to a greater degree than overall mortality!

Thus, the data from the Framingham Study, the longest-running project examining the connection between cholesterol and CHD, has shown that declining cholesterol does not increase longevity, but instead increases one's risk of death from all causes, including cardiovascular disease! This fact should have brought the entire cholesterol campaign to a screeching halt, but of course, it didn't. After 30 years of vigorously pushing the idea that elevated cholesterol levels promoted heart disease, attacking animal fats with unbridled venom, and convincing generations of people to drastically alter their diets and even take lipid-lowering drugs, proponents of the lipid hypothesis apparently could not find it within themselves to admit to the public that they might have been wrong.

Instead, they went into denial.

Witness the following statement in the study's conclusion: *"We believe those who would argue that low serum cholesterol levels should be avoided--because they pose an increased risk from cancer or other causes--cannot support such a stand when the pattern of mortality during a 30-year follow-up period is considered"*.

According to the authors, it is unreasonable to infer from their study that cholesterol lowering may increase mortality, even though that is exactly what their results indicated. The establishment's irrational, reality-evading tendencies were also manifest in a joint statement by the American Heart Association and the NIH's National Heart, Lung, and Blood Institute (the Framingham project's sponsor) entitled *The Cholesterol Facts,* where one finds the following claim, supported by a citation from the above study: *"The results of the Framingham study indicate that a 1% reduction...of cholesterol [corresponds to a] 2% reduction in CHD risk"*(25). This, evidently, was their interpretation of a study that showed an eleven percent increase in total mortality and a fourteen percent increase in CVD mortality for every 1mg/dl reduction in cholesterol! The extreme lengths to which our 'trusted' guardians of public health will go to preserve the status quo are nothing short of mind-boggling!

Healthy Hearts in Honolulu: Low Versus High Cholesterol

Proponents of the lipid hypothesis love citing the Japanese, a population that eats less animal fat and displays lower average cholesterol levels than most Western nations. According to many 'experts', it is these qualities that largely explain the greater longevity and lower rates of CHD in Japan. I also like citing the Japanese, but for starkly different reasons. The Japanese experience actually helps to illustrate why the claims of anti-cholesterol campaigners are totally false.

The Honolulu Heart Program is a long-running epidemiological study of cardiovascular disease that began in 1965 with 8,006 Japanese/American men living on the island of Oahu, Hawaii. The men were born between 1900 and 1919, and were therefore aged 45 to 68 years old at the start of the study. Since the late sixties, this group has undergone several check-ups. The fourth of these was performed in the early nineties and involved over 3,700 men aged 71-93.

After this fourth examination, the researchers decided to examine data obtained from the deceased and surviving participants to see if there was any relationship between cholesterol and mortality. There was indeed a relationship, but it was the exact opposite of what promoters of the lipid hypothesis would have us believe. The worst outlook for all-cause mortality was seen among men who maintained a *low* serum cholesterol between the early seventies and early nineties! In contrast, the lowest mortality risks were seen among those who maintained an intermediate cholesterol level and among those whose cholesterol *increased from the low to the high category* during this 20-year period!(26)

There's no need for Japanese folks to migrate to Hawaii in order to avoid the alleged dangers of high cholesterol; an abundance of research from Japan itself shows that low-cholesterol levels are inimical to the goal of living a long, healthy life. In 1975, Japanese researchers began studying the relationship between cholesterol levels and mortality among over 12,000 Osaka residents aged 40-69. After an average of 8.9 years of follow-up, they found that every 34mg/dl drop in blood cholesterol was associated with a twenty-one percent *increased* risk of overall mortality. While higher cholesterol levels were weakly and insignificantly associated with CHD mortality, low cholesterol levels were accompanied by a far greater risk of cancer death. This association was seen in both males and females, and held even after accounting for age, weight, hypertension, occupation, cigarette smoking, and alcohol intake. The harmful relationship between low cholesterol and cancer also held after researchers excluded cancer deaths occurring during the first five years of the study(27).

The Japanese Lipid Intervention Trial was a six-year study of over 47,000 patients treated with the cholesterol-lowering drug simvastatin. Those with a total cholesterol level of 200-219 mg/dl enjoyed a *lower* rate of coronary events than those whose levels were above or below this range. More importantly, the lowest overall mortality rate was seen in the patients whose total cholesterol levels were between 200-259 mg/dl, and whose LDL levels were between 120-159 mg/dl. The highest death rate in the study was observed among those whose cholesterol levels were below 160 mg/dl(28).

So much for the claim that the Japanese experience proves the value of cholesterol lowering. What about the gigantic MRFIT study which, with over 360,000 participants, was one of the largest cholesterol investigations ever conducted?

MRFIT--Or Anti-Cholesterol MISFIT?

Between 1973 and 1975, over 360,000 men aged between 35-57 years were screened in eighteen cities across the U.S.A. for possible inclusion in MRFIT, a clinical trial examining the effect of dietary and pharmaceutical interventions on CHD. From this massive group, just under 13,000 men were eventually selected to participate in the trial. Researchers did not simply forget about those excluded from the official trial; their vital statistics, including blood cholesterol levels, were filed away and any deaths occurring amongst this group over the ensuing years were duly recorded.

After six years of follow-up, the MRFIT researchers decided to look at just how many of these screenees had died, and why. When the results were tallied, they showed that CHD mortality among the MRFIT screenees tended to increase with each successively higher category of initial cholesterol concentration. In November 1986, the MRFIT researchers excitedly reported their findings in one of the nation's most prominent medical publications, the *Journal of the American Medical Association*(29). Of course, *the "strong, continuous and graded"* relationship between blood cholesterol and CHD was detected in a cohort of men aged 35-57, a group among whom only a minority of CHD deaths occur.

The 1986 *JAMA* report failed to report on overall mortality. A few years later, however, Dr. Hiroyasu Iso and his colleagues took the MRFIT data, divided the participants into ten separate categories according to their blood cholesterol levels, and presented the figures for not only CHD mortality, but also *overall* mortality. In stark contrast to the CHD mortality curve, which showed a steady gradual climb with each increasing category of blood cholesterol, the trend-line for overall mortality displayed an unmistakably U-shaped curve. Those in the lowest cholesterol category (<140mg/dl) had a higher all-cause death rate than all but the very highest category! As shown in Figure 2b, the lowest mortality was seen across the 160-219 mg/dl range(30).

While the stated goal of studies such as MRFIT is to monitor trends associated with CHD death rates, for the majority of us the most telling data is that for overall mortality. After all, most of us wish to avoid CHD so that we can live as long as possible, not merely to have our lives cut equally short by some other deadly event.

There exists another vitally important reason for reporting overall mortality data accurately. Determining the exact cause of death can be a very subjective matter, and numerous studies have shown great variability in the diagnoses issued by different physicians examining the same post-mortem information(31-33). There can be a great deal of overlap, for example, in the symptoms suffered by coronary and non-coronary heart disease victims. When a group of doctors recently analyzed 2,683 death certificates issued in Framingham, it was observed that the original physicians were twenty-four percent more likely to assign coronary heart disease overall, and more than twice as likely to assign it in over-85's(34).

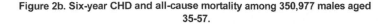

Figure 2b. Six-year CHD and all-cause mortality among 350,977 males aged 35-57.

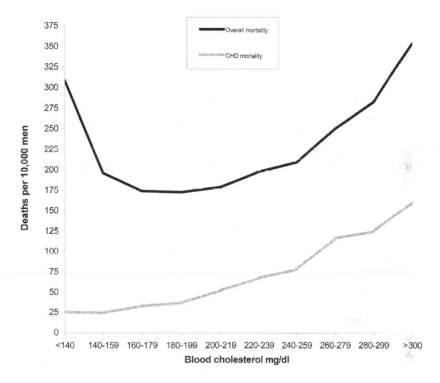

Adapted from: Iso H, et al. Serum cholesterol levels and six-year mortality from stroke in 350,977 men screened for the Multiple Risk Factor Intervention Trial. *New England Journal of Medicine*, Apr, 1989; 320 (14): 904-910.

In another study, a group of physicians was asked to assess six standardized, written case reports of death in order to assess the accuracy of death certificate completion. Researchers reported only fifty-six percent agreement between the underlying causes of death offered by physicians and the correct standardized diagnoses published by the National Center for Health Statistics. The exact level of agreement varied from fifteen to ninety-nine percent, depending on the complexity of the case(35).

While the exact diagnosis of death can vary widely, the results for total mortality are final. One can debate endlessly about the precise cause of death, but in the end, the point is moot--the patient is dead. Obviously, overall mortality data is of extreme importance when considering the results of long-term investigations like Framingham and MRFIT.

Those who self-assuredly cite the enormous MRFIT project as if it were definitive proof of the relationship between cholesterol and CHD not only ignore the young age of the participants and the heightened overall death risk of those with low cholesterol levels--they flippantly disregard the results of the MRFIT clinical trial itself, which was the reason the MRFIT study ever came to fruition in the first place!

In the official trial, half of the almost 13,000 participants were randomized to receive anti-hypertensive medication, encouragement to quit smoking, and intensive counseling on reducing their fat and cholesterol intake. The remainder were not given any special intervention, but simply told to follow the usual advice provided by their personal doctors. After an average seven years' follow-up, those receiving the intervention treatment experienced slightly greater reductions in blood pressure and cholesterol levels. Despite this, there was no difference in cardiovascular or all-cause mortality between the two groups. The only noteworthy reduction in mortality was seen among those who stopped smoking, irrespective of whether they belonged to the treatment or control groups(36).

Finnish Redemption?

Very few people have been made aware of the harmful association between low cholesterol and mortality observed in the above studies. However, mainstream media outlets were quick to report on a study appearing in the September 2004 issue of the *Journal of the American College of Cardiology* which, at first glance, suggested that low cholesterol levels increased longevity(37). Researchers in this study had measured the blood cholesterol of over 3,000 healthy Finnish men aged 30-45 during the sixties, then recorded their mortality during an average follow-up period of thirty-five years.

They found that men with blood cholesterol levels at or below 194 mg/dl were less than half as likely to develop heart disease and had a twenty-five percent lower overall mortality rate than those with cholesterol levels above this limit. However, only eight percent of the population had a cholesterol level of 194 mg/dl or lower, and when this group was split in two, those in the lower half, with cholesterol levels at or below 182 mg/dl, actually had a ten percent higher mortality rate than the upper half. While the small number of men with low cholesterol precludes any firm conclusions, this result is concordant with a collective analysis of other population studies showing that overall mortality begins to rise when blood cholesterol drops below 180 mg/dl(38). The Finnish study also contained no data on the fate of those whose cholesterol levels *fell* during the follow-up period.

Neglecting the Negative

It is interesting to note the stark contrast in publicity awarded to the aforementioned Finnish project and that given to a non-supportive study also published in 2004. The latter, a massive fifteen-year follow-up by Austrian researchers, clearly confirmed yet again the harmful relationship between low cholesterol and overall longevity.

The researchers had followed over 67,000 men and 82,000 women aged 20-95 years during the period 1985-1999. It was observed that high cholesterol was associated with a higher risk of CHD death in men of all ages and in women under the age of 50. However, low cholesterol was significantly associated with increased all-cause mortality in men across the entire age range, and in women from the age of 50 onward. Low cholesterol showed significant associations with death from cancer, liver diseases, and mental diseases. The researchers remarked that: *"the low cholesterol effect occurs even among younger respondents, contradicting the previous assessments among cohorts of older people that this is a proxy or marker for frailty occurring with age."*(39)

The 'Supportive' is Non-Supportive!

Upon closer inspection, the very studies most commonly used to support the lipid hypothesis actually show that low cholesterol levels are predictive of *increased* mortality! The studies discussed in this chapter are by no means the only ones that have shown cholesterol reduction to be a potentially dangerous undertaking. In the next chapter, we will examine the association between low cholesterol levels and increased illness and death a little more closely.

Chapter 3

*"Everybody is entitled to his own opinion, but no one is entitled to his own
facts. The data is the data."*
Spiropulu

Lower is Not Better

Your longevity versus the mainstream cholesterol agenda

Over the last forty-odd years, we have been bombarded with messages urging
us to drive down our cholesterol levels as far as we can with Spartan diets and
lipid-lowering drugs. As we learnt in the previous chapter, however, the largest
and longest-running CHD investigations ever conducted clearly show that by
following such advice, all we succeed in doing is to place ourselves in a group
at risk of *increased* overall mortality!

Whilst eagerly downplayed by advocates of the lipid hypothesis, the association
between low cholesterol and increased total mortality was of sufficient concern
to the NHLBI that it convened a special conference in 1992 to discuss the
problem. Evidence from a multitude of studies was presented linking low blood
cholesterol levels to an increase in various cancers, hemorrhagic stroke,
respiratory and digestive diseases, and violent death. The conference
participants could not explain the mechanisms behind the association, but
decreed that further research into the matter was warranted(1).

The public, of course, was left out of the loop. Disclaimers about the increase in
total mortality that is often seen with low cholesterol levels are conspicuously
absent from the barrage of cholesterol-lowering announcements issued by
health authorities. The problem might be ignored, but it isn't going away--a
French study published in 1997, involving over 6,000 men followed for an
average of seventeen years, found that those with the highest decline in
cholesterol displayed an excess risk for most types of cancers(2). A 2002 study
with heart failure patients found that those with the lowest levels of cholesterol
were more than twice as likely to succumb to a fatal event than those with the
highest cholesterol levels(3).

It has been proposed by defenders of the lipid hypothesis that the association
between falling cholesterol levels and increased cancer risk is in fact due to a
cholesterol-lowering effect of cancer, rather than any causal contribution of low
blood cholesterol to the risk of cancer(4). At present, there exists no conclusive
clinical evidence to support either argument. What is interesting, though, is
how the anti-cholesterol hierarchy have eagerly embraced the argument that

low-cholesterol is simply a side effect of the cancer process, yet steadfastly refuse to entertain the notion that elevated cholesterol levels are a product, rather than a cause, of the coronary disease process.

Low Cholesterol and Mental Health

In 1990, Professors Matthew Muldoon, Stephen Manuck, and Karen Matthews performed an analysis of violent death rates among the almost 25,000 male participants of six major cholesterol-lowering clinical trials. They found that, while the death rate from violence and suicide in the control groups was equivalent to that of the entire U.S. population, the rate for those in the treatment groups--that is, those who were receiving cholesterol-lowering diets or drugs--was double the national average.

The authors noted that low blood cholesterol levels occurred more often amongst criminals, individuals diagnosed with violent or aggressive conduct disorders, homicidal offenders with histories of violence and suicide attempts related to alcohol, and people with poorly internalized social norms and low self control(5).

Beatrice Golomb and her colleagues from the University of California, San Diego, have been conducting a large-scale study of statin side effects. Unlike most statin studies, the UCSD project is not funded by drug company money. In a 2004 journal article, Golomb and her colleagues recounted the experience of six patients presenting with irritability and short temper whilst on cholesterol-lowering statin drugs. In each case these negative personality changes were sustained until statin use was discontinued and resolved promptly with drug cessation. Four of the patients resumed statin therapy, and in each of these the problems reappeared. Among the manifestations of severe irritability in these patients were homicidal impulses, threats to others, road rage, generation of fear in family members, and damage to property(6). Supporting Golomb's observations was a clinical trial involving 120 healthy men with high cholesterol who took twenty milligrams of simvastatin for a twelve week period and a placebo for another twelve weeks; a significant increase in depression scores occurred while the men were taking simvastatin(7).

Low Fat Diets Make People Moody

Unlike cancer, the link between violent death and low cholesterol is supported by experimental evidence, and cannot therefore be explained away so easily by authorities. In 1998, U.K. researchers reported the results of an experiment involving twenty healthy male and female volunteers. One group was placed on a forty-one percent fat diet, while the other group consumed a twenty-five percent fat diet. After four weeks had passed, the groups were swapped around so that those originally on the low-fat diet were consuming the high-fat diet, and vice-versa. Throughout the study, all meals were prepared by the university conducting the study and supplied to the participants. Both diets were specially designed to be as palatable and similar in taste as possible.

At the beginning and end of each diet period, every subject underwent a battery of psychological assessments, including various mood state questionnaires and an interview by a psychiatrist who was blinded to the participant's dietary status. The study was tightly controlled and adherence to the diets appears to have been high. HDL cholesterol levels declined during the low-fat period, a typical response on low-fat, high-carbohydrate diets, indicating that subjects ate the foods as supplied.

What the researchers found was that, while ratings of anger-hostility slightly declined during the high-fat diet period, they significantly increased during the low-fat, high-carbohydrate diet period! Similarly, ratings of depression declined slightly during the high-fat period, but increased during the low-fat period, mainly due to two of the low-fat subjects reporting significantly greater depression-dejection ratings. Levels of tension-anxiety declined during the high-fat period, but did not change during the four weeks of low-fat eating. As the researchers stated, the study participants were *"a psychologically robust group who had never previously suffered from depression or anxiety, and who were not going through any 'stressful' events during the study."* They further speculated that: *"The alterations in mood observed in the present study may have been greater if subjects were feeling more stressed or were more susceptible to mental illness."*(8)

These observations raise some interesting questions. Could the low-fat, high-carbohydrate diets that have been so heavily promoted over the last thirty years be at least partially responsible for increases in anti-social behavior witnessed during the same period? Worrying insight into this question can be gained from research performed with our close primate cousins.

Monkey Business Turns Nasty on Low-Fat Diets

When adult male monkeys were fed a 'luxury' diet (43% calories from fat) or a 'prudent' diet (30% calories from fat, and 85% less cholesterol than the luxury diet), researchers observed that the low-fat diet monkeys were more irritable and initiated more aggression than the luxury diet animals. The prudent diet resulted in lower total serum cholesterol levels, and while most health authorities would automatically assume this is a good thing, the researchers noted: *"These results are consistent with studies linking relatively low serum cholesterol concentrations to violent or antisocial behavior in psychiatric and criminal populations and could be relevant to understanding the significant increase in violence-related mortality observed among people assigned to cholesterol-lowering treatment in clinical trials."*(9)

Recent studies have shown a significant increase in the frequency and severity of depression amongst middle-aged and elderly men with low cholesterol levels when compared to those with higher levels(10,11).

When mortality data during 1993 was obtained for over eleven thousand participants in the 1970-1972 Nutrition Canada Survey, those with a total cholesterol level of less than 4.27 were more than six times as likely to commit suicide as subjects with a cholesterol reading greater than 5.77. These results were adjusted for age and sex, and persisted even after excluding the first five years of follow-up, those who were unemployed, and those who had been treated for depression(12).

When it comes to cholesterol, lower is *not* better.

Unforeseen Effects

An article appearing in the same journal as the original paper by Muldoon and his colleagues stressed that the most widespread consequence of increased violent behavior from cholesterol-lowering efforts would remain undetected by clinical studies(13). The author of the article, David Horrobin, pointed out that increased aggression leads to increased child-abuse, wife beating, violent confrontations, and problems at work. In other words, more anti-social behavior that leads to unhappiness and social incohesion. Unfortunately, the damage caused by this aspect of cholesterol-lowering will never be fully elucidated by published intervention studies, as they only record deaths due to violence, not the degree of misery or number of non-fatal violent incidents. While it is a boon to those who market low-fat foods and lipid-lowering drugs, cholesterol reduction appears to be anathema not only to those who would like to live a long, healthy, life, but also to those of us who would prefer to live in a civil, benevolent and cohesive society.

Low Cholesterol Slows You Down

As if an increased risk of depression and violent death is not bad enough, low cholesterol levels can also impair normal brain function. After testing over four thousand men and women aged twenty to fifty-nine, Muldoon and his colleagues found that as cholesterol concentrations in males decreased, so too did visuomotor speed. If you're wondering why you should care less about visuomotor speed, this is one of the qualities that determines whether you react quickly enough in emergency situations to save yourself from permanent extinction. When some kamikaze driver runs a red light and speeds into your direct line of travel, a deficit in reaction time could quite literally mean the difference between getting home safely or being fatally maimed beyond recognition.

Muldoon and his team tested the subjects' visuomotor speed by repeatedly having them press a button as quickly as possible whenever a solid square was displayed in the center of a blank computer screen. The researchers found that the mean total reaction time of men in the lowest category of blood cholesterol (average 152 mg/dl) was 12.7 milliseconds slower than that of men in the highest category (average 242 mg/dl).

In order to put these results into better perspective, the researchers decided to compare this difference with the decline in reaction time that occurs during normal aging. They found that, on average, visuomotor speed increased 0.09 milliseconds for each year of aging. Therefore, between ages thirty and fifty-nine, the cumulative increase in reaction time would be around three milliseconds. In other words, the difference in reaction time between the highest and lowest cholesterol categories was several times greater than that caused by three decades of aging!(14)

This is in no way the first time that low cholesterol levels have been associated with poorer cognitive performance. In a previous study, Muldoon and his team found that individuals with low total and LDL cholesterol levels performed poorer in a test that involved putting sets of blocks together to match patterns on cards(15).

A UK study published in 1995 found that low blood cholesterol levels in college students were associated with slower movement and slower decision times(16).

As part of the NHLBI's Twin Study, researchers measured the blood cholesterol of forty-four sets of twins, then followed their cognitive status over the next five years. Among monozygotic twins displaying a discordant decline in a test of information processing speed, the decliners had lower serum cholesterol levels than their non-declining siblings(17).

In eastern Finland, an examination of 980 men and women aged sixty-nine to seventy-eight found that low cholesterol levels were significantly associated with Alzheimer's disease(18).

Cause or Effect?

The question that begs to be asked, of course, is whether the relationship between low cholesterol and poorer cognitive function is one of direct causality or merely a statistical association. To answer this question, one would need data from controlled clinical trials in which cognitive function was measured before and after cholesterol-lowering treatments.

Luckily, researchers have conducted several such studies.

In one of these, healthy subjects were randomized to receive either a low-fat or standard diet for twelve weeks. Performance on a sustained attention task was significantly worse among those who reduced their cholesterol during the trial(19).

A 1992 double-blind, placebo-controlled trial found that healthy young men randomized to receive the popular cholesterol-lowering drug lovastatin (Mevacor) displayed significant deterioration in divided attention (the ability to simultaneously focus on multiple tasks and stimuli), vigilance (the ability to sustain attention) and global performance (a more general assessment of cognitive function). These changes were seen after only three weeks of treatment(20). As with visuomotor speed, the ability to maintain divided attention is essential for safe driving.

In 2000, Muldoon and his colleagues reported the results of a double-blind, placebo-controlled trial that assessed cognitive function and psychological well-being in healthy adults randomly assigned to receive either lovastatin or a placebo. At the start and at the conclusion of the study, subjects were given a battery of tests assessing attention, psychomotor speed, mental flexibility, working memory, and memory retrieval. After six-months' month follow-up, the placebo group had improved significantly in all five domains of cognitive function, but the lovastatin group improved only on memory recall tests(21). When Muldoon and his team subsequently performed another study, this time using simvastatin, they obtained similar results. Failure to improve on cognitive tests was observed with both ten and forty milligram doses of simvastatin(22).

The ability of cholesterol-lowering treatments to impair reaction time and mental focus goes a long way towards explaining the well-documented increase in accident risk among individuals with low cholesterol levels(21).

Meddling Where One Shouldn't

At the end of the day, the association between low cholesterol and increased mortality should not come as a big surprise to anyone with even a smidgen of knowledge in the areas of physiology and biochemistry. There is an optimal range for just about every substance in the body, be it minerals such as potassium and sodium, vital hormones like testosterone and estrogen, or even water. Both excessive *and* insufficient amounts of these substances can disturb the body's finely tuned symphony of metabolic processes, increasing the likelihood of illness and disease. Growth hormone, for example, is vital for optimal health, but individuals who secrete excess amounts are at higher risk of experiencing abnormal bone growth, the development of Neanderthal-like facial features, organ enlargement, diabetes, cardiovascular disease and colon cancer. A deficiency of growth hormone, on the other hand, leads to accelerated aging, organ atrophy, poor immune function, impaired growth and recovery, and body fat gain.

Witness also the disruption caused by abnormal levels of thyroid hormones. Excessive thyroid hormone secretion is often characterized by jitteriness, shaking, increased nervousness and irritability, rapid heart beat and palpitations, increased sweating, weight loss, fatigue and exhaustion. Insufficient thyroid output, in contrast, results in weight gain, dry skin and hair, lowered body temperature that causes one to continually feel cold, heavy menstrual periods, constipation, forgetfulness and other signs of mental impairment.

Clearly, interfering with the levels of fundamentally important substances in the body is not a matter to be taken lightly. Advocates of the lipid hypothesis appear to have given little thought to this elementary fact before embarking on their fanatical quest to lower the population's cholesterol, even though this substance is a vital component of every single cell in the human body, forms the raw material for some of our most important hormones, and plays a vital role in digestion and mental function.

In the next chapter, we'll find out why autopsy studies and animal experiments further highlight the spurious nature of the lipid hypothesis.

Chapter 4

"What luck for the rulers that men do not think."
Adolf Hitler

Irrelevant Rabbits and the Ungrateful Dead

Why autopsy and animal studies do not support the lipid hypothesis.

The medical profession would have us believe that high blood cholesterol causes heart disease by triggering the build-up of atherosclerotic plaque along the arterial wall. This plaque then allegedly grows to the point where it blocks blood flow to the heart, at which point we receive our just punishment for the heinous crime of eating butter, whole eggs and untrimmed meats.

If cholesterol did indeed cause atherosclerosis, then one would logically expect post-mortem examinations of heart attack victims to find a strong correlation between blood cholesterol levels and the degree of plaque build-up in their coronary arteries.

The first post-mortem study to examine this possibility was conducted in 1936, by Kurt Landé and Warren Sperry. In a thorough and methodical investigation, they analyzed the blood cholesterol content of individuals who had died suddenly from violent death, and compared them to the degree of atherosclerosis in the aorta. Responsible for channeling blood as it leaves the heart, the aorta is the biggest artery in the body, and a common site of atherosclerosis. After excluding all cases where there was any sign of pre-existing organ damage, apart from that caused by the fatal injury or atherosclerosis, they were left with one hundred and twenty-three individuals ranging in age from eleven to eighty. Landé and Sperry could not find any relationship between the level of blood cholesterol and the lipid content of the aorta. They wrote: *"No relationship was evident, and it is concluded that the incidence and severity of atherosclerosis are not directly affected by the level of cholesterol in the blood serum per se"*(1).

In the early sixties, as the anti-cholesterol, anti-animal fat campaign gathered steam, similar studies were performed confirming Landé and Sperry's findings. In India, researchers examined 200 autopsied individuals who had died suddenly, who had no recent history of illness, who showed no evidence of organic disease, and for whom blood samples were available within sixteen hours of death. Again, no correlation could be found between serum cholesterol values and the amount and severity of atherosclerosis. The Indian researchers also compared cholesterol readings from blood taken before and after death, and found that both were closely correlated as long as the post-mortem sample was taken within sixteen hours of death(2). This was an important validation of Landé and Sperry's work, whom critics had tried to discredit by claiming that post mortem cholesterol levels were not a reliable reflection of those seen prior to death.

In 1963, the results of post-mortem examinations performed on forty-two war veterans residing at the Westminster Hospital in London, Canada were published(3). Cholesterol values obtained soon after death were again shown to correlate accurately with those obtained before death. And once again, there was no correlation between serum cholesterol and the severity of atherosclerosis in the coronary arteries. Nor was there any correlation between serum cholesterol levels and the cholesterol content of either coronary or cerebral arteries. In fact, when the authors searched for features of CHD that were demonstrable at autopsy, such as blood clots, death of heart muscle and coronary insufficiency, they found those displaying these characteristics actually had a lower mean cholesterol level than those in whom these features were absent.

The authors were compelled to make mention of one of the patients, who over a nine-year period displayed a mean cholesterol level of 111mg/dl. Despite this extremely low value, he exhibited severe coronary atherosclerosis and a very high lipid content in the artery wall (the third highest value amongst all those autopsied). The fact that this individual possessed cholesterol levels that would bring forth a reassuring smile from the average physician was of little consolation--his arteries were in terrible shape!

The Westminster Hospital researchers are not the only ones to have observed severe cardiovascular disease among those sporting extremely low cholesterol levels. In his book *Heart Frauds*, Charles T. McGee, MD. cites the case of a patient who had suffered a stroke and a heart attack shortly before consulting with him--despite a cholesterol level of only 115 mg/dl. Ironically, this very low cholesterol reading automatically prompted the pathology lab's computer to print out:

"THIS PATIENT IS AT VERY LOW RISK FOR ATHEROSCLEROSIS".(4)

In 1962, an autopsy study by Polish researchers found that two-thirds of those who died with confirmed atherosclerosis had serum cholesterol levels in the normal to low ranges. When the researchers dissected the patients' arteries, they could find no relationship between blood cholesterol and the cholesterol content of arterial plaque. The factor showing the strongest association with atherosclerosis was age(5). As we grow older, even the fittest amongst us accumulate at least some plaque build-up in our arteries. The key is to prevent this plaque build-up from developing to the point where it can severely obstruct arteries and initiate a coronary event. Because they have no correlation with the severity of atherosclerosis, nor the cholesterol composition of plaques, fretting over blood cholesterol levels does not in any way assist the attainment of this goal. Subsequent autopsy studies from Gautemala and the U.S.A. have further underscored this fact(6,7).

Of the post-mortem studies that have claimed a relationship between serum cholesterol and athcrosclerosis, the best correlation coefficient any of them could muster was a meager 0.36 (8-11). For those not mathematically inclined, a correlation coefficient is a measure of the strength of the relationship between two variables (in this case, serum cholesterol and athcrosclerosis). The correlation coefficient scale ranges between -1 to 1, with 1 being a perfect correlation. A correlation coefficient of 0.36 is desperately weak and can hardly be used to support claims for a 'significant' association.

The Irrelevance of Animal Studies

Many readers arc no doubt wondering how cholesterol originally came to be implicated in the development of CHD. The earliest seeds of the lipid hypothesis were sown in 1908, when Russian researcher M.A. Ignatovsky fed a diet of protein-rich animal foods to rabbits. When the rabbits developed cholesterol-rich deposits in their arteries, he speculated that dietary protein may have been responsible. Just a few years later, fellow Russians N.W. Wesselkin and Nikolai Anitschkov decided to examine the possibility that dietary cholesterol, not protein, was the cause of the arterial plaque seen in Ignatovsky's rabbits. Instead of high protein foods, they added cholesterol to the rabbits' diet, and noted that their blood cholesterol levels rose dramatically. Examination after autopsy again revealed the formation of fatty deposits in the animals' arteries(12).

Subsequent studies over the years have shown that high fat diets cause similar arterial deposits in such species as chickens, guinea pigs, pigeons, parrots, goats, rats and mice. The problem is that these animals are either totally or primarily *herbivorous* creatures that have evolved on low-fat plant-based diets, and it is quite a leap of faith to extrapolate results from such species to omnivorous human beings. Studies with carnivorous animals such as cats, dogs and foxes have failed to reproduce the results obtained in the early rabbit studies. Cholesterol-feeding experiments with dogs completely fail to induce arterial deposits unless their thyroid glands are either removed or neutralized with thyroid-suppressing drugs beforehand(13). High amounts of cholesterol appear to be readily metabolized by carnivorous animals, whereas herbivorous animals may not be equipped to metabolize large amounts of dietary cholesterol or animal fat, both of which are absent from plant foods.

In addition, the fatty deposits seen in susceptible animals' arteries are similar but not identical to the atherosclerotic lesions seen in human CHD patients. Rabbit lesions resemble those of early stage human arteriosclerosis, but they do not develop more advanced types of plaques. The distribution pattern of these lesions also differs considerably from humans, occurring at locations in the aorta that are uncharacteristic of human arteriosclerosis.

Perhaps most telling of all is the fact that when rabbits are force-fed cholesterol and fat-rich animal foods, their blood cholesterol values skyrocket to astronomical levels, far higher than those ever seen in human beings. Cholesterol does not just accumulate in their arteries but permeates the organs, causing fatty build-up in the kidneys and liver, yellowing of the eyes, and loss of fur. Unless sacrificed beforehand, these animals die from a loss of appetite that leads to emaciation and starvation, not from a heart attack. The fallacy of extrapolating the results of such studies to humans was extensively highlighted by one critical scientist way back in 1935(14), but many researchers continue to cite these irrelevant animal studies as 'proof' that saturated fat and cholesterol are damaging to humans!

In human beings, cholesterol consumption does not cause the astronomical blood cholesterol elevations seen in rabbits. In fact, dietary cholesterol has hardly any effect on blood cholesterol at all because the body readily accommodates changes in dietary cholesterol intake simply by increasing or decreasing its own output as required. An extensive review of 167 cholesterol-feeding studies confirms that the increase in blood cholesterol induced by dietary cholesterol is negligible and has no association with CHD risk(15).

Drop the Monkey

Some lipid theorists eagerly point to experiments that have shown saturated fat feeding to produce atherosclerosis in monkeys. Because primates are our closest animal cousins, these folks believe any agent which causes atherosclerosis in monkeys must surely do the same in humans.

Wrong.

In experiments with African Green monkeys, researchers have repeatedly found that omega-6-polyunsaturated fats cause less atherosclerosis than saturated and monounsaturated fats(16-18). If monkey experiments were a valid proxy for humans, this would mean that we should all start cutting monounsaturated and saturated fats from our diets, replacing them instead with polyunsaturated omega-6 fats. As you will learn in coming chapters, evidence from studies involving real live humans indicates that such a strategy can have disastrous consequences, by actually *increasing* the risk of heart disease and cancer!

When researchers pulled cholesterol from the diets of rhesus monkeys, but did not reduce the high level of saturates they were consuming, they observed a significant drop in cholesterol and regression of atherosclerosis in the animals(19). This indicates that the cholesterol-raising and atherogenic factor was cholesterol itself, not saturated fat. In humans, however, dietary cholesterol has almost no effect on serum cholesterol, so why should we believe it has any effect on atherosclerosis--especially when dietary cholesterol restriction, just like saturated fat restriction, has completely failed to lower CHD mortality in humans? (See Chapter 8). Clearly, these monkey experiments have little relevance to humans.

What these animal studies do prove is that every species should consume the diet it evolved to eat. For optimal health, herbivorous animals should eat a herbivorous diet while carnivores should subsist on meat; left to their own devices in their natural habitat, that is exactly what they do. Humans are a unique species. We are omnivorous creatures that have evolved over the last 2.4 million years to eat fresh, minimally processed animal and plant foods, yet thanks to industrial processing and the promotional efforts of food companies and health authorities, we willingly eat all manner of highly refined and processed foodstuffs, often in the erroneous belief that by doing so we are benefiting our health.

Even Lipid Hypothesists Have Poor Regard For the Lipid Hypothesis!

The complete failure of autopsy studies to reveal any noteworthy correlation between cholesterol and atherosclerosis lends further support to the contention that cholesterol is not a cause of heart disease. Any relationship between cholesterol and CHD cannot be anything more than a secondary association. Even leading proponents of the lipid hypothesis, during rare moments of candor, admit as much. Writing in the prominent medical journal *Lancet*, William Kannel (director of the Framingham Study) and Tavia Gordon (who headed another large-scale CHD study) stated that: *"Serum cholesterol is not a strong risk factor for CHD, in the sense that blood pressure is a strong risk factor for stroke or cigarette smoking is a risk factor for lung cancer"*(20).

Frederick Stare, a former AHA member who, via his syndicated column in the *Los Angeles Times,* wholeheartedly recommended the liberal use of cholesterol-lowering polyunsaturated oils to millions of Americans, wrote in a 1989 letter to the *Journal of the American Medical Association: "The cholesterol factor is of minor importance as a risk factor in cardiovascular disease. Of far more importance are smoking, hypertension, obesity, diabetes, insufficient physical activity, and stress."* He further stated that *"the cholesterol content of the diet has only a minor effect on the total cholesterol content of the blood",* and that the National Cholesterol Education Program was *"most unfortunate, because it gives undue emphasis to a minor risk factor in cardiovascular disease and thus false hope to millions of individuals."*(21)

Of course, these statements appeared in medical journals rarely read by journalists, the public and--sadly--a significant portion of medical professionals. Such statements are *never* included in the enthusiastic press releases, public announcements and advertisements that help keep the anti-cholesterol juggernaut steaming along.

Chapter 5

"There are liars, damn liars, and then there are statisticians."
Kurt Oster, M.D.

The Vilification Of Saturated Fat

How selective science gave birth to the anti-fat theory

Most of the evidence supposedly incriminating saturated fat as an instigator of heart disease comes from *epidemiological*, or population-based, studies. Advocates of the lipid hypothesis are extremely fond of pointing to populations that eat diets low in animal fats and whom experience low rates of CHD. For some strange reason, their enthusiasm suddenly fades when it comes to discussing the numerous populations that consume high-saturated fat diets yet enjoy low rates of CHD.

Epi-*what*?

The field of *epidemiology* examines the statistical relationship among populations between the prevalence of a phenomenon, in this case CHD, and the occurrence of those factors that are hypothesized to cause the phenomenon. If, for example, we notice that CHD is consistently more common in populations that eat large amounts of saturated fat, and less frequent in populations with low saturated fat consumption, then we have established an *epidemiological association*. This association would give us reasonable grounds for suspecting that saturated fat may be a *possible* culprit in the causation of CHD.

Suppose for a moment we did find a consistent relationship between CHD and saturated fat consumption. No matter how strong the association appeared to be, it still does not in any way 'prove' that saturated fat causes CHD. There always exists the very real possibility that some other as yet-unidentified confounding factor is the true culprit. After all, it is no secret that populations consuming higher amounts of saturated fat also tend to consume more refined carbohydrates, vegetable oils, hydrogenated fats, processed foods, and contain a larger proportion of sedentary and chronically stressed individuals. As we shall learn in later chapters, all of these factors have been implicated in the development of CHD. How do we know whether it is saturated fat or these other factors that is responsible for any observed relationship between diet and CHD?

Epidemiological evidence can provide useful leads and point to areas where further study is warranted, but because of the multitude of possible confounding influences, it should *never* be taken as conclusive proof of anything. To be accepted as causal, a relationship must have a plausible explanation and be readily and repeatedly demonstrable in carefully controlled clinical trials (which are fully discussed in Chapter 8). When it comes to fulfilling these important criteria--consistency, plausibility, and clinical demonstrability--the epidemiological evidence linking saturated fat with CHD fails on all counts.

The Birth of the Anti-Animal Fat Movement

The Twentieth Century saw CHD emerge from relative obscurity to become the leading cause of death in America and most other modernized nations around the world. Researchers, governments, the medical profession, and the general public all desperately wanted to know why.

Researchers knew that dietary cholesterol had produced dramatic blood cholesterol elevations in early animal experiments, and that these cholesterol elevations were accompanied by the build-up of 'fatty deposits' in the animals' arteries. Some of these researchers began to speculate that the same process could be occurring inside humans. One such investigator was a gentleman by the name of Ancel Keys.

It was during the 1950's that the late Keys first proposed that saturated fat and cholesterol were responsible for the widespread prevalence of heart disease in modernized nations such as America. He set out to 'test' his hypothesis by comparing the correlation between fat intake and coronary mortality in various countries. Although reliable food intake data was available for twenty-two countries at the time, Keys chose a mere six of these to examine the link between fat, cholesterol and heart disease. Using this limited data, Keys was able to demonstrate a perfectly curvilinear correlation between coronary mortality and fat intake(1).

The fact that Keys ignored data from sixteen other countries did not go entirely unnoticed--numerous researchers criticized the Minnesota researcher for allegedly selecting countries that fit his hypothesis, and conveniently ignoring those that did not. George Mann, a University of Vanderbilt researcher highly critical of the lipid hypothesis, discovered that Keys had deleted countries from his study where the data supported physical activity as the most accurate predictor of heart disease risk.

When researchers analyzed all twenty-two countries that had nutrient intake information available at the time of Keys' analysis, the correlation between fat, cholesterol and heart disease disappeared(2). Instead of a perfectly uniform pattern, the resultant graph looked more like the holes on an old dartboard--all over the place!

Professor John Yudkin from the University of London also decided to examine the strength of the epidemiological association between dietary fat and CHD. Using data from fifteen countries, he examined the link between various dietary factors and CHD. Yudkin's suspicion that proponents of the lipid hypothesis were *"quoting only those data which support their view"* was readily confirmed by his analysis, which appeared in a 1957 issue of *The Lancet*(3).

The British researcher found that countries with similar fat intakes exhibited a marked divergence in CHD mortality. West Germany, for example, had a similar per capita fat intake to Finland, while residents of the Netherlands and Switzerland had a slightly higher fat intake than the Finns. CHD mortality, however, was three-fold higher in Finland than in the aforementioned countries. A similar disparity was seen when the U.S.A., Canada and Australia were compared to Sweden and Norway. Despite almost identical per capita total fat intakes, coronary mortality in Canada and Australia was almost three times higher than in the two Scandinavian countries. In the U.S., CHD mortality was four times higher! The notion that fat was the over-riding determinant of heart disease risk appeared rather fanciful in the face of such extreme variations in CHD mortality.

Yudkin's analysis was far more extensive than Keys'--he examined not only total fat intake, but also fat as a percentage of calories, the influence of different types of fats, and the possible role of carbohydrates and protein. Despite claims that animal fats were particularly harmful, he found that their association with CHD was even weaker than that observed for total fat. Out of all the dietary factors that Yudkin examined, the one showing the strongest association with CHD was sugar.

Yudkin did not limit his analysis to dietary factors. He also examined the association between CHD and various markers of prosperity. He found that the strongest predictor of coronary mortality among countries was the level of TV and radio ownership, followed closely by car ownership. It goes without saying that electrical appliances and motor vehicles do not, in and of themselves, cause heart disease, but their widespread use among a population does reflect the adoption of a predominantly sedentary lifestyle pattern. We now know that physical inactivity directly promotes heart disease via accelerated degeneration of the cardiovascular system. Indeed, statistics available at the time showed increased CHD incidence among those engaged in professional, sedentary-type occupations.

Yudkin noted that CHD appeared to be a disease of affluence, increasing with rising per capita income. He also observed that affluent countries tended to have higher per capita total calorie intakes, a phenomenon that served to amplify the negative effects of physical inactivity. Yudkin concluded that the overwhelming focus on dietary fat was highly inappropriate, because CHD was a multi-factorial disease, caused not by one single dietary agent, but a combination of deleterious influences that were most prevalent among residents of modernized, prosperous nations.

Some years later, in 1978, Professor Michael Marmot analyzed forty years' worth of mortality trends in England and Wales and found that mortality from coronary heart disease had become progressively more common in working-class men and women than in those from the middle and upper classes. The change in social-class distribution correlated with relatively more smoking, and a shift towards greater refined carbohydrate consumption, as reflected by higher consumption of sugar in the lower classes. There was no correlation between the shift in heart disease mortality and change in the social-class pattern of fat consumption(4).

In 1992, the *International Journal of Epidemiology* published data from the Food and Agriculture Organization and the World Health Organization showing the relationship between animal fat consumption in twenty-seven countries around the world. Of the eighteen countries that displayed increased per capita animal fat consumption during the period 1961 through to 1985, eleven experienced *declines* in CHD mortality between 1972 and 1984!(5)

Just Getting Started

Despite attracting much criticism for his highly questionable research methods, Keys' six-country analysis of 1953 proved to be but a mere warm-up. In 1958, he launched a massive follow-up project known as the Seven Countries study, which further explored the proposed link between fat, cholesterol, and heart disease. Once again, the seven countries (Finland, Greece, Italy, Japan, Yugoslavia, the Netherlands, and the U.S.A.) were selected by Keys. Groups of men residing in all these countries were examined at the start of the study then followed for ten years.

Comparisons between these handpicked countries showed that saturated fat was the best predictor of heart disease risk. *Within* countries however, the alleged association disappeared. This is an important point, because comparisons within nations, where the residents experience similar environmental, cultural, economic and political conditions, are less likely to be swayed by confounding variables than those between different nations.

Inside countries, cardiovascular mortality varied widely between regions, despite similar dietary habits and risk factors. In Finland, CHD deaths were four times higher in Karelia than in Turku, even though similar diets were consumed in both regions. In Greece, Cretans experienced a far lower incidence of CHD than residents of Corfu, despite similar saturated fat intakes. ECG readings also showed no correlation between diet and heart disease risk. Unlike the clinical diagnosis, which was conducted by local doctors with varying degrees of competence, all electrocardiograms were analyzed in the American study center.

The study also claimed an association between serum cholesterol levels and heart disease. The lowest cholesterol levels were found amongst the Japanese, who experienced a far lower incidence of coronary deaths than the U.S. and Finland, the two countries with the highest mean serum cholesterol readings. However, the lowest rates of heart disease in the study occurred amongst the residents of Crete, in Greece, whose average cholesterol levels were positioned right between the middle of the two extremes. The Cretans, in fact, were the healthiest participants in the entire study, experiencing the lowest death rates not just from heart disease, but all causes.

The Cretans had an average serum cholesterol of 202; across Greece, on the island of Corfu, cholesterol levels were 198, yet coronary deaths were five times higher than those seen in Crete. In Crevalcore and Montegiorgio, two different districts in Italy, mean serum cholesterol levels were identical, yet death rates from heart disease were 2.5 times higher in the former than the latter. In Rome, Croatia and the Netherlands, serum cholesterol also showed no relationship with CHD mortality. As with saturated fat, cholesterol levels *within* nations were not a reliable indicator of heart disease risk(6).

Despite these findings, Keys claimed his study showed that low cholesterol levels and a low fat intake, especially from saturates, reduced heart disease risk. Numerous researchers challenged his conclusions, but Keys' low fat theory received much wider publicity. Keys was a nutrition advisory committee member of the highly influential American Heart Association, and his erroneous theories were officially incorporated into AHA dietary guidelines in 1961(7), heralding a long tradition in which mainstream authorities would selectively cite epidemiological research of questionable validity.

As it turns out, the fifties gave birth to a whole lot more than rock'n'roll; it is Keys who is widely credited with beginning the anti-saturated fat movement, despite the many inconsistencies in his arguments.

Customizing the Statistics

Dr. Malcolm Kendrick, a researcher and physician from the UK, points out that if Keys had chosen to use:

1. Finland
2. Israel
3. Netherlands
4. Germany

5. Switzerland
6. France
7. Sweden

instead of:

1. Italy
2. Greece
3. Former Yugoslavia
4. Netherlands
5. Finland
6. U.S.A.
7. Japan

--he would have obtained the exact opposite result--namely, the more saturated fat and cholesterol consumed, the lower the risk of CHD!(8)

So why did Keys choose to conduct such a highly selective and misleading analysis? The answer may lie in events that transpired in 1954, when the World Health Organization held its first Expert Committee on the Pathogenesis of Atherosclerosis to consider the flourishing 'epidemic' of CHD. Many leaders in the field of CHD research had assembled in Geneva, including such notables as Paul Dudley White of Boston, Gunnar Björk of Stockholm, Noboru Kimura of Japan, George Pickering of Oxford, and one Ancel Keys of Minnesota.

Ancel Keys, known for his sharp, blunt, and biting commentary, was reportedly true to form at the conference. But when the outspoken Minnesotan confidently put forth his dietary theory of heart disease at this hallmark gathering, he was greeted with considerable skepticism. Henry Blackburn, a long time collaborator of Keys, recalls that the researcher was *"flabbergasted to find that his ideas were not accepted on the spot"*.

British professor George Pickering interrupted Keys' presentation with a query something along these lines: *"Professor Keys, would you be kind enough to cite for us the principle piece of evidence that you think supports this diet-heart theory of yours?"*

At this crucial moment, Keys, not usually at a loss for words, was caught off guard. Blackburn recounts: *"...Ancel fell into a trap, he made a mistake; he cited a piece of evidence and they were able to destroy it. Instead of citing 'well, this theory's based on a body of evidence that we've seen here and here from the clinic, from the laboratory, and from comparing populations', he didn't make his case. He cited a piece--destroyed. He got up from being knocked to the ground and went out saying, 'I'll show those guys,' and designed the Seven Countries Study"*(9).

Keys was reportedly *"so stung by this event that he left the Geneva meeting intent on gathering the definitive evidence needed to establish or refute this Diet-Heart theory"*(10).

To avenge the humiliation and ridicule he received at the World Health Organization conference, it appears that Keys became hell-bent on proving his theory at all costs. A massive cross-country study, featuring only countries whose data confirmed his hypothesis, was just the ticket to the supportive evidence he so desperately needed. And so the Seven Countries study was born.

It is absolutely reprehensible that one man's misguided quest for personal redemption was allowed to irrevocably alter the entire course of modern medicine. As Kendrick points out, if someone approached a research council today to seek approval and funding for a study as limited and biased as the Seven Countries study, they would be laughed into oblivion. And rightly so. Personal vendetta or not, good science involves arriving at a conclusion only after one has considered all the available evidence, not just that which supports one's predetermined conclusions.

Chapter 6

"History is the version of past events that people have decided to agree upon."
Napoleon Bonaparte

The Studies You Weren't Told About

The research linking saturated fat with low rates of CHD and stroke.

While proponents of the lipid hypothesis incessantly claim that populations with the lowest saturated fat consumption enjoy the lowest rates of heart disease, numerous epidemiological investigations have revealed just the opposite. Researchers have provided us with examples of populations the world over that enjoy extremely low rates of heart disease yet consume large amounts of saturated fat. They have also shown that low saturated fat intakes do not in any way explain the lower incidence of cardiovascular disease in Japan and the Mediterranean.

The Mediterranean Diet: Fact Versus Fiction

The observation that certain Southern European countries experience lower than average rates of heart disease has created considerable interest in the so-called 'Mediterranean Diet'. Being the product of Italian parentage, my curiosity was naturally aroused by the growing publicity awarded to this concept, and I read with interest the descriptions of an allegedly typical Southern European diet. Fresh fruit, vegetables, olive oil, red wine, and legumes, it was stated, were common staples of the diet, and I knew this to be true at least of Italian diets. But when I read claims that a typical Southern European resident ate a low fat diet, with minimal consumption of saturated fat-containing animal foods, I simply rolled my eyes and shook my head.

Anyone even remotely familiar with Italian, French or Greek food knows it is anything but lean. I vividly recall childhood visits to my Grandparents' farm, where my loving Nonna (Italian for Grandma) would feed us sausages, made from pork or veal, and freshly laid eggs. Homemade cheese and salami were also a regular part of my grandparents' diet, as were chickens, pheasants and pigeons. Beef, pork and poultry were eaten in their entirety - surgically trimming the fat from meat or removing skin from poultry was unheard of, and no doubt would have been frowned upon as both strange and wasteful. Lard was frequently used when cooking, and in addition to all this animal fat, generous amounts of olive oil were frequently added to sauces, salads and vegetable dishes.

My grandparents were not an isolated case, for virtually all of their generation, who had migrated from the same area of Italy, ate pretty much the same way. This was not an eating pattern they spontaneously developed after emigrating-- it was the staple diet they had consumed back home in their native Calabria, in Southern Italy. Far from being riddled with illness, Italians of this generation tended to be hardy, robust and long-lived. It was amongst the following generation, who took to sugar, refined flour, polyunsaturated oils and other processed foods with far more vigor than their elders, that heart disease occurred with much more frequency, and at an increasingly younger age.

Southern Italians are not the only Mediterraneans with a taste for fat-rich foods. Across the Adriatic, high fat foods like lamb, pork and feta cheese are a central feature of Greek cuisine, while the French are well known for their generous consumption of saturated fat. The so-called 'French Paradox' describes the fact that high saturated fat consumption in France is accompanied by an especially low rate of heart disease mortality, an extremely puzzling observation to those inculcated with the low fat doctrine. Saturated fat consumption in France is almost double that seen in the U.S., yet CHD death rates in the former are less than half of those in the latter.

Avid consumption of antioxidant-rich red wine by the French has frequently been cited as an explanation for this alleged paradox, but does not satisfactorily explain the difference. After all, the Italians are also fond of red wine, with a per capita wine consumption similar to that of the French. Yet CHD death rates in Italy, while notably lower than those in the USA, are still significantly higher than those seen in France.

So what else do the French do differently when it comes to diet? Well, compared to Americans, the French consume, on average, seventy-eight percent less calories from nutritionally void, blood sugar-boosting sweeteners such as table sugar. They consume four-and-a-half times as much butter, whereas Americans consume far higher amounts of unsaturated vegetable oils, mostly in the form of polyunsaturated soybean oil and margarine. While other Mediterranean countries with low rates of CHD, including Greece, Italy, Portugal and Spain, also consume high amounts of unsaturated fats, these come mostly from monounsaturate-rich olive oil. While all these countries have lower rates of CHD than the USA, none can match France, where saturated fat consumption is the highest.

In all of the aforementioned Southern European countries, the consumption of animal fat rose significantly between 1961-2000. Total fat intake also rose substantially during this period, contradicting popular depictions of the Mediterranean as some sort of low-fat nirvana. The increase in both total and animal fat consumption has been accompanied by an increase in CHD mortality in Spain and Greece, but a reduction of such deaths in France, Italy and

Portugal(1). The notion that a low-saturated fat diet contributes to the low rate of heart disease seen amongst inhabitants of southern Europe appears to be nothing more than wishful thinking.

The East African 'Paradox'

The famous Masai tribes people of Kenya are yet another refutation of the lipid hypothesis. These nomads are a lean people who have survived as shepherds for thousands of years. Most of us in the West would consider their diet to be, well, a little extreme. The Masai thrive on fat-rich milk, with male tribesmen consuming over three liters of full cream milk daily. To say the Masai also enjoy a good steak now and then would be something of an understatement; on market days or occasions of celebration, Masai males have been observed to devour huge amounts of meat--between two to five kilograms (4.5-11 pounds) each of fatty beef in a single sitting!

While young and elder Masai do eat some plant foods, custom dictates that Masai males between the ages of twelve and thirty adhere strictly to this diet of milk and meat, which may be supplemented with fresh cattle blood during the dry season. The fat intake of these young men would have most low-fat gurus choking on their rice cakes; thanks to their substantial intake of fatty milk and meat, Masai warriors average a hefty 300 grams of animal fat daily(2).

In the 1960's, Professor George Mann decided to visit Kenya and examine the effect of such a diet on the cardiovascular health of the Masai. According to prevailing wisdom, heart disease should have been rampant amongst the Masai people, but Mann encountered a slim and extremely fit population virtually free of CHD(3). When he examined their blood cholesterol he found one of the lowest average levels ever measured in any population. Most Masai males had serum cholesterol values below 160, a striking contradiction to the assertion that high animal fat diets automatically lead to elevated cholesterol levels(2).

Supporters of the cholesterol hypothesis speculated that this must have been due to some sort of genetic aberration, so researchers decided to compare serum cholesterol values between rural and urban Masai. Examination of Masai males who had moved to the city of Nairobi, exposed to a more 'refined' urbanized diet and sedentary lifestyle, showed an average serum cholesterol level twenty-five percent higher than their cattle-herding counterparts(4). Genetic factors could not solely explain the Masai's low-cholesterol levels, for they appeared to be just as prone to environmental influences on cholesterol levels as the rest of us.

When Mann examined the hearts and aortas of deceased Masai males and compared them to age-matched autopsied Americans, he found that atheromas (advanced arterial plaques) were almost non-existent in the former and commonplace in the latter. Mann could also find no evidence of myocardial infarction in the Masai hearts he studied(5). An athletic people in outstanding physical condition, Mann believed an important factor in the absence of CHD amongst the Masai was the above average size of their coronary arteries. Mann observed that in males aged between fifteen and thirty, fibrous plaque build-up in the arteries tended to stabilize and remain at a constant level, before continuing to advance after age thirty.

It is interesting to note that the period between twelve to thirty years of age is the period where both fat intake and physical activity are at their highest amongst the Masai. Whilst men in this age bracket are bound to a diet of milk and meat, Mann noted that young and elder Masai outside of this group were both less active and did partake, to a small extent, in processed food items such as flour, sugar, confectionery and shortening. Mann's first-hand observations of the Masai convinced him that the lipid hypothesis was *"the public health diversion of this century . . . the greatest scam in the history of medicine."*(6)

A few years later, another group of American researchers performed similar autopsy examinations on deceased Masai and confirmed *"the paucity of atherosclerosis"* documented by Mann(7).

Shortly before Mann's visit to Kenya, Dr Gerald Shaper from the Makerere College Medical School in Uganda studied another tribe a little further north, the Samburus. Like the Masai, the Samburus have little regard for plant foods and consume an extreme high fat, high protein diet of milk and meat. Whilst they eat less meat than the Masai, the Samburus tend to consume far more milk. Samburu warriors and elders may consume between four-and-a-half to seven liters of high fat milk in a single sitting. During the wet season when grass is abundant and their cattle consequently produce more milk, they will do this twice a day. This amount may drop to a 'mere' two to three-and-a-half liters daily during the dry season.

As a result of their copious milk intake, the slender Samburus are anything but lightweights when it comes to fat consumption, with males consuming up to four hundred grams of animal fat daily. Again, if the lipid hypothesis had any merit, the record-breaking fat intake of the Samburus would be accompanied by sky-high cholesterol levels and astronomical rates of heart disease. Shaper found the exact opposite. Similar to the Masai, the slim, athletic Samburus displayed both low serum cholesterol levels and a notable absence of CHD(8).

You may be thinking that a high level of physical activity was responsible for the low rates of CHD among these east African nomads, who walked up to thirty miles a day. That no doubt helped, but not because it was countering any purported harmful effects of saturated fat. After all, heavy physical activity did not help the population of North Karelia, Finland in the 1960's. Despite a high proportion of lumberjacks and farmers, residents of this isolated community suffered one of the highest CHD rates in the world. The population of St. Helena, where motorized transport was rare and the residents were forced to transverse the hilly landscape by foot, was also observed to suffer from a high rate of CHD during the sixties. Fat consumption was relatively low in St. Helena, but sugar consumption was high(9).

Coconuts and Cholesterol: The Pacific Island 'Paradox'

During the 1960's researchers also began studying the inhabitants of Pukapuka and Tokelau, two tiny atolls in the South Pacific. The most abundant staple of the Pukapukan and Tokelaun diet is coconut, which is eaten at just about every meal. Coconut is unique among plant foods in that it is very high in saturated fatty acids, even more so than animal fats. Researchers found that the Pukapukans and Tokelauans obtained thirty-five percent and fifty-three percent, respectively, of their daily calories from fat, which, due to their high coconut consumption, was almost entirely saturated. The islanders consumed a diet that went against everything advocated by the lipid theorists--and were all the better for it. Researchers noted a complete lack of cardiovascular disease amongst the Pukapukans and Tokelauans(10). In fact, degenerative disease of any type was remarkably low amongst the islanders.

It is interesting to note the average serum cholesterol level amongst the Tokelauans was 240, excessively high according to current guidelines. Despite their exemplary health, if the Tokelauans walked into a doctor's surgery today for a routine check-up they would likely be urged to commence lipid-lowering therapy to reduce their 'elevated risk' of CHD!

Again, those who believe in the cholesterol theory may be tempted to rationalize away the good health of the islanders as a genetic phenomenon. However, observations of islanders who had moved to New Zealand, where they consumed a western diet high in refined foods, showed unfavorable blood lipid changes, increased blood pressure, and far higher rates of ailments like diabetes and gout. The incidence of these illnesses increased the longer the islanders remained in New Zealand(11-14).

Animal Fat and CHD in India

Dr. S.L. Malhotra, of Bombay, India, studied the incidence of coronary heart disease amongst more than a million male Indian railway employees. He found the highest rate of heart disease (135 per 100,000 employees) occurred in Madras in southern India, whilst the lowest rate (20 per 100,000) occurred in Punjab in northern India. Compared to Punjab, fat intake was far lower in CHD-prone Madras, and came primarily from polyunsaturated-rich vegetable sources. In Punjab, saturated fats from milk and other dairy products made up a significant portion of the diet, with polyunsaturates comprising only two percent of the total fat intake.

Despite a far higher rate of smoking, employees from Punjab consuming their saturated fat-rich diet were seven times less likely to die from heart disease than those in Madras. In addition, the average life span of Punjab employees who died during the study was eight years longer than those from Madras(15). Like most non-supportive research, Malhotra's gargantuan study is all but ignored by those recommending low fat diets.

What About the Japanese?

The Japanese, who experience relatively low rates of heart disease, are frequently cited in support of the lipid hypothesis. A large study of Japanese emigrants by Dr. Michael Marmot and colleagues showed that after migration to the United States, their chances of dying from a heart attack rose significantly, almost on a par with Americans. Because the Japanese diet typically contains less fat than the average American diet, low fat advocates have seized upon this study as 'proof' of the lipid hypothesis. These folks obviously have not read Marmot's study in full; neither diet nor serum cholesterol levels were associated with the increased mortality from heart disease amongst the emigrants(16).

In a follow-up study, Marmot found the strongest indicator of risk was the degree to which Japanese emigrants retained their traditional culture. Japanese-Americans who were most faithful to their native cultural traditions experienced an incidence of heart disease as low as that seen back in Japan. The group that adopted Western culture most extensively, however, was two-and-a-half to five times more likely to suffer from CHD. In order to disentangle the relationship between culture and diet, Marmot and his colleagues proceeded to further divide the traditional and non-traditional groups on the basis of their dietary habits. They discovered that those who adhered to Japanese cultural traditions but ate higher fat American foods, were far better protected than those who adopted the American lifestyle but ate lower fat Japanese fare(17).

Marmot's study suggests that the low incidence of CHD amongst the Japanese may be due largely to cultural and social, rather than dietary, influences. Marmot noted that the Japanese tend to place high emphasis on group cohesion and social stability, and this supportive social structure may provide an important buffer against stress. As we shall learn in Chapter 14, stress is an extremely powerful antagonist of cardiovascular health.

Not only do Japanese citizens experience low rates of heart disease, they currently enjoy the longest average life expectancy in the world. Low fat proponents again claim this is due to low animal fat consumption. The historical data tells a different story.

In 1961 it was Greece, not Japan, that held the longevity title. By the year 2000, total fat and animal fat intake in Japan had risen over 250 percent from its 1961 levels. If saturated fat is unhealthy, someone forgot to tell the Japanese, for their ascendancy to the top of the longevity ladder does not appear to have been harmed in any way by increasing animal fat consumption. It is interesting to note that Sweden, where animal fat consumption is high, currently ranks second behind Japan on the life expectancy scale: Swedish men fall short of the average Japanese male life expectancy by a mere two months(18).

In the 1960s, stroke was the leading cause of death in Japan, but in the ensuing decades both stroke mortality *and* incidence decreased dramatically in Japan, particularly during the high economic growth period from 1960 to 1975. During this period, animal fat and protein intake markedly increased, blood cholesterol levels increased, while dietary salt intake and blood pressure levels decreased(19,20).

The decline in stroke is unlikely to have been an artifact of changing diagnostic methods because long-term follow-up studies show high animal protein and fat intakes to markedly reduce stroke risk among men and women of Japanese ancestry. For example, when Japanese researchers followed over 3,700 men and women aged 35 to 89 years from 1984 to 2001, they found those with the highest intake of animal fat had a sixty-two percent lower risk of ischemic stroke death!(21)

A much larger study involving over 40,000 Japanese adults found that, during sixteen years of follow-up, those who ate the most eggs, dairy products, and fish had a twenty-eight percent lower risk of stroke than those who ate the least(22). Yet another study of almost 5,000 Japanese men and women found that, over a fourteen-year period, those in the highest quartile of saturated fat intake had a seventy percent lower risk of hemorrhagic stroke than those in the lowest quartile!(23) The Japanese enjoy long life and low cardiovascular mortality, not because of their low fat diet, *but in spite of it!*

Back to Framingham

We have already discussed the alleged association between cholesterol and CHD claimed from the Framingham Heart Study, but what about saturated fat? Did the longest running of all CHD studies detect any link between saturated fat and CHD? In a 1992 editorial in the *Archives of Internal Medicine*, the study's director, Dr. William Castelli, admitted: *"...in Framingham, Mass, the more saturated fat one ate, the more cholesterol one ate, the more calories one ate, the lower the person's serum cholesterol...we found that the people who ate the most cholesterol, ate the most saturated fat, ate the most calories, weighed the least, and were the most physically active."*(24)

Another research paper that has been used to support low-fat, high-carbohydrate diets appeared in the March 1981 edition of *Circulation*. A dietary questionnaire was given to over 16,000 men participating in three different cardiovascular studies--the aforementioned Framingham study, the Honolulu Heart Study and the Puerto Rico Heart Health Program. The data showed that in Honolulu and Puerto Rico, those who suffered a heart attack ate less grams of starch (carbohydrates from foods such as breads, pasta, potatoes and rice) than those who remained free of CHD, whilst in Framingham the opposite was noted. The results from Honolulu and Puerto Rico, claimed the authors, suggested that starchy foods afforded protection from CHD. However, those who experienced CHD also ate fewer grams of fat and protein, but no protective role was discussed for these two macronutrients!

One thing that stands out when perusing the data from this report is that all three populations showed an inverse relationship between total calories and CHD incidence. The more people ate, the less likely they were to suffer a heart attack. Those who remained healthy also had the lowest average bodyweight, despite their higher energy intake. This strongly suggests that higher levels of physical activity, not starchy foods, were the most important protective factor, for if all participants were equally active (or inactive), those with the highest caloric intakes would be expected to weigh more, not less.

The researchers emphasized how CHD victims in Honolulu and Puerto Rico ate a higher percentage of fat than those who remained free from heart disease. The increase was a miniscule 2.2 percent in the former and 1.7 percent in the latter, and consisted mostly of supposedly 'heart-healthy' unsaturated fats, a point that was not discussed by the authors.

According to the authors, none of the studies' results *"would lead to an alteration of currently recommended preventive diets that emphasize lowering fat intake"*(25). Well, that's one way of looking at it; it would have been more accurate to point out that the results from Honolulu and Puerto Rico failed to support such diets, and that the Framingham study completely contradicted the anti-fat theory!

"Monica? We Don't Know Any Monica!"

Few people have ever heard of the MONItor trends in CArdiovascular diseases (MONICA) project, even though it is by far the largest investigation into the relationship between diet, lifestyle, and cardiovascular mortality ever conducted. Born in the early 1980s, MONICA was a collaborative effort involving thirty-two centers in twenty-one countries around the globe, monitoring a whopping ten million men and women aged between 25-64 years. The participants were followed for a period of ten years.

MONICA must have been a huge disappointment for supporters of the lipid hypothesis; the highest cardiovascular mortality was observed in Central and Eastern Europe, despite the fact that these regions exhibited blood cholesterol levels and dietary saturated fat intakes similar to those seen in Western Europe and the U.S.A.(26). Central and Eastern Europe did differ from the West in other important ways; the intake of dietary antioxidants from domestic and imported fruits, vegetables, nuts was substantially lower, while struggling economical and political systems gave rise to greater psychological stress. Alcohol abuse was also widespread in the Eastern bloc countries(27).

While MONICA was a far larger and more through investigation than Ancel Key's shamelessly biased and selectively interpreted Seven Countries study, and despite the fact that the MONICA results have been known for over a decade, health authorities rarely mention this massive investigation. CHD researchers, meanwhile, mindlessly continue to use what is known as the Keys' Equation, supposedly *"the most precise way to predict the effect of diet on the blood cholesterol levels of individuals and populations, and thus, their risk of coronary heart disease"*,(28) even though it is based on some of the shabbiest, one-sided research ever conducted in the field of epidemiology.

The INTERHEART project was another large, international study which compared the dietary and lifestyle habits of over 12,000 heart attack victims with those of over 14,000 controls who had no previous diagnosis of heart disease or angina. The participants in this study were recruited from 262 centers from fifty-two countries in Asia, Europe, North and South America, the Middle East, Africa, and Australia.

The INTERHEART researchers found that smoking, a raised apolipoprotein B/apolipoprotein A1 ratio, history of hypertension, diabetes, abdominal obesity and psychosocial stress all significantly raised the risk of heart attack, while daily consumption of fruits and vegetables, regular alcohol consumption and regular physical activity were all protective. These associations were noted in men and women, old and young, and in all regions of the world. Collectively, these nine risk factors accounted for ninety percent of the identifiable risk in men and ninety-four percent in women(29).

Interestingly, the INTERHEART investigators did not even bother to measure blood cholesterol levels, instead opting to ascertain the ratio of apolipoprotein B to apolipoprotein A1. ApoB and ApoA1 are blood lipids that other researchers have found to be significantly better predictors of acute myocardial infarction than total cholesterol and LDL-cholesterol (raised ApoB is associated with an increased risk of heart attack, while elevated ApoA1 is linked to a reduced risk)(30).

In an attempt to gain further insight into the alarmingly high cardiovascular death rate in Central and Eastern Europe, a group of U.S. researchers decided to analyze food intake and mortality data for various nations around the world. They created four groups with different cultural patterns; Central and Eastern Europe; Western Europe and the U.S.A.; Mediterranean; and Asian. Data on coronary mortality was available for all countries with the exception of three Asian nations.

Coronary mortality in Central and Eastern Europe was six to seven times higher than in Japan, three to four times higher than in the Mediterranean countries, and one and one-half times higher than in Western Europe and the U.S.A. These differences could not be explained by dietary cholesterol and saturated fat intakes, as these were similar among all the groups (excepting Japan, where saturated fat consumption was below average).

Instead, the researchers found that the majority of variation in coronary mortality was best explained by differing intakes of folate and carotenoids (beta-carotene, lutein and zeaxanthin), and omega-6 and omega-3 fatty acids. Higher intakes of folate, carotenoids and omega-3 fatty acids were protective, while higher intakes of omega-6 fatty acids were associated with increased CHD mortality(31) (the importance of dietary antioxidants, omega-6 and omega-3 fatty acids, fruits and vegetables, and stress will be discussed extensively in Section Two).

Ignoring Contradictions, Inventing Paradoxes

Proponents of the lipid hypothesis repeatedly fail to tell us about the numerous populations in which high saturated fat consumption has never been shown to increase CHD risk, nor the studies in which saturates have actually been associated with low rates of CHD. On the rare occasion when they do mention these populations, it is only to dismiss them as 'paradoxical' (in the case of the French), or to falsely claim that they in fact demonstrate the value of a low-saturated fat diet (as in the case of the Japanese)!

Hopefully, readers are now starting to realize the importance of verifying information for themselves, rather than uncritically accepting conventional dietary 'wisdom'. To further facilitate such awareness, the next chapter will uncover even more studies that the anti-saturated fat establishment would prefer you did not know about.

Chapter 7

"When all think alike, no one is thinking very much."
Walter Lippmann

More Studies You Weren't Told About!

Yet more conflicting epidemiological evidence.

We learnt in the previous chapter how population studies quoted in support of saturated fat restriction have been selectively cited, and how non-supporting evidence has consistently been misquoted and even completely ignored. In this chapter, we will decisively deliver the final and fatal blow to the epidemiological argument against saturated fat. Before we do that, though, it is imperative that we briefly summarize the various types of epidemiological evidence and their inherent pitfalls.

Epidemiology 101

Epidemiological evidence generally falls into three main categories, all of varying reliability:

1) *Ecological data*, which is based on cross-country comparisons. Because it involves comparing apples with oranges--that is, countries with widely varying cultural, social, political and physical environments--ecological data is the least reliable of all epidemiological evidence. It is also the type most frequently used in support of the lipid hypothesis.
2) *Case-control studies*, which compare the past dietary habits of individuals who have recently experienced a CHD event with those of 'control' subjects from the same geographic area who are free of CHD.
3) *Prospective studies* (also referred to as *cohort* or *follow-up* studies), in which a population sample living in a selected geographic location is recruited, interviewed about their dietary habits, and then followed for a given period of time to see who develops CHD and who remains healthy.

Of case-control and prospective studies, the latter--while far from perfect--is generally considered to be the most reliable. Case-control studies require patients to recall their past dietary intake, often as far back as childhood. Given that many folks have trouble remembering what they ate last week, let alone decades earlier, it is easy to see how the findings of case-control studies could be skewed by incorrectly recalled data.

Furthermore, patients' recall of certain foods can be biased in favor of those believed to have contributed to their condition. For example, in an atmosphere where saturated fat and cholesterol are believed to cause CHD, heart attack patients may place greater emphasis on their past consumption of fat-rich foods during questioning than other items.

Prospective studies, on the other hand, obtain dietary data at the start of an investigation before any coronary or other health episodes occur, and are therefore far less susceptible to recall bias. One problem with prospective studies, though, is that they ascertain food intake for periods that can span up to decades from questionnaires given to participants at the start of the study. These studies operate on the premise that the dietary pattern recorded on the survey form is representative of the subject's usual intake for years on end.

Some of these questionnaires quiz respondents about their food intake for periods as brief as one day--too bad if the dietary intake recorded on that day was not typical of the subjects' usual eating habits, or if the subject changed their diet during the follow-up period! Some of the better-designed studies attempt to at least partially circumvent this problem by having the participants fill out additional questionnaires every few years throughout the study.

Prospecting For an Association

Do prospective studies, generally considered the most reliable of epidemiological studies, give any support to the assertion that saturated fats cause CHD?

Table 7a summarizes the results of twenty-six prospective studies of the relationship between dietary fat intake and CHD published between 1963 and 2005(1-26). These projects involved a collective total of over 268,000 subjects who were followed for periods ranging from four to twenty- three years. After making allowances for potential confounding factors, individuals who went on to develop fatal and/or non-fatal CHD had eaten 'significantly' higher amounts of saturated fat in only four of these studies(9,11,19,25), and 'significantly' less in another(21).

Just How Significant is 'Significant'?

Before we continue, it behooves me to explain just what researchers mean when they use the word 'significant'. When you or I use this term, we usually do so in reference to something large or pronounced, but when researchers use the same word they are talking about *statistical significance*.

When it can be demonstrated that the probability of obtaining a difference solely by chance is relatively low, then the difference is said to be 'statistically significant', regardless of the actual size of the difference. Researchers routinely

Table 7a. Prospective studies examining link between saturated fats & CHD					
Authors	Follow-up period (years)	Gender distribution (M/F)	Baseline age range	Number of participants (CHD/no CHD)	Increase in CHD risk detected for saturated fat?
Paul et al 1963 (1)	4	100% M	40-55	88/1797	NO
Gordon 1970 (2)	16	49%/51%	37-69	47/799	NO
Medalie et al 1973 (3)	5	100% M	45-64	431/9764	NO
Morris et al 1977 (4)	20	100% M	40-69	45/292	NO
Yano et al 1978 (5)	6	100% M	45-68	179/7411	NO
Garcia-Palmieri et al 1980 (6)	6	100% M	45-64	286/7932	NO
Gordon et al 1981 (7)	4-6	100% M	45-64	629/15720	NO
Shekelle et al 1981 (8)	20	100% M	40-55	215/1900	NO
McGee et al 1984 (9)	10	100% M	45-68	456/6632	YES
Kromhout & de Lezenne Coulander 1984 (10)	10	100% M	40-59	30/827	NO
Kushi et al 1985 (11)	20	100% M	30-69	110/891	YES
Lapidus et al 1986 (12)	12	100% F	38-60	28/1424	NO
Khaw & Barrett-Connor 1987 (13)	12	41%/59%	50-79	65/794	NO
Farchi et al 1989 (14)	15	100% M	45-64	58/1536	NO
Posner et al 1991 (15)	16	100% M	45-65	213/600	NO
Dolecek 1992 (16)	10.5	100% M	35-57	175/5728	NO
Fehily et al 1993 (17)	10	100% M	45-59	137/2197	NO
Goldbourt et al 1993 (18)	23	100% M	40+	1098/8961	NO
Esrey et al 1996 (19)	12 / 12	53%/47% / 45%/55%	30-59 / 60-79	52/3873 / 40/581	YES / NO
Ascherio et al 1996 (20)	6	100% M	40-75	734/43757	NO
Pietinen et al 1997 (21)	6.1	100% M	50-69	635/21930	NO
Hu et al 1997 (22)	14	100% F	34-59	939/80082	NO
Tanasescu et al 2004 (23)	10.8	100% F	30-55	451/5674	NO
Laaksonen et al 2005 (24)	14.6	100% M	42-60	78*/1551	NO
Walker et al 2005 (25)	18	100% M	34-80	71/430	YES
Leosdottir et al 2005 (26)	6.6	39% / 61%	45-73	339*/27759	NO

*Figure includes all cardiovascular deaths; separate figures for CHD not provided in published paper.

calculate the statistical significance of their findings, that is, the probability that any differences noted in their investigations are not simply due to chance.

A closer look at the prospective studies that detected 'statistically significant' differences in fat intake between CHD patients and healthy subjects reveals just how misleading this whole concept can be. Take the dietary data from the Ireland-Boston Heart study, where the difference in average saturated fat intake between the two aforementioned groups was a measly 0.5 percent of calories! In the Lipid Research Clinics Prevalence Follow-Up study(19), the difference among CHD patients and healthy subjects aged 30 to 59 was a paltry 1.7 percent (in those aged 60-79, the CHD-free subjects ate 0.5 percent *more* saturated fat calories). In the Baltimore Longitudinal Study of Aging, those who went on to develop CHD reported eating an average 1.5 percent more saturated fat calories than those who remained free of coronary problems(25).

To put these figures in perspective, a 0.5 to 1.7 percent increase in energy from saturated fat intake for someone eating a 2,500 calorie per day diet amounts to a measly 1.4 to 4.7 grams of extra saturated fat daily.

In the ten-year report of the Honolulu Heart Program(9), the authors claimed that, after adjustment for confounders, saturated fat intake was significantly associated with fatal CHD. The difference in daily saturated fat intake between those who remained free of CHD and those who died of a heart attack was a measly *half of one gram* (31.9 versus 32.4 grams, respectively)! A statistically significant difference? Yes. Physiologically significant? You've got to be joking!

Even if you choose to believe that such microscopic differences could truly mean the difference between suffering a fatal heart attack or remaining CHD-free, then you should know that McGee and his colleagues found saturated fat intake was lower in the group that included those with fatal *and* non-fatal CHD than in the group that remained free of CHD (31.7 versus 31.9 grams, respectively). Saturated fat intake was also lower among the group that experienced the non-fatal outcomes of angina or coronary insufficiency (30.4 versus 31.9 grams). If these results are to be taken at face value, then it means that such miniscule increases in saturated fat intake paradoxically decrease the risk for non-fatal CHD while increasing the risk for fatal CHD!

Similarly illogical findings were obtained in the Baltimore Longitudinal Study of Aging, where men who reported eating less than twelve percent of calories as saturated fat were thirty-six percent less likely to die from CHD than those obtaining over twelve percent of calories as saturates. In the same study, however, those in the lower bracket of saturated fat consumption did not enjoy any noteworthy protection against overall CHD incidence!

A far more logical and plausible conclusion is that the infinitesimal differences in saturated fat intake between the various groups in the above studies had absolutely no causal relationship with CHD whatsoever. Strongly supporting this contention is the fact that--apart from one study that found a protective association--none of the remaining studies detected any statistically significant association between saturated fat intake and increased CHD mortality.

So yes, the prospective data can be used to confirm a link between saturated fat and CHD, but only if you focus on the four studies that yielded 'statistically significant' supportive results and turn a blind eye to the twenty-two that did not!

Looking Below the Surface

In Chapter 4, we learnt how autopsy studies have failed to demonstrate a relationship between blood cholesterol concentrations and the extent of atherosclerosis in deceased victims' arteries. What about saturated fat intake-- has this shown any relationship with severity of atherosclerosis at autopsy?

Two prospective studies have examined the possibility of such a relationship. Saturated fat was not associated with the degree of post-mortem atherosclerosis in either of these(27,28). Another study, in which the dietary habits of 253 deceased New Orleans men were ascertained by interviewing respondents who had lived with the men for an average of eighteen years, found no relationship between reported saturated or unsaturated fat intake and severity of atherosclerosis(29).

Stroke and Fat

After searching the literature, I found five prospective studies reporting the relationship between stroke and dietary fat. The most recent of these involved almost 44,000 male health professionals aged forty to seventy-five years who were free from cardiovascular diseases and diabetes in 1986. After fourteen years of follow up, there was no relationship between the amount or type of dietary fat and the risk of developing ischemic or haemorrhagic stroke(30).

The largest prospective project examining stroke and fat intake was the Nurses' Health Study, which found after fourteen years' follow-up that the risk of intraparenchymal hemorrhage (bleeding in the superficial surface of the brain) was 2.36 times higher among women in the *lowest* category of saturated fat intake than those at all higher levels of intake. Dietary fat was not related to other types of stroke(31).

A fourteen-year prospective study of 4,775 Japanese folks aged forty to sixty-nine years found that the risk of intraparenchymal hemorrhage increased as saturated fat and animal protein intake *decreased*(32). A similar inverse relationship between animal fat and intracerebral hemorrhage was seen in the Hiroshima/Nagasaki Life Span Study among over 15,000 men and 25,000 women followed for sixteen years(33).

In Framingham, a twenty-year follow-up of 832 men, aged forty-five to sixty-five years and free of cardiovascular disease at baseline, found that the risk of ischemic stroke *declined* with increasing intakes of total fat, saturated fat, and monounsaturated fat, but not polyunsaturated fat(34).

On the Case With Case-Control

What about case-control studies? We know they are considered inferior to prospective studies, but what the heck, let's check them out anyway.

Two case-control examinations found that intake of total fat was significantly higher among CHD patients, but no difference in saturated fat intake was noted(35,36). The remainder failed to detect any statistically significant differences in saturated *or* total fat intake(37-41).

Epidemi-hogwash

Epidemiological evidence is cited with almost boring predictability by those who would have us believe saturated fat causes CHD. Such evidence remains supportive only so long as one:

- Uses artistic license in reporting the results;
- Neglects to quote the numerous reports of healthy populations eating high saturated fat diets, and;
- Conveniently ignores the fact that the overwhelming majority of prospective and case control studies have completely failed to find any association between saturated fat and the development of CHD or stroke.

The lack of association between saturated fat and CHD evident in epidemiological studies raises a very important point: whatever explains the elevated cholesterol levels that have been accompanied by increased CHD mortality in some studies, it cannot be saturated fat!

Clearly, the epidemiological data gives us no reason whatsoever to swap the sizzle of mouth-watering steak for the rubber-like taste of tofu, but what about clinical evidence? Haven't carefully controlled clinical trials shown that low-animal fat diets reduce the risk of CHD? That is the topic we shall discuss in the next chapter.

Chapter 8

"About almost any subject, there are the facts 'everyone knows' and then there are the real ones."
Ernest G. Ross.

The Cholesterol Theory On Trial

The fallacy that clinical trials have proven saturated fat is harmful.

Imagine, for a moment, that we want to prove beyond all reasonable doubt that saturated fat causes CHD. As we have already learnt, epidemiological data, no matter how supportive, is at best circumstantial. In order to begin to establish a definite relationship between saturated fat and CHD, we need to conduct what is known as a randomized, controlled clinical trial.

Such a trial would compare a group of subjects of similar sex, age and health status, who have been randomly assigned to eat diets that are identical in every respect, except that one contains a significant amount of saturated fat (the control group), while the other contains a greatly reduced amount (the treatment group). Ideally, this trial would be 'double-blind', meaning that both researchers and participants would be unaware of who is in the treatment group and who is in the control group, a safeguard that would help prevent researcher bias and the possibility of a placebo effect amongst the subjects.

Because they provide the best available protection against such factors, double-blind studies are the gold standard of clinical research. Unfortunately, double-blind conditions are very hard to achieve when it comes to dietary experiments. People will quickly notice that their meat has been trimmed, that their milk tastes watery, and that they are being fed vegetable oils instead of butter. A very small number of studies have achieved double-blind conditions through the use of specially prepared foodstuffs, but most dietary trials have been only partially blinded. This means that the people taking part in the trial were aware of which type of diet they were following, but the researchers ascertaining the cause of death were not.

The issue of blinding is not a trivial one, as even the most objective scientist can be subconsciously swayed by ingrained convictions. Despite the best of intentions, a researcher who believes that saturated fat really does cause heart disease may be less likely to assign the cause of death to CHD if he knows that the subject in question was consuming a low-saturate diet. As early as 1969, researchers observed that dietary CHD intervention trials which were not blinded were far more likely to achieve results supportive of the lipid hypothesis than those which were either double- or partially-blinded(1).

When we talk about a clinical trial being 'randomized', this means that the participants have been randomly assigned to the treatment and control groups. Randomization prevents subjects with a more favorable prognosis from being channeled to the researchers' preferred dietary regimen. For example, if a larger proportion of smokers or diabetic subjects are assigned to the control group, this provides the treatment group with a significant advantage. As it relies largely on lady luck, this process is not perfect; sometimes the treatment and control groups in randomized clinical trials differ markedly in their baseline CHD risk, despite randomization.

Another reason randomization is employed is to avoid the potential influence of 'self-selection bias'. This is the phenomenon whereby subjects who are more health-conscious and motivated are inclined to choose the treatment diet because it is perceived, rightly or wrongly, as 'healthier'. If the treatment group is characterized by a greater proportion of such individuals, then it may again possess a significant advantage. Any favorable outcomes subsequently experienced by this group may have little to do with the studied intervention. They may, however, have everything to do with other favorable dietary or lifestyle characteristics practiced by the especially conscientious members of the group. For these reasons, most tightly controlled clinical trials now utilize the process of randomization.

Crunch Time

At the conclusion of our clinical trial, we would tally up the total number of coronary incidents and, more importantly, the number of CHD deaths that occurred in each dietary group. It would also be imperative for us to record total mortality, that is, the number of deaths not just from CHD but from *all* causes. As most people wish to avoid heart disease in order to live a longer life, we would need to make sure that any observed reduction in CHD mortality was not merely countered by a similar-sized increase in death from other causes.

Let us assume that upon completing our trial we did indeed record a higher prevalence of CHD and overall mortality amongst the subjects on the high-saturated fat diet. Was it a chance occurrence or was it real? If our study were blinded, tightly controlled, involved a large number of subjects who strictly adhered to their prescribed diets, and was conducted over a substantial period of time, the possibility that the difference was due to chance alone would be greatly diminished. Even so, we would still need to await the results of other studies to confirm our suspicion that the culprit was indeed saturated fat.

If a string of subsequent high-quality studies produced similar findings, we could confidently conclude that saturated fat restriction would be beneficial in reducing the death rate from CHD. However, if these subsequent studies failed to confirm our findings, or produced contradictory results, then we could not legitimately claim that saturated fat restriction offered any benefits in terms of decreasing CHD. The evidence simply would not support such an assertion.

Keeping all this in mind, let us now turn our attention to Table 8a, which presents the results of CHD dietary intervention trials conducted since 1946. Take a good, long, hard look at this table; it represents six decades of clinical research, costing hundreds of millions of taxpayer dollars and countless hours of scientific manpower. Most of this outlay was spent in an attempt to prove that a low saturated fat diet could lower the incidence of CHD. As one browses through the table, it quickly becomes obvious why advocates of the lipid hypothesis rely so heavily on selectively cited and notoriously unreliable epidemiological evidence; clinical trials designed to prove the benefits of saturated fat restriction have been an abysmal failure!

Let the Trials Begin!

The first clinical trial that sought to examine the effects of fat restriction on cardiac mortality was conducted by Lester M. Morrison, M.D., and began in 1946. The Los Angeles physician took 100 heart attack patients and placed half of on a high-protein, low-fat diet and a regimen of nutritional supplements that included calcium, phosphorous, wheat germ, and brewer's yeast. After eight years, thirty- eight of the fifty control patients had died, compared to only twenty-two of the treatment patients(2).

Some of the more outspoken advocates of the lipid hypothesis, such as Dean Ornish, have cited this study in support of low-fat nutrition. However, Morrison's intervention was multi-faceted; in addition to fat restriction, it also incorporated overall calorie restriction that resulted in weight loss, increased protein intake and the use of nutritional supplements.

Excess weight has long been linked to higher rates of CHD, while weight loss has been clinically demonstrated to improve various measures of cardiovascular health. Epidemiological evidence shows that higher protein intakes are linked to reduced CHD mortality(3). The wheat germ and brewer's yeast were administered because of their high B-vitamin content, the latter also containing the important antioxidant mineral selenium. It is now well-recognized that certain B-vitamins lower blood levels of a potentially atherogenic substance known as homocysteine (See Appendix E), while a small pilot trial found a marked reduction in mortality among CHD patients taking selenium-rich yeast on a daily basis(4,5).

Table 8a. CHD Dietary Intervention Trials

Trial	Intervention used	CHD mortality diet/control (%)	Total mortality diet/control (%)	Statistically significant total mortality benefit from intervention?
Morrison LM. 1955 Non-blind/non-randomized, 8 years	High-protein/low-fat diet & nutrition supplements	-	44/76	YES
Rose et al. 1965 Semi-blind/randomized, 2 years	Replaced animal fat with corn oil	17.8/3.8	17.8/3.8	NO
Ball et al. 1965 Semi-blind/randomized, 3 years	Decreased total & saturated fat	8/9.3*	16.2/18.6	NO
Hood et al. 1965 Non-blind/non-randomized, 5-17 years	Replaced animal fat with polyunsaturated vegetable fat	-	14/47	YES (NE)
Anti-Coronary Club 1966 Non-blind/non-randomized, 4 years	Replaced animal fat with polyunsaturated vegetable fat	1.1/ 0	3.3/1.4	NO
Bierenbaum et al. 1967 Non-blind/randomized, 5 years	Compared polyunsaturated fat-rich diet with saturated fat-rich diet	-	10/8	NO
National Diet-Heart Study 1968 Double-blind/randomized, 2 years	Replaced animal fat with polyunsaturated vegetable fat	No data given for mortality, only total CHD incidence (for which there was no significant difference between groups).		NO
Medical Research Council 1968 Semi-blind/randomized, 2-7 years	Replaced animal fat with soya-bean oil	12.6/12.9	14/16.5	NO
Los Angeles Veterans Admin. Study 1969* Double-blind/randomized, 8 years	Replaced animal fat with polyunsaturated vegetable fat	9.7/11.8	41/42.2	NO
Oslo Diet-Heart Study 1970 Semi-blind/randomized, 5 years	Replaced animal fat with polyunsaturated vegetable fat. Increased fish, fruit & vegetable intake.	18/25**	20/27	NO (NE)

*Percentage of deaths from first cardiac incident only.
** Figure includes all cardiovascular deaths; separate figures for CHD deaths
not provided in published paper.

Table 8a (cont). CHD Dietary Intervention Trials

Trial	Intervention used	CHD mortality diet/control (%)	Total mortality diet/control (%)	Statistically significant total mortality benefit from intervention?
Finnish Mental Hospitals 1972 Non-blind/non-randomized, 12 years	Replaced animal fat with soybean oil & margarine	*Hospital K* 1.3 / 2.4 *Hospital N* 2.3 / 5.7	*Hospital K* 5.8 / 6.7 *Hospital N* 14 / 19.7	**YES** *(NE)*
Medical Research Council 1968 Semi-blind/randomized, 2-7 years	Replaced animal fat with soya-bean oil	12.6/12.9	14/16.5	**NO**
Sydney Diet-Heart Study 1978 Non-blind/randomized, 5 years	Replaced animal fat with polyunsaturated vegetable fat	-	17.6/11.8	**NO**
Minnesota Survey 1989 Double-blind/randomized, 384 days	Replaced animal fat with polyunsaturated vegetable fat	1.3/1.2	5.9/5.5	**NO**
DART 1989 Semi-blind/randomized, 2 years	Reduced fat intake *or* increased fish intake *or* increased fiber intake	*Fat* 9.5/9.6 *Fiber* 10.7/8.4 *Fish* 7.7/11.4	*Fat* 10.9/11.1 *Fiber* 12.1/9.9 *Fish* 9.3/12.8	*Fat* **NO** *Fiber* **NO** *Fish* **YES**
STARS 1992 Semi-blind/randomized, 3 years, 3 months	Reduced processed food & total fat intake/ increased omega-6 & omega-3 fat, fruit, vegetable, & complex carbohydrate intake	3.7/10.7	3.7/10.7	**YES**
Lyon Diet Heart Study 1994 Semi-blind/randomized, 2 years, 3 months	Increased omega-3 fat, fruit, vegetable, legume & bread intake/ decreased saturated fat	1/5.4**	2.6/6.6	**YES**
Women's Health Initiative 2006 Semi-blind/randomized, 8 years, 1 month	Reduced total fat intake, increased grain, fruit, and vegetable consumption.	0.08/0.08	4.9/5.0	**NO**

** Figure includes all cardiovascular deaths; separate figures for CHD deaths not provided in published paper.

Morrison's trial was a non-blinded, non-randomized affair; the first published randomized, blinded, clinical trial examining the effect of saturated fat restriction upon CHD involved eighty subjects and was conducted by London scientists, who compared the effect of substituting corn oil for saturated fat. The results were dismal. CHD incidents, deaths and total deaths were all increased in the corn oil group, despite the fact that serum cholesterol levels were, on average, 23 mg/dl lower in this group throughout the study. A group using olive oil also fared much worse than those eating saturated fat. A similar trend was observed in patients who were followed for a further twelve months. The researchers concluded, *"under the circumstances of this trial corn oil cannot be recommended in the treatment of ischaemic heart disease. It is most unlikely to be beneficial, and it is possibly harmful."*(6)

Also published in 1965 was the trial conducted by Bell and colleagues, who found no difference in CHD incidence, CHD mortality, or total mortality among 252 subjects assigned to either low-fat or high-fat diets during an average of three years' follow-up. Again, mean serum cholesterol levels were consistently lower in the low-fat group throughout the trial, with a difference of 25 mg/dl. The researchers noted that the intervention diet was poorly tolerated and concluded: *"A low-fat diet has no place in the treatment of myocardial infarction."*(7)

The 1965 study by Hood and co-workers in Sweden was a non-randomized, non-blinded affair involving 460 patients. The authors observed a large decrease in total mortality in the dietary intervention group, who followed a low-saturated fat, high-polyunsaturated fat diet. There were however, some glaring discrepancies. The percentage of individuals in the most CHD-prone age category (sixty-one years and older) was significantly higher in the control group. Furthermore, the one hundred and twenty-one subjects who followed the 'strict' diet were closely monitored, whereas the control subjects *"went mostly out of our field of vision"*, according to the researchers(8).

What this study was in effect comparing was a group that not only modified their fat intake but also received close medical supervision, with a group that made little change to their fat intake and did not enjoy close medical follow-up. Was it the diet or the more intense medical supervision that made the difference? There's no way of knowing for sure, but a comparison of 112 intervention subjects and 112 controls that were matched for age and initial symptoms provided a clue; while the incidence of heart attacks was similar between the two groups, mortality decreased only in the intervention group, strongly suggesting a favorable effect from close supervision. Also, males in the control group actually lowered their cholesterol levels to a greater degree than those in the diet group, so whatever caused the lower mortality in the latter, it most certainly was not a dietary-induced drop in serum cholesterol.

The Anti-Coronary Club study was the first of the American dietary trials to be published, and heralded a long and irritating tradition of downplaying and even ignoring negative findings that contradicted the lipid hypothesis. In this particular trial, more than 800 men were placed on the 'Prudent Diet', where animal fat consumption was dramatically reduced and replaced by liberal use of polyunsaturated oils. A further 463 men eating their normal diet served as the control group. The authors were quick to highlight the reduction in non-fatal CHD events in the treatment group, and repeatedly praised the Prudent Diet's ability to lower serum cholesterol levels. After four years, subjects in the diet group had lowered their cholesterol levels to an average of 225, while those in the control group remained at their initial level of 260.

After reading the summary of the study, which made no mention of death rates, one could easily conclude that the Prudent Diet was an outstanding success. One had to read the paper carefully to discover that while none of the subjects in the control group experienced a fatal coronary event, nine subjects in the treatment group died from CHD! Death from all causes tallied twenty-seven in the Prudent group and only six in the control group. These figures were casually mentioned in a throw-away line embedded in the midst of the study paper, the bulk of the text instead devoted to the 'impressive' reductions in serum cholesterol seen in the treatment group(9).

In 1967, Dr. Marvin Birenbaum and his colleagues from St. Vincent's Hospital in Montclair, New Jersey, published the results of a five-year trial that examined the effects of two different low-fat diets in CHD patients aged twenty to fifty. They began by randomly assigning 100 men to follow a twenty-eight percent fat diet in which the predominant source of fat was either a 50/50 mix of polyunsaturated corn and safflower oils, or a 50/50 mix of polyunsaturated peanut oil and highly saturated coconut oil. The group receiving coconut oil had twice the saturated fat intake of the corn/safflower oil group, but after five years, the death rate in the two groups was almost identical. Blood cholesterol levels among those who died and those who survived were also virtually identical (239 versus 235, respectively)(10).

The National Diet-Heart Study was a 'feasibility' project comparing the average American diet with various diets in which polyunsaturated oils had replaced animal fats. It was originally intended as a prelude to a highly anticipated national super-trial involving up to 100,000 men. Double-blind conditions were achieved by the weekly distribution of specially prepared foodstuffs to the study participants. The modified foods given to the treatment group were lower in saturated fats but higher in polyunsaturated fats, but had no detectable impact whatsoever upon the incidence of CHD among the 2,032 participants. After the poor results of the Diet-Heart trial, the proposed mega-trial was quietly abandoned due to 'reasons of cost'(11).

Throughout the London soybean oil study, involving 393 participants, cholesterol levels in the diet group ranged between 24-46 mg/l lower than those in the control group. Regardless, there was no mortality benefit from substituting polyunsaturated fat for saturated fat, the authors stating, *"the results of this trial alone lend little support…to the suggestion that a diet of the kind used should be recommended in the treatment of patients who have suffered a myocardial infarction."*(12)

The Los Angeles Veterans Administration Study compared the effect of a diet high in polyunsaturated oils and low in saturated fat with that of a control saturate-rich diet among 846 institutionalized veterans. The researchers observed a reduction in CHD deaths amongst those eating the polyunsaturated-rich diet. However, a significant increase in cancer deaths amongst the diet group entirely negated the reduction in CHD mortality. After eight years, the overall death rate in both the diet and control groups was almost identical.

The Veterans Administration Study was, in fact, the only double-blind study to have found any noteworthy decrease in the incidence of CHD in the diet group. But was the difference due to diet? When autopsies were performed on the deceased subjects the researchers found that there was very little difference in the degree of atherosclerosis between the two groups. If anything, those in the soybean oil diet group, despite having lower serum cholesterol levels, had slightly more plaque build-up in the aorta, the main artery carrying blood away from the heart.

When one examines the tabulated data for the Veterans Administration Study, one sees that there were more non-smokers in the diet group, and a significantly higher number of heavy smokers in the control group(13). Researchers have shown that the arteries of smokers are far more susceptible to undergo blood-stopping spasm than those of non-smokers, even when their coronary angiography findings are normal(14). This could easily explain the lower incidence of CHD among the diet group. Cancer incidence on the other hand, was highest in the diet group, and showed no association with the number of cigarettes smoked. In animal studies, polyunsaturated vegetable oils consistently increase the incidence of cancer and accelerate tumor growth(15). One has to wonder what the mortality result would have been in the Veterans Study had there been a similar proportion of heavy smokers in both treatment and control groups…

The Oslo Diet-Heart Study involved over 400 men aged between thirty to sixty-four who, one to two years after their first heart attack, were randomized to either a diet or control group(16,17). Those in the diet group were advised to eat a low saturated fat, high polyunsaturated fat diet. The experimental group experienced lower CHD incidence, lower cardiovascular mortality, and lower all-cause mortality (the magnitude of the latter being statistically insignificant).

Was it the saturated fat restriction among those in the diet group that accounted for the improvement in cardiovascular outcomes? Or was it due to other potentially confounding factors?

While the diet group was handicapped by a higher number of hypertensive men at the start of the trial, the control group featured a higher number of subjects aged sixty years or older. The control group was also burdened by a higher number of overweight men at baseline, a disparity that was exaggerated further by weight loss in the diet group shortly after beginning the trial. Overweight is strongly associated with higher susceptibility to CHD and premature mortality, and even moderate loss of excess fat improves cardiovascular health. If weight loss was protective, then it should be remembered that--all propaganda from low-fat food manufacturers aside--saturated fat restriction is *not* a prerequisite for fat loss. In fact, as clinical researchers have shown, and as millions around the world have discovered for themselves, high-animal fat, low-carbohydrate diets are extremely effective for fat loss. As for smoking habits, at the start of the trial both groups had a similar number of heavy smokers; by the end of the study, there were almost twice as many heavy smokers in the control group.

Let us be exceedingly generous and assume for a moment that none of the above factors had any influence on the observed cardiovascular or total mortality outcomes, that the men in the diet group indeed owed their improved fortunes to the dietary intervention. It should be noted then that the replacement of animal fats by cholesterol-lowering polyunsaturated vegetable fats was only one of several dietary interventions employed. Those in the diet group were also instructed to increase their fruit, vegetable and nut intake, which would have served to increase the intake of antioxidants and many other cardio-protective nutrients (see Section Two). They were also told to eliminate the consumption of margarine which, because of its high trans fatty acid content, has been implicated as a possible contributor to CHD. Men in the diet group were also encouraged to consume more fish and were supplied, free of charge, with large quantities of sardines canned in cod liver oil. Both sardines and cod liver oil are rich in heart-protective 'long-chain' omega-3 fatty acids. According to the researchers, the complementary sardine and cod liver oil combination proved popular as a bread spread among the dieters.

So which of the dietary interventions would most likely have contributed to the observed cardiovascular benefits? Given the dismal results seen in the seven studies discussed previously, it was highly unlikely that saturated fat restriction was the beneficial agent. In fact, the replacement of animal fat with ungodly amounts of soybean oil (up to 500 ml per week) was likely counterproductive; such a high intake of this oxidation-prone and linoleic acid-rich oil may well explain why the diet group did not experience the far more dramatic reductions in cardiovascular and all-cause mortality seen in later trials involving increased fish/fish oil, fruit and vegetable intake.

The Finnish Mental Hospital Study was conducted in two different institutions, situated in the towns of Kellokoski and Nikkila(19). The study was not blinded, nor was it randomized. The researchers decided upon a 'crossover' design, where between 1959 and 1965 Hospital N used the cholesterol-lowering diet and Hospital K followed a normal diet. In 1965 the diets were reversed and again followed for six years. CHD, as with most other degenerative diseases, is not an ailment that develops overnight; it is a gradual process that occurs over many years. When we examine the death rates from the second phase of the study, are we observing the consequences of the diet followed during that particular period, or the one before? Note that the only noteworthy difference in total mortality was obtained in Hospital N, where the normal diet was preceded by the cholesterol-lowering diet. Is this increase due to the control diet, or the fact that patients spent the preceding six years eating a high-polyunsaturated fat diet?

Such questions assume that diet was in fact an influence on mortality in this study, an assumption that is highly questionable. In addition to its bizarre design, the ongoing scientific conduct of this trial was atrocious; patients who stayed at the hospital for as little as one month were included in the results, as were patients who were discharged from the hospital and re-admitted at a later date. To claim any benefits from such a poorly designed, loosely controlled study, as the authors did, cannot be viewed as anything other than a very bad joke.

The Finnish Mental Hospital Study was so badly conducted that even NHLBI staff criticized it at length in a 1973 edition of the prominent British journal *The Lancet*(18). In fact, the northern European studies (marked 'NE') have generally been such atrocious aberrations of the scientific process that Russell L. Smith, Ph.D. author of *Diet, Blood Cholesterol and Coronary Heart Disease: a Critical Review of the Literature,* the largest critical scientific evaluation of the lipid hypothesis ever published, wrote: *"... it is completely bewildering how some of the trials were ever approved by funding agencies because they probably could not be designed more poorly if the researchers purposely tried to do so."*(20)

In Australia, 458 men with CHD, aged thirty to fifty-nine, took part in the Sydney Diet-Heart Study. Of these, 221 were counseled to increase the polyunsaturated fat content of their diet to fifteen percent of calories per day, but to reduce saturated fat to approximately ten percent of calories and dietary cholesterol to 300 milligrams or less. The control group was given no specific dietary instruction *"apart from restriction of calories if thought to be overweight" and "... to use polyunsaturated margarine instead of butter if they wished".* After five years, death rates were higher in the intervention group (17.6 percent) than in the control group (11.8 percent), even though cholesterol levels were five percent lower in the former(21).

The double-blind Minnesota Coronary Survey was described by its authors as *"an outgrowth of the National Diet-Heart Feasibility Study"*. It involved over 9,000 male and female patients at six mental hospitals and a nursing home in the state of Minnesota. Around half of the patients were placed on a high-polyunsaturated, low-saturated fat diet, while the remainder followed a low-polyunsaturated, high-saturated fat diet. The average patient follow-up was 384 days. Cholesterol levels fell to a greater degree in the treatment group than in the control group (175 mg/dl versus 203 mg/dl, respectively), but there was no difference in CHD incidence, CHD deaths, or total mortality between the two groups(22).

After decades of stubbornly flogging a dead horse, researchers finally began investigating dietary strategies other than those centered on saturated fat-restriction. The Diet And Reinfarction Trial (DART) allocated over 2,000 men to each receive or not receive the following advice:

1. Increase fish intake (men who disliked fish were permitted to use fish oil supplements instead);
2. Reduce total fat intake while simultaneously increasing the ratio of polyunsaturated to saturated fat;
3. Increase cereal fiber intake.

When the results came in, no overall mortality change was seen in the fat advice group, a small mortality increase was observed in the cereal fiber advice group, and a significant reduction of total mortality was seen in the fish advice group. The authors suggested the failure of fat reduction was due to an insufficient decrease in serum cholesterol levels--a most unconvincing line of argument considering that the fish advice group experienced a significant decrease in mortality whilst simultaneously *increasing* their average cholesterol levels!(23)

In the St. Thomas Atherosclerotic Regression Study (STARS), thirty patients were instructed to decrease their intake of vegetable oils and *trans* fat-rich margarines. The intervention group was also instructed to eat more fruits and vegetables and more starchy complex carbohydrate foods like bread, pasta and potatoes. They were additionally advised to reduce their consumption of processed foods--including such refined carbohydrate-rich junk as *"cookies, pastry, cakes"*. The dietary guidelines given to the patients also called *for "strictly limiting"* their intake of meats, fish and dairy products. Dietary records, however, showed a higher intake of decosahexaenoic acid (DHA) among the treatment subjects, indicating that at least some of them had in fact increased their fish consumption.

At the conclusion of the study, one person in the treatment group died, compared to three in the thirty-subject control group. Coronary angiographies revealed that ten of the diet group subjects experienced widening of their arteries, compared to only one in the control group(24). These favorable results have been cited in support of saturated fat restriction, but this study effectively examined the influence of several different but simultaneous dietary interventions. Which of these was responsible for the greater improvements seen in the intervention group? Was it saturated fat reduction? *Trans* fatty acid reduction? Decreased intake of nutrient-poor junk foods? Or the increase in antioxidant-rich fruits and vegetables?

The authors did not address this question in their original paper, but four years later they published a further analysis of the study showing that reduced dietary intake of saturated fat, *trans* fatty acids and monounsaturated fats was significantly associated with the improved angiography results(25). An accompanying editorial even hailed this observation as *"decisive"* proof that *"foods containing saturated and trans fatty acids enhance coronary occlusion..."*(26) The authors of the paper themselves claimed that a causal role for these fats was supported by favorable outcomes in two other angiographic trials which involved low-fat diets(27,28). The intervention groups in both of these other trials, however, also participated in regular exercise and/or stress reduction. Exercise is well known for its ability to widen arteries, while stress has been shown to do the opposite!

In reality, this retrospective analysis of dietary fat intake among the STARS participants does not even begin to prove causality. All it shows is that compliance with the prescribed diet--which involved several different dietary modifications--was associated a greater incidence of angiographically-determined arterial widening. The study, it was noted, *"did not find any other dietary factors that are protective against coronary disease"*--hardly surprising, considering that the authors failed to examine a whole host of other potential confounding dietary factors. They did not report on the effect of refined versus unrefined carbohydrates, and with the sole exception of vitamin E, appear to have made no attempt to analyze dietary or blood levels of any of the protective nutrients commonly found in fruits and vegetables.

The authors of the small STARS study are fully justified in stating that their prescribed dietary regimen, in which saturated fat reduction was merely one of numerous major dietary changes, was associated with a favorable outcome. They cannot, by any objective standard, state that saturated fat reduction was a *"decisive influence"* in achieving such an outcome--the multi-factorial design of their study makes such a claim impossible.

As part of the Lyon Diet Heart Study, 605 patients who had recently suffered a first heart attack were randomly assigned to one of two groups. The control group received no specialized dietary advice apart from that which may have been given by their physicians or hospital dieticians. In contrast, the experimental group was advised to eat a Mediterranean-type diet, where consumption of root vegetables, green vegetables, fish and bread were to be increased, and poultry was to be eaten at the expense of beef, lamb and pork. Experimental subjects were instructed to eat fruit daily, and advised to replace butter with olive oil and a canola-based margarine that was higher in monounsaturated and omega-3 fatty acids than regular margarine.

The study was originally intended to follow the patients for four years, but death rates diverged so dramatically early on that researchers decided it would be unethical to continue and called an end to the trial. After an average follow-up of twenty-seven months, CHD and overall mortality in the treatment group were slashed by a massive eighty-one percent and sixty percent, respectively. Yet again, the difference could not be explained by cholesterol lowering, as both the total and LDL blood cholesterol levels of the treatment and control groups were virtually identical throughout the entire study(29).

What the researchers did find were significantly higher blood levels of omega-3 fatty acids and reduced concentrations of omega-6 fatty acids in the experimental group subjects. This observation is in accord with the findings of other researchers who have compared heart attack victims with healthy controls and observed higher blood levels of omega-3 and lower levels of omega-6 fatty acids in the latter(30-32). In controlled clinical research, the administration of omega-3's from fish oil has produced significant reductions in cardiac mortality(33). Blood levels of vitamin C and E were also increased in the experimental group. Along with vitamin A, these were the only vitamins measured, but it is not unreasonable to assume the diet raised levels of other important antioxidants supplied in greater quantity by the increased fruit and vegetable intake.

The Lyon Diet Heart Study is important because it underscores the fact that ensuring regular intake of vital fatty acids and important antioxidants is far more beneficial than the mindless pursuit of low blood cholesterol levels. But when the Lyon Study paper was originally submitted to the *New England Journal of Medicine* for publication, it was rejected because the *"intervention induced no changes in serum lipids"*. This 'paradoxical' finding left the journal's reviewers, faithful followers of the cholesterol dogma that they were, *"wondering how such a large mortality reduction could have possibly been achieved"*(34). Thankfully, the reviewers at the British journal *The Lancet* were a little more open-minded, and the Lyon Diet Heart Study report was finally published in 1994.

In February 2006, the *Journal of the American Medical Association* published the results of the largest ever trial to examine the effect of dietary intervention upon CHD incidence. The giant Women's Health Initiative involved almost 49,000 women aged fifty to seventy-nine, followed for an average of 8.1 years. Those in the intervention group were intensively counseled to reduce their daily fat intake to twenty percent of calories, to increase their intake of fruits and vegetables to at least five servings daily, and to increase grain consumption to at least six servings daily. By year six, the intervention group was consuming, on average, twenty-nine percent of calories as fat, compared to thirty-seven percent in the control group. The corresponding figures for saturated fat were 9.5 percent and 12.4 percent, respectively. The intervention group was also consuming 0.5 more servings of grains and a measly 1.1 more servings of fruits and vegetables each day. By now, readers should hardly be surprised to learn that there were no significant differences in CHD or stroke incidence, CHD or stroke mortality, or total mortality. Among the 3.4 percent of trial participants with pre-existing cardiovascular disease, the relative risk of non-fatal and fatal CHD was *increased* by twenty-six percent(35). The Women's Health Initiative researchers also examined the effect of the low-fat diet on cancer rates; there was no reduction in the incidence of, or mortality from, breast cancer, colorectal cancer, or total cancer(36,37).

Multiple Intervention Trials

The trials discussed in this chapter are those that were designed to test the impact of dietary change upon CHD incidence and mortality. Before leaving the subject, it is worth mentioning the numerous 'multiple intervention trials' that utilized, in addition to dietary change, such strategies as hypertensive medication, smoking cessation and stress relief. Similar to the diet-only trials, these multiple intervention efforts, which included the massive MRFIT and WHO European Collaborative studies, failed dismally to show any reduction in CHD or overall mortality(38-41).

The Bottom Line

If saturated fats caused even a portion of the damage for which they are frequently blamed, their negative effects should be readily and repeatedly demonstrable in controlled clinical trials. However, after excluding the results of the poorly designed and sloppily-conducted northern European studies, it quickly becomes apparent that there does not exist a single tightly-controlled trial which shows that saturated fat restriction can save even a single life.

Some of these trials, in fact, suggest the exact opposite. The Rose et al, Anti-Coronary Club and Sydney Diet Heart studies all showed significant increases in overall mortality from replacing animal fats with omega-6-rich vegetable fats. The longest-running study focusing on saturated fat restriction (the Los Angeles Veterans study) showed a significant increase in cancer mortality among the intervention subjects--despite their lower rate of smoking!

The only well-conducted dietary intervention studies to have produced any real decrease in coronary and overall mortality are those that involved an increase in omega-3 intake, increased antioxidant-rich vegetable and fruit consumption, nutrient supplementation, restriction of highly-processed foods and/or weight loss.

It must also be pointed out that saturated fat restriction failed miserably to reduce CHD mortality even though it significantly reduced serum cholesterol levels in almost all of the intervention groups. Defenders of cholesterol lowering have complained that these trials could not have reduced serum cholesterol to a large enough degree. Not only does their argument reek of wanting to shift the goal posts after failing to score, it directly contradicts their cherished and oft-repeated dogma that a one percent reduction in serum cholesterol translates to a two percent reduction in CHD risk.

It also blatantly disregards the fact that in the successful trials--i.e. those involving interventions apart from saturated fat restriction--large reductions in mortality occurred even though there was little difference in HDL, LDL or total cholesterol levels between the treatment and control groups!

It must again be emphasized that the dietary intervention studies discussed in this chapter represent sixty years' worth of intensive research, the expenditure of hundreds of million of dollars in public funds, and an enormous amount of time and effort. The reason this massive undertaking has failed miserably to find any causative role for highly saturated animal or tropical fats in the development of CHD should by now be obvious--*there is none!*

Chapter 9

"The medical profession has, after more than 30 years of excellent propaganda, successfully created the wholly iatrogenic-'pseudo-disease' dubbed 'hypercholesterolemia' and the associated malady 'cholesterol neurosis'. After decades of dismal failure to cure this 'disease' of numbers with low fat diets and a host of cholesterol lowering drugs, the medical profession stumbled upon the magic bullet, the cure for this dreaded artificial disease--statins."
Peter H. Langsjoen, MD.

Diet, Drugs, And Wishful Thinking

Erroneously equating the effects of diet and cholesterol-lowering drugs.

After decades of failed dietary and drug intervention trials(1), the cholesterol hypothesis that the health orthodoxy had invested so heavily in was beginning to look like a total bust. It is not surprising, then, that when the positive results from intervention trials using lipid-lowering 'statin' drugs started rolling in during the mid-nineties, the powers-that-be could barely contain themselves. Finally, proof that cholesterol reduction really worked!

Statins were quickly dubbed 'miracle drugs', became a physician favorite, and were transformed into the world's best-selling drug category. The current number one selling pharmaceutical item in the world, amassing a staggering 10.9 billion dollars of sales in 2004, is atorvastatin, manufactured by Pfizer and marketed under the name Lipitor(2). In second place is Merck's Zocor (simvastatin), with sales of 5.2 billion dollars in 2003(3).

Statins: Saviors of the Lipid Hypothesis?

Studies with lipid-lowering drugs prior to the mid-nineties proved to be a source of continual frustration for the anti-cholesterol cartel because any reduction they produced in CHD mortality was usually countered by a corresponding increase in non-CHD mortality, usually from violent death and cancer. Successful trials with statin drugs, on the other hand, have actually shown decreases in total as well as CHD mortality.

Some supporters of the lipid hypothesis have made a rather huge leap of faith and claimed that the positive results seen in some statin trials support the value of cholesterol-lowering diets. This is shady extrapolation at its worst. First of all, lipid -lowering drugs reduce blood cholesterol to a far greater degree than most individuals could ever achieve through diet alone, which, of course, is the main reason for their widespread use.

Secondly, we have seen how blood lipid levels are hardly a consistent, reliable forecaster of CHD, and that any association between serum cholesterol and CHD is at best secondary. As a result, one must consider the possibility that lipid-lowering drugs may affect CHD through some mechanism other than merely lowering cholesterol. Numerous studies have established that this is exactly the case.

Statins: No Benefit From Cholesterol-Lowering

While heavily promoted, the claim that the CHD reductions seen in clinical trials with statins are due to their potent cholesterol-lowering action is scientifically baseless. A close look at the data from the major controlled, randomized clinical trials with statin drugs reveals that in most instances there was no association between the degree of total cholesterol lowering and the CHD survival rate. In other words, the risk of a fatal heart attack was similarly reduced whether cholesterol levels were lowered by a small or large amount. The same applies to LDL cholesterol, which we have been brainwashed into believing is the 'bad' cholesterol; death rates in those with the highest and lowest LDL levels are virtually identical(4-10).

There are at least two statin trials that *have* shown a relationship between cholesterol lowering and survival--one that directly contradicts mainstream dogma. In the PROSPER trial, which involved high-risk elderly subjects, the highest survival rates in both the treatment and control groups were seen among those with the *highest* LDL cholesterol levels(11). In the Japanese Lipid Intervention Trial (J-LIT), a six-year study of over 47,000 patients treated with simvastatin, those with a total cholesterol level of 200-219 mg/dl had a lower rate of coronary events than those whose levels were above or below this range. The lowest overall mortality rate was seen in the patients whose total and LDL cholesterol levels were between 200-259 mg/dl and 120-159 mg/dl. The highest death rate in the study was observed among those whose cholesterol levels were below 160 mg/dl(12).

If statins exert a favorable effect on coronary health, it most certainly isn't through cholesterol reduction!

How Statins Really Work

Statin drugs exert their lipid-lowering effect by blocking *3-hydroxy-3-methylglutaryl coenzyme A reductase,* an enzyme in the liver that is involved in the early stages of cholesterol synthesis. Statins inhibit the synthesis not only of cholesterol, but a whole host of important intermediate metabolites including, but not limited to, *mevalonate pyrophosphate, isopentanyl pyrophosphate, geranyl-geranyl pyrophosphate* and *farnesyl pyrophosphate*. Inhibition of these compounds means that statins exert a plethora of effects unrelated to cholesterol lowering. Below are numerous examples of how these lipid-independent effects can indeed impact positively upon the cardiovascular system:

- *Impairment or reversal of atherosclerotic plaque formation.* Statins reverse or impede the progression of atherosclerosis in rabbits, without any accompanying change in serum cholesterol(13,14).
- *Improvements in arterial function.* In elderly diabetic patients, cerivastatin increased dilation of the brachial artery after only three days, before any change in cholesterol levels had occurred(15). In healthy young males with normal cholesterol, improved endothelial function was observed within twenty-four hours of treatment with atorvastatin; again, this improvement preceded any drop in serum cholesterol levels(16). Longer-term improvements in arterial function by statins are also unrelated to the degree of cholesterol reduction. In human volunteers with slightly elevated cholesterol, researchers found that four weeks of simvastatin therapy significantly enhanced forearm blood flow. The improvement increased with continued administration of simvastatin despite no further reduction in serum cholesterol, and there was no relation between the decrease in cholesterol and improvement in endothelial function(17).
- *Anti-clotting effects.* Statins have been shown to reduce blood platelet production of thromboxane, an eicosanoid that encourages blood clotting. This effect was not seen with older drugs that lowered total or LDL cholesterol such as cholestyramine, cholestipol, and fibrates(18). Italian researchers observed that simvastatin, atorvastatin, and fluvastatin reduced platelet reactivity before significant reductions in LDL cholesterol occurred(19,20).
- *Anti-inflammatory effects.* As will be discussed further in Section Two, atherosclerosis is an inflammatory disorder. In research with mice, statins markedly reduce measures of both inflammation and atherosclerosis, despite little change in serum cholesterol levels(21). In humans, statin therapy produces significant reductions in C-reactive protein (CRP), a marker of inflammatory activity that has repeatedly been associated with increased cardiovascular risk. This statin-induced reduction in CRP levels is not correlated with any decrease in LDL cholesterol levels(22-25). *Adhesion molecules* and *chemoattractants* are key players in this inflammatory process. They promote adhesion and migration of leukocytes into the arterial wall, furthering the development of atherosclerotic plaque(26). In an important experiment, Swiss researchers produced a specially modified form of lovastatin (Mevacor) with no inhibitory effect on HMG-CoA reductase. This 'designer statin' still possessed potent anti-adhesive, anti-

chemoattractant effects, despite complete disablement of its cholesterol-lowering actions(27).

- *Antioxidant effects.* Free radical damage, also known as oxidative damage, plays a key role in the development of atherosclerosis. In animal studies, statins reduce various measures of oxidative stress even when cholesterol levels remain unchanged(28-30). In humans, a mere nine days of atorvastatin administration (20 mg/day) significantly decreased platelet levels of oxidized LDL. These changes were observed before any noteworthy drop in LDL cholesterol was evident(20). In patients randomly assigned to receive ten milligrams of pravastatin or twenty milligrams of fluvastatin for twelve weeks, significant reductions in oxidized LDL cholesterol occurred in both groups. The reduction was significantly higher in the fluvastatin group than in the pravastatin group (47.5 versus 25.2 percent, respectively). Reductions in total and LDL cholesterol, however, did not differ between the two groups(30).

- *Inhibition of the migration and proliferation of smooth muscle cells that is seen during atherosclerotic plaque formation*(31,32). That this phenomenon occurs independently of lipid-lowering was first confirmed when researchers observed that addition of mevalonate, geraniol, farnesol and geranylgeraniol, but not LDL cholesterol, prevented the anti-proliferative effect of statins(33-35). Animal research also shows a disconnect between the lipid-lowering and anti-proliferative effects of statins. When collars were placed around one of the carotid arteries in rabbits, treatment with lovastatin, simvastatin and fluvastatin significantly reduced intimal lesion formation, despite no change in the animals' cholesterol levels(14).

- *Prevention of atherosclerotic plaque rupture.* Plaque rupture is believed to be the instigating factor in a significant portion of coronary events(36). In patients with symptomatic carotid atherosclerosis, forty milligrams per day of pravastatin reduced the lipid and oxidized LDL cholesterol content but increased the collagen content of plaques as compared to control subjects. These changes are commensurate with those seen in stable plaques that are less prone to rupture(37). In experiments with mice, simvastatin significantly *increased* serum cholesterol levels but induced a forty-nine percent reduction in the frequency of intraplaque hemorrhage and a fifty-six percent reduction in the frequency of calcification, both markers of advanced and unstable atherosclerotic plaques(38). Compared to controls, adult male monkeys fed an atherogenic diet and given pravastatin or simvastatin showed significantly reduced inflammatory activity in plaques, while markedly increasing their collagen content. This effect was totally independent of cholesterol reduction; blood lipid levels in the animals were kept stable by manipulating dietary cholesterol intake(39).

- *Prevention of cardiac hypertrophy.* Takemoto and co-workers demonstrated the ability of statins to prevent cardiac hypertrophy in mice.

This benefit occurred despite no change in serum cholesterol levels. Research by these and other researchers suggests the anti-hypertrophic effect of statins may derive from their antioxidant properties(40,41).

- *Increased nitric oxide activity.* Nitric oxide synthase (NOS) is the enzyme that stimulates the production of nitric oxide, a substance that plays a critical role in maintaining healthy arteries (see Chapter 21). Rats pretreated for one week with either cerivastatin or placebo underwent thirty minutes of coronary artery occlusion followed by 180 minutes of reperfusion--a procedure that mimics the metabolic stress encountered during a heart attack. Cerivastatin decreased infarct size (the damaged portion of heart muscle) by forty-nine percent--without reducing plasma cholesterol levels. Cerivastatin did this by increasing the activity of NOS by over fifty percent. Another group of rats given an NOS inhibitor along with cerivastatin did not experience increased NOS activity nor any cardiac protection(42).

Cholesterol Camouflage

The evidence that statins exert a multitude of favorable cardiovascular effects independent of cholesterol reduction is incontrovertible. Nonetheless, the medical mainstream continues to claim that LDL cholesterol reductions largely explain the lowered coronary mortality seen in some statin trials. Increasingly aggressive statin therapy is now being heavily promoted on the basis that greater reductions in LDL cholesterol will lead to far more favorable coronary mortality outcomes. Let's take a closer look at the studies being used to support this highly dubious contention...

PROVE-IT Didn't Prove Diddly

The PROVE-IT trial randomized 4,162 patients who had recently been hospitalized for an acute coronary event to either forty milligrams of pravastatin or eighty milligrams of atorvastatin daily. During the trial, the median LDL cholesterol levels achieved on the forty-milligram pravastatin and eighty milligram atorvastatin doses were 95 mg/dl and 62 mg/dl, respectively. After an average follow-up period of two years, the high dose atorvastatin group enjoyed a thirty percent reduction in CHD mortality and a twenty-eight percent decrease in overall mortality(43). In response to these results, the establishment almost wet itself with delight. According to the barrage of media publicity that accompanied publication of the PROVE-IT results, this trial established once and for all that the lower the LDL cholesterol level, the better!

Actually, PROVE-IT proved no such thing.

That statins exert a whole host of biochemical effects beyond mere lipid lowering is incontestible; how do we know it was not a magnification of some other beneficial action of statins that produced the favorable mortality outcomes? Furthermore, the PROVE-IT trial not only tested two different statin dosages, but *two different statins!* As a result, the trial violated one of the most fundamental rules of clinical research: *Control all your variables!* Statin drugs might belong to the same family, but they are hardly identical clones. Even slight variations in a drug's structure can dramatically alter its pharmacologic actions. Indeed, a comparison of atorvastatin with fluvastatin, lovastatin, pravastatin, and simvastatin found that the former not only lowered LDL cholesterol to a greater extent--it also produced greater reductions in CRP and another inflammatory marker known as lipoprotein-associated phospholipase A2 (Lp-PLA2)(44). Such differences could easily have contributed to the divergent mortality outcomes.

Given the multiple actions of statins, it is most illogical to claim that any mortality benefit was due to LDL reduction. Such incongruity proved little hindrance to a group of NCEP panelists from using the PROVE-IT results to promptly revise official guidelines in July 2004, endorsing even more aggressive LDL lowering(45). Overnight, these revised NCEP guidelines created millions of new patients qualifying for cholesterol drug 'therapy'. Jaded observers were hardly surprised when most of the panelists were subsequently revealed to have financial ties with statin drug manufacturers(46).

Interestingly, the fanfare awarded to the PROVE-IT trial was not extended to the subsequent A to Z trial, a randomized, double-blind study of coronary patients receiving either forty milligrams daily of simvastatin for one month followed by eighty milligrams daily thereafter, or placebo for four months followed by twenty milligrams daily of simvastatin. Among the patients in the placebo plus low-dose simvastatin group, the median LDL cholesterol level achieved was 77 mg/dl after eight months. In the high dose simvastatin group, LDL cholesterol levels were reduced to 63 mg/dl at eight months. Cardiovascular death occurred in 5.4 and 4.1 percent of the patients in the low and high-dose groups, respectively. All-cause mortality was 6.7 and 5.5 percent, respectively, but the difference was not statistically significant. What's more, there is no guarantee that greater LDL cholesterol reductions were responsible for the less-than-spectacular trend towards lower mortality in the high dose group. C-reactive protein values became significantly lower in the high dose simvastatin group only, indicative of an increased anti-inflammatory effect(47).

TNT Bombs Out

While the uninspiring results of the A to Z trial were quietly ignored, a subsequent trial that appeared to support the results of PROVE-IT was warmly welcomed in March, 2005. This was the TNT study, which randomly assigned 10,001 CHD patients with LDL cholesterol levels of less than 130 mg/dl to either ten or eighty milligrams of atorvastatin daily. Those receiving low-dose atorvastatin reduced their mean LDL cholesterol levels to 101 mg/dl, while those taking the high dose brought their LDL readings down to 77 mg/dl. After a median follow-up of 4.9 years, 2.5 percent of the low-dose group had died from coronary causes, compared to 2 percent in the high dose group, a twenty percent relative risk reduction. Media reports enthusiastically hailed these supportive results as triumphant confirmation of the PROVE-IT findings. According to the hype, the *"lower is better"* era of LDL cholesterol reduction had officially arrived.

Not so gleefully embraced was perhaps the most important TNT finding of all-- namely, the fact that there was no difference between the two treatment groups in overall mortality. The total death rates in the low- and high-dose atorvastatin groups were 5.6 and 5.7 percent, respectively. Cancer deaths were thirteen percent higher on the eighty-milligram dose of atorvastatin, while non- traumatic deaths from causes other than cancer were increased by over a third. Despite all the commotion, those taking the high dose atorvastatin did not experience a single day of increased life span, although they did suffer a greater risk of adverse side effects (5.8 versus 8.1 percent in the low- and high-dose groups, respectively--a forty percent relative risk increase). And again, there is no support whatsoever for the claim that LDL cholesterol reductions were in fact responsible for the decline in coronary mortality; markers of anti- inflammatory, vasodilatory and anti-clotting activity were not reported in the TNT paper(48).

The official response to concerns about the lack of reduction in overall mortality were a shining example of how the medical orthodoxy focuses on what it wants to believe and rationalizes away that which it does not. According to head researcher of the TNT study, Dr. John LaRosa, *"We need to make the assumption that mortality has been proven, that LDL lowering does in fact lower total mortality rates"*. To assume from a study showing absolutely no reduction in overall mortality that higher statin dosages do in fact lower overall mortality requires a complete abandonment of one's rational faculties.

Dr Roger Blumenthal, from Johns Hopkins University Medical Center, in Baltimore, Maryland, said that the TNT mortality finding was *"unfortunate"* and *"a bit surprising,"* but that the increase in non-cardiovascular mortality was likely due to chance. According to Blumenthal, *"The totality of evidence does not suggest that lowering LDL cholesterol to very low levels is associated with non-cardiovascular mortality"* (Chapters Two and Three of this book explain at length why such an assertion is absurd). Meanwhile, Steve Nissen, a prominent researcher and advocate of statin drugs, was quoted as saying that *"If you don't die of coronary heart disease, you're going to die of something else"*(49). Gee, to have such enlightened commentators at the helm of modern coronary care sure fills me with a sense of confidence and relief!

Cut the CRP

The effect of statins upon CRP levels is worthy of further mention. In January 2005, the *New England Journal of Medicine* published two studies examining the interplay between statin use, CRP levels, and subsequent coronary events. The first, using data from the PROVE IT study, found: *"Patients who have low CRP levels after statin therapy have better clinical outcomes than those with higher CRP levels, regardless of the resultant level of LDL cholesterol."*(50) In the second study, researchers used intravascular ultrasonography to examine the association of LDL and CRP with the continued development of atherosclerosis in 502 CHD patients. They found *"Atherosclerosis regressed in patients with the greatest reduction in CRP levels, but not in those with the greatest reduction in LDL cholesterol levels."*(51)

Another study demonstrating the primary importance of statins' anti-inflammatory effects was the CARE trial, where recent heart attack patients with average cholesterol levels were randomized to forty milligrams of pravastatin per day or placebo. The CARE results clearly show that the risk of major coronary events was reduced to a similar degree among those taking pravastatin regardless of their baseline total or LDL cholesterol level. There was one exception; those with baseline levels of LDL below 125 mg/dl experienced a four percent relative *increase* in major coronary event risk during the trial(6). So much for the *"lower is better"* paradigm...

The picture changed dramatically when the authors subsequently pored through the CARE data for evidence of an anti-inflammatory effect. They found that participants with the highest baseline levels of CRP and Serum Amyloid A (another protein that serves as a marker of inflammatory activity) experienced a reduction of fifty-four percent in the incidence of recurrent coronary events compared with a reduction of twenty-five percent in those with low CRP and SAA. This was despite the fact that baseline cholesterol values almost identical in the two groups!(52)

Also worthy of mention is the PRISM study. In this trial, the effect of statin therapy on coronary event rates was evaluated in over 1,600 patients with proven coronary artery disease and a history of chest pain during the 24 hours prior to hospital admission. At thirty days, statin therapy significantly reduced mortality and the incidence of nonfatal myocardial infarction compared with patients who did not receive statins. The need for revascularization, and the length of hospitalization was also decreased by statin therapy. The benefits were independent of cholesterol-reduction--total cholesterol levels were similar between treatment groups throughout the study!(53)

Because atherosclerotic heart disease is an inflammatory ailment, it is hardly surprising that reductions in inflammatory markers like CRP are accompanied by significant reductions in atherosclerosis progression and CHD risk. Science has yet to determine whether CRP itself is just a secondary risk factor, or whether it plays a directly causal role in cardiovascular disease. Regardless of what future research reveals, the good news is that one need not resort to potentially toxic drugs like statins in order to lower CRP levels.

In a controlled clinical trial, subjects consuming a diet high in fruits, vegetables and nuts experienced reductions in CRP similar to those observed in participants randomized to receive twenty milligrams per day of lovastatin; CRP was reduced by twenty-eight and thirty-three percent in the diet and lovastatin group, respectively(54). Another randomized trial found that those assigned to a calorie-restricted low-fat diet experienced only a five percent drop in CRP levels; in contrast, those assigned to a calorie-restricted higher protein, higher fat, lower carbohydrate diet void of fruit juices and other foods high in quickly absorbed carbohydrates experienced a hefty 48 percent drop in CRP levels(55). Exercise, weight loss, and supplementation with omega-3-rich fish oils have also been shown to produce substantial reductions in CRP levels(56-60). More importantly, all the aforementioned interventions have been shown in clinical trials to lower cardiovascular mortality.

The Truth Comes Out...At Last!

In late 2006, two prominent medical journals published articles that broke the established trend of automatically ascribing any benefit of statin therapy to LDL reduction. In September, the American Medical Association's *Archives of Internal Medicine* featured a pooled analysis of thirteen randomized controlled trials comparing intensive statin therapy with a control treatment (no statins, lower dose statins, or usual care) in patients recently hospitalized for acute coronary syndromes. When the results of these trials were collectively analyzed, at twenty-four months there was a nineteen percent reduction in the composite endpoint of overall cardiovascular events (recurrent myocardial infarction or ischemia, and cardiovascular death). But this risk reduction was independent of LDL cholesterol reduction. The authors acknowledged the importance of statins' pleiotropic effects, and stated clearly in their paper: *"There is no significant evidence that reduction in LDL-C level explains these beneficial effects."*(61)

In the October 2006 issue of the *Annals of Internal Medicine*, researchers reviewed all controlled trials, cohort studies, and case–control studies that examined the independent relationship between LDL cholesterol and major cardiovascular outcomes in patients with LDL cholesterol levels less than 130 mg/dl. The NCEP considers LDL under 130 mg/dl as desirable and in their 2004 guidelines, the NCEP "expert" panel recommended physicians titrate lipid therapy to reach an LDL cholesterol level less than 70 mg/dl in very high risk patients. The panel stated that consistent and compelling evidence showed a strong relationship between LDL cholesterol level and cardiovascular risk. When the researchers went searching for this "compelling" evidence cited by the NCEP "experts" (most of whom were the beneficiaries of drug company money) they found "...*no clinical trial subgroup analyses or valid cohort or case–control analyses suggesting that the degree to which LDL cholesterol responds to a statin independently predicts the degree of cardiovascular risk reduction.*"(62)

So much for the theory that statins owe their efficacy to cholesterol lowering! Now, what about their safety record?

The Steep, Steep Downside of Statins

A visit to any of the numerous health-oriented forums on the internet will quickly reveal hundreds of posts from dissatisfied statin users, describing an alarming array of side-effects: the most common being extreme fatigue, nausea, gastrointestinal problems, and muscle weakness and pain(63). Complaints from patients about their doctors' inability to link recent health problems with statin use are frequent. In many instances, users report that they put two-and-two together themselves, stopped taking the drugs, and experienced significant or even complete remission of their symptoms. Frequent side effects are no doubt a major reason why up to seventy-five percent of people taking statins discontinue their use(64,65).

When questioned about these safety concerns, those who defend statins repeatedly and enthusiastically point to the low incidence of adverse effects reported in controlled, randomized clinical trials. These trials, it is claimed, clearly demonstrate that statins are safe, effective and extremely well tolerated drugs. Don't you believe it! As proof of their alleged safety among the general population, the clinical trial experience with statins is next to useless.

Why?

Because when researchers recruit participants for statin clinical trials, they carefully screen for--and exclude--a wide range of individuals including women of childbearing age, those with a history of drug or alcohol abuse, poor mental function, heart failure, arrhythmia, and other cardiac conditions, liver and kidney disorders, cancer, *"other serious diseases",* and *"hypersensitivity"* to statins. Thus, the disparity between the widespread 'real-world' prevalence of side effects from statin use and the low prevalence of side effects in clinical trials is hardly surprising. These trials exclude groups that comprise a significant proportion of the real world population, and can hardly be taken as a realistic barometer for the expected incidence of side effects in the general population.

This sort of careful screening is par for the course with clinical trials, so it's little wonder that fifty-one percent of prescription drugs are subsequently found to have serious adverse effects not detected prior to regulatory approval!(66) And even with these strict exclusion criteria, there is evidence to show that the clinical experience with statins has been far from trouble-free. Data from the largest statin trial, the Heart Protection Study (HPS), suggest that the daily forty-milligram dose of simvastatin used was nowhere near as well tolerated as the authors would have us believe. A substantial number of patients did not enter the trial after a six week run-in period on simvastatin before randomization; of the 32,145 who participated in the run-in phase, 11,609 patients--over one third--dropped out before the official start of the trial

Of these 11,609 patients who did not proceed to the trial, sixty-five percent *"chose not to continue"* for reasons that were not specified, seventeen percent *"did not seem likely to be compliant long-term"*, thirteen percent *"were considered by their own doctor to have a clear indication for (or contraindication to) statin therapy after review of the screening lipid results provided"*, ten percent *"had abnormal screening blood results"*, nine percent *"reported problems associated with the run-in treatment"* (which comprised forty milligrams of simvastatin, plus vitamins E, C and beta-carotene), and one percent had *"other reasons for not continuing"*(67). These figures suggest that the incidence of adverse reactions to simvastatin among those who did not enter the HPS trial ran into the thousands, a stark contrast to the handful of adverse reactions reported among the fastidiously-screened patients who participated in the official trial.

The results of the ALLHAT trial, published in December 2002, provide yet more evidence that statin side effects are far more frequent than typically claimed. ALLHAT was unique in that it included populations that had been excluded or underrepresented in previous statin trials, particularly older persons, women, racial and ethnic minority groups, and persons with diabetes. While most of the other usual exclusion criteria, such as evidence of liver or kidney dysfunction, were still enforced, the broader range of participants, and the non-blinded nature of the study, meant that it approximated real life conditions a little more closely than most other statin trials. Extending for a period of six years, ALLHAT was also one of the longest-running statin trials.

By the sixth year, twenty-three percent of the ALLHAT participants randomized to receive pravastatin had stopped taking their medication. About half of these subjects did so without citing a specific reason, while the remainder cited *"adverse effects and other medical and nonmedical reasons."* Unfortunately, we'll never know the exact type and frequency of side effects among the ALLHAT participants; specific adverse effects data were not collected during the study(68).

Absent from the glowing media reports results of the PROVE-IT trial was the fact that liver enzymes were elevated in 3.3 percent of the group taking eighty milligrams of Lipitor, compared to 1.1 percent of the group taking forty milligrams of Pravachol (when liver enzyme levels rise, patients must be advised to stop taking the drug or reduce the dose). Even more telling were the study's withdrawal rates: thirty-three percent of patients discontinued Pravachol and thirty percent discontinued Lipitor after two years due to adverse events or other reasons(43).

Statins Can and Do Kill

Regardless of what the medical orthodoxy would have us believe, the dangers from statin use are very real, as illustrated by the tragic death of Mrs. Elnoisa Calabio. Mrs. Calabio's story was presented at an FDA public hearing in May 2000: *"On October 7, 1999, at the age of 48, registered nurse, wife and mother, Elnoisa Calabio, succumbed to the end stages of irreversible dermatomyositis and interstitial pulmonary fibrosis directly caused by her use of a prescribed cholesterol-lowering medication, simvastatin (Zocor). Mrs. Calabio had no substantial risk factors for heart disease. Her blood pressure was controlled. Her cholesterol was slightly high, but not considered dangerous. Tragically, in her last days she knew that the cholesterol lowering drug her doctor had recommended to extend her life was in fact the cause of her fatal illness."*(69)

Contrary to decades of anti-cholesterol propaganda, the mere presence of elevated cholesterol does not constitute a 'disease'. In any sane world, prescribing potentially deadly drugs to individuals free of heart disease, simply because they failed to meet some arbitrary level of serum cholesterol, would be considered nothing less than a cut-and-shut case of medical malpractice.

Sadly, Mrs Calabio's family is hardly alone in grieving the needless, statin-induced loss of a loved one. In August 2001, pharmaceutical giant Bayer AG was forced to withdraw Baycol (cerivastatin) from the market, after at least fifty-two deaths had been linked to the drug. Baycol was causing rhabdomyolysis, a condition characterized by severe muscle damage. This rare disorder occurs when a large number of skeletal muscle cells die, subsequently releasing massive amounts of muscle protein into the bloodstream. This muscle protein saturates the kidneys, effectively overwhelming their filtration capacities. At last count, over one hundred deaths and 1,600 injuries had been linked to Baycol. Bayer has reportedly paid 477 million dollars to settle over 1,300 Baycol cases out of court in the U.S., and still faces around 11,000 cases for which the company has refused to acknowledge legal liability(70).

Indeed, kidney failure was reportedly a major cause of death amongst the Baycol victims. Baycol is not unique in its ability to damage muscle--all the statins have been shown to produce muscle disorders in susceptible patients, and muscle pain is one of the most common reasons for patients being taken off statin drugs(71). It is also now known that some patients may suffer muscle deterioration caused by statins while still maintaining normal levels of creatine kinase, the most commonly used indicator of muscle damage(72).

Despite these findings, many researchers continue to endorse the official party line that muscle damage in statin users is a rare occurrence. However, in June 2006, Swedish scientists published research indicating that the prevalence of statin-induced muscle damage may be far more common than that previously predicted by even the staunchest statin critics. The researchers had taken muscle biopsies from fourteen statin-treated and eight non-statin-treated patients, none of whom had a previous history of rhabdomyolysis or myalgia. Upon examining the biopsied tissue samples, they found clear evidence of muscle damage in ten of the statin-treated patients, but only one of the eight controls. The muscle damage in the statin users was present despite their being asymptomatic. Though the degree of overall damage was slight, it exhibited a characteristic pattern that included damage to the cholesterol-rich components of muscle fibers known as *T-tubules* and *sarcolemma*. To determine whether or not these findings were mere coincidence, the researchers then took isolated muscle fibers and depleted them of cholesterol. When they placed these cholesterol-depleted fibers under the microscope, they observed the same structural abnormalities found in the damaged muscle fibers of statin-treated patients!(73)

Those who need further proof of the disparity between side effect rates in carefully controlled clinical trials and the real world should carefully consider the findings of the PRINCESS study. This study was scheduled to enroll 3,605 heart attack patients who were to be randomized to either Baycol or placebo for three months. The trial was supposed to have had a two-year follow-up, but when cerivastatin was pulled from the market in 2001, the trial was stopped, and the data acquired after 4.5 months was tallied. Among those who had already completed 4.5 months of cerivastatin use, there was little evidence of increased myopathy or rhabdomyolysis risk, with adverse events similar in the treatment and placebo groups. If trial data was relied upon to ascertain the risk profile of Baycol, one would conclude that it was a remarkably safe drug, rather than the deadly menace it quickly proved itself to be in general practice!(74)

Those who have been taken in by the extravagant hyperbole lavished upon statins would also be wise to consider the experience of Auckland, New Zealand resident Brian Barker. In April of 2002, Barker was a healthy and physically fit fifty-four year old who watched his diet and walked twenty-five kilometers each week. He did take some medication for mild hypertension, but otherwise showed no sign of any heart trouble. His younger brother, however, had not been so fortunate, having already endured a heart attack and triple bypass surgery.

As a result of his brother's premature heart problems, it had been suggested to Barker that he visit his doctor for a precautionary examination. His physician arranged an exercise stress test, which Brian passed with flying colors. His recovery after the treadmill session was excellent, and ultrasound images showed no sign of blockage to his arteries. Blood testing also showed his cholesterol to be within 'normal' limits at 200mg/dl. To any rational observer, Barker would hardly have seemed like a suitable candidate for powerful cholesterol-lowering drug therapy. However, despite his highly positive test results, Barker 's doctor decided that-- *"as an extra precaution"*--he should start taking simvastatin on a daily basis. Barker dutifully obeyed and started taking twenty milligrams of the widely prescribed statin every night.

On the morning of June 23, 2002, Barker sat eating his breakfast and reading the Sunday paper, just as he had done countless times before. It was after finishing his second piece of toast that he felt a sudden pain shoot through the base of his spine. He started shaking and began feeling extremely cold. His legs felt weak, his complexion turned gray, his speech became incoherent, and his eyes became glassy. His wife Heather wrapped him in a winter jacket, put a duvet around him, and turned the heater on, but Barker still continued to shake. Twenty minutes later, he got up and staggered towards the toilet, where he proceeded to vomit violently. Barker was about to discover that his health problems were as severe as they were sudden. Five days after becoming abruptly ill, the drained and dehydrated Kiwi was hospitalized with acute kidney failure. He was suffering from life-threatening rhabdomyolysis, courtesy of the simvastatin that had been prescribed *"as an extra precaution"* against heart disease.

As of mid-2004, Barker has been able to stop dialysis, although his doctors have explained it may still be a possibility in the future. He still has continual pains in his muscles and joints. He still gets nauseous, and has even had an operation for the hiatus hernia caused by his continual vomiting. Cognitive difficulties have made it impossible for Barker to continue doing his previous job. By early afternoon every day, fatigue gets the better of him and he falls asleep. His speech is impaired, he has traumatic nightmares, a frequent and urgent need to urinate, a raised PSA level, and neuropathy. Barker's wife Heather explained to me that *"there are many other unexplained and concerning phenomena which we hope will resolve in the not too distant future. He has had various therapists, a psychologist, and many excellent physicians. But very few answers."*

Statins and Coenzyme Q10 Depletion

Statins have also been shown to deplete the body of a vital substance known as Coenzyme Q10 (CoQ10)(75). CoQ10 is a crucial component of mitochondria, the intracellular "engines" responsible for producing almost all of a cell's energy requirements. In addition to this fundamental role in energy production, CoQ10 acts as a potent antioxidant. Not surprisingly, CoQ10 is extremely important for cardiovascular health, with high levels being found in healthy heart tissue.

Ironically, while statins can reduce the risk of atherosclerotic heart disease, their CoQ10-robbing effects have been linked to an increased risk of congestive heart failure. The first statin (lovastatin) appeared on the market in 1987. Figures from the National Center for Health Statistics show that since the early nineties--several years after statin drugs began hitting pharmacy shelves--the incidence of congestive heart failure (CHF) has risen sharply(76). CHF, in fact, is the fastest growing cardiovascular disorder in the United States. Sadly, there is no cure for CHF short of a heart transplant.

Approximately 4.8 million Americans are diagnosed with CHF. Each year, there are an estimated 400,000 new cases, and around half of these patients will die within five years. Although the causes of this epidemic are unknown, statin-induced CoQ10 deficiency has been implicated as a possible contributing factor. Peter H. Langsjoen, MD, a foremost authority on the use of coenzyme Q10 in the treatment of heart disease, has little doubt as to the culprit behind this sharp rise in CHF: *"In my practice of 17 years in Tyler, Texas, I have seen a frightening increase in heart failure secondary to statin usage, "statin cardiomyopathy". Over the past five years, statins have become more potent, are being prescribed in higher doses, and are being used with reckless abandon in the elderly and in patients with "normal" cholesterol levels. We are in the midst of a CHF epidemic in the US with a dramatic increase over the past decade. Are we causing this epidemic through our zealous use of statins? In large part I think the answer is yes."*(77)

Because all large-scale statin trials have excluded patients with established heart failure, the long-term safety of statins in such patients is not known. Clinical research gives little cause for optimism; Langsjoen recently studied fourteen patients with completely normal heart function, and found that after three to six months on twenty milligrams of Lipitor a day, ten of the subjects developed abnormalities in the heart's diastolic phase (when the heart muscle fills with blood)(78). Diastolic dysfunction is believed to be responsible for between thirty to fifty percent of congestive heart failure cases in older people(79).

The deleterious effects of statins on CoQ10 levels are hardly news to drug company manufacturers. In 1989, Merck & Co., Inc. filed two patents for the use of CoQ10 with statins in order to prevent CoQ10 depletion and attendant side effects. The patent applications, which can be viewed online at the United States Patent and Trademark Office website, clearly show that the statin manufacturer was aware of the link between CoQ10 depletion and heart failure(80). One of the Merck patent applications states that: *"Since Coenzyme Q10...is of benefit in congestive heart failure patients, the combination with HMG-CoA reductase inhibitors (statin drugs) should be of value in such patients who also have the added risk of high cholesterol."*

Research has shown that statin-induced CoQ10 deficiency can be prevented with supplemental CoQ10, without adverse impact on the drugs' cholesterol-lowering or anti-inflammatory properties(75). Amazingly, even though both of the Merck patents were granted in 1990, the company has neither exercised the patents nor educated physicians or patients about the necessity of taking coenzyme Q10 along with statin drugs. The end result is that most doctors and their patients remain completely ignorant that failure to supplement statin drugs with coenzyme Q10 may have potentially life-threatening consequences.

CoQ10, by the way, is not the only important antioxidant depleted by statin use. A three-month trial found that twenty milligrams daily of simvastatin decreased blood levels of alpha-tocopherol (a form of vitamin E) by 16.2 percent, beta-carotene by 19.5 percent, and CoQ10 by 22 percent as compared to placebo(81).

This Your Brain on Statins

Along with along with muscular symptoms, cognitive dysfunction is one of the most frequently reported side effects of statin use. Numerous case reports of statin-associated cognitive impairment and memory loss have appeared in the medical literature, and clinical trials have found that statins can indeed induce negative mental changes(82). A 1992 double-blind trial found that healthy young men given lovastatin displayed significant deterioration in cognitive function after only three weeks of treatment, whereas no change was noted in those receiving a placebo(83). In another trial, lasting six months, the placebo group improved significantly in all of five assessments of cognitive function, while the lovastatin group improved only in one(84).

Total Global Amnesia (TGA) is a transient form of memory loss that can last anywhere from fifteen minutes to half-a-day. Duane Graveline, M.D., a former astronaut, aerospace medical research scientist, flight surgeon and family doctor, experienced this normally rare phenomenon in 2001 shortly after doctors at the Johnson Space Center placed him on Lipitor. Six weeks later his cholesterol had plummeted from 240 to 150, much to the delight of his doctors. *"All was well until several days later",* Graveline recalls, *"when my wife found me aimlessly walking about the yard after my usual walk in the woods that morning."* Graveline did not recognize her, and while he reluctantly accepted cookies and milk, he refused to go inside the 'unfamiliar' building that was in fact his home. Graveline's wife eventually convinced him to take a ride to their family doctor, and then to a neurologist who made the diagnosis of TGA, *"cause unknown"*. While sitting in the neurologist's office, about six hours after the onset of his TGA, Graveline's memory abruptly returned.

Because his MRI results were normal, and since Lipitor was the only new medicine he was taking, Graveline quickly suspected that he was suffering an unforeseen side effect and promptly stopped taking the drug. During the next year, he experienced no further episodes of TGA. At his next astronaut physical the following year, his NASA doctors were aghast that he had stopped taking the cholesterol-lowering drug they prescribed, and adamantly insisted that it was in no way related to his TGA episode. Graveline relented, and again began taking Lipitor at one-half the previous dose.

"Six weeks later I again descended into the black pit of amnesia, this time for twelve hours and with a retrograde loss of memory back to my high school days. During that terrible interval, when my entire adult life had been eradicated, I had no awareness of my marriage and four children, my medical school days, my ten adventure-filled years as a USAF flight surgeon, my selection as scientist astronaut or of my post retirement decade as a writer..."

Graveline was mortified by the sudden onset of his TGA episodes: *"What if I had been flying my taildragger at the time? My flight instruction had come during my ten years as a USAF flight surgeon. If my ability to pilot an aircraft had been eradicated by this event, what might have been my reaction? How could I ever have brought it in for a safe landing?"*

Graveline again went off his Lipitor, this time permanently. Again, his doctors refused to even consider that the popular statin could have had anything to do with his TGA. In desperation, he sent an email to the writers of *People's Pharmacy*, a syndicated column appearing in newspapers throughout the US. His letter, in turn, was passed on to researchers conducting an ongoing statin study at the University of California, San Diego. The principal investigator of this study, Beatrice Golomb, contacted Graveline and reassured him that she knew of several cases just like his. The real break came several days later when his e-mail was reprinted in *the People's Pharmacy* column. Both Graveline and the column's writers were flooded with e-mails, containing hundreds of reports of statin-related amnesia, memory loss, confusion, and disorientation.

Graveline launched himself into an intense investigation of the phenomenon of statin-induced TGA, discovering in the process just how crucial cholesterol is for efficient brain function. Laboratory evidence suggests that cholesterol is essential for the creation of the all-important synapse, the gap between nerve cells that allows neurotransmitters to carry nervous system messages(85). While cholesterol is the most common organic molecule in the brain, this organ cannot tap the blood cholesterol supply because the lipoproteins that carry cholesterol are too large to cross the blood-brain barrier. Statins, it would appear, directly interfere with cholesterol production in the brain, just as they do in the liver.

Graveline uncovered enough startling facts about statins, cholesterol, and nervous system function to fill a book--which is exactly what he did. The end result, *Lipitor: Thief of Memory,* should be mandatory reading for anyone taking statins and for the doctors who prescribe them. As Graveline warns: *"Statin drug use is not all glamour and risk-free patient benefit as strongly implied in the monumentally effective direct patient advertising of Pfizer and other drug giants."*(86)

Statins and Cancer

In 1996 the *Journal of the American Medical Association* published an extensive review of the research studying the link between cholesterol-lowering drugs and cancer. The authors, Dr Thomas Newman and Dr. Stephen Hulley, stated: *"All members of the two most popular classes of lipid-lowering drugs (the fibrates and the statins) cause cancer in rodents, in some cases at levels of animal exposure close to those prescribed to humans."* In light of their findings, the authors recommended that: *"lipid-lowering drug treatment, especially with the fibrates and statins, should be avoided except in patients at high short-term risk of coronary heart disease."*(87)

Newman and Hulley's recommendation has been all but ignored. Statins are being recommended and prescribed, not just to people at high short-term risk, but to perfectly healthy people who show no clinical manifestations of CHD whatsoever, except for the non-disease of hypercholesterolemia. Drug companies and health authorities repeatedly assure us that statins are wonderful low-risk drugs that are well tolerated in most people. They claim that clinical trials have shown no increase in cancer incidence with statin use, but most of these studies ran for only six years or less. Cancer is a chronic disease that may take decades to manifest itself as a life-threatening illness--can we really conclude from trials lasting five to six years that statins are safe for lifetime use? Even heavy smokers are highly unlikely to develop cancer within six years of taking their first puff; most continue for decades before they come to realize the true value of those little warnings adorning cigarette packets.

Because rodent studies routinely use far higher dosages of drugs than those prescribed to humans, some have questioned the relevance of Newman and Hulley's findings. In many studies, rodents have been shown to eliminate drugs much faster than humans, necessitating higher dosages to maintain constant blood levels of the drug. The authors noted, however, that when the drug exposure was considered in terms of blood levels, carcinogenicity occurred at levels close to those seen in humans. In the same journal in which this review appeared, a commentary critical of Hulley and Newman claimed that higher dosages used in rodents placed inordinate stress on their gastrointestinal tracts, and that most of the cancers seen in rodent studies were malignancies of the gastrointestinal tract and liver(88). Given that gastrointestinal distress and liver toxicity are among the most frequently reported side effects in patients prescribed statins, this proffered explanation provides little reassurance.

Cancer Incidence in Human Statin Trials: A Closer Look

There are two trials whose follow-up periods have extended for longer than the usual four-to-six years. The first is the EXCEL trial, which showed an increase in total mortality after one year of lovastatin use, and for which no subsequent mortality data has ever been released(89)). The second is the Scandinavian Simvastatin Survival Study (4S), the ten-year follow-up data of which was published in a 2004 issue of *The Lancet*. The 4S trial officially ran for five years, but researchers continued to monitor mortality outcomes after this double-blind portion of the study ended. In the years following the trial's closure, over eighty percent of the subjects in both the original simvastatin *and* placebo groups reported that they were taking cholesterol-lowering drugs, usually statins. When researchers tallied up the number of cancer deaths after ten years, they found that cancer mortality was 4.5 percent in the placebo group and 3.8 percent in the simvastatin group(90). While the small difference favoring the simvastatin group did not reach statistical significance, the lack of increased cancer incidence seen in this trial was encouraging.

Not so reassuring were the results of the PROSPER trial, which found a twenty-five percent increase in newly diagnosed cancers among elderly individuals treated with pravastatin. While there were twenty less deaths from CHD and stroke in the treatment group, twenty-four more deaths from cancer were observed, and, in an ominous confirmation of animal findings, one of the highest increases was observed for gastrointestinal cancers(11).
The PROSPER authors dismissed these findings by referring to a pooled analysis they performed of eight statin trials that lasted three or more years, which showed no statistically significant difference in cancer incidence between the placebo and statin groups (6.9 versus 7.1 percent, respectively). However, all of these other trials involved younger subjects. Because cancer risk increases with age, such a comparison bears little relevance to the PROSPER results. Due to their heightened risk, elderly subjects may act as a far more sensitive barometer to any cancer-promoting capacity possessed by statins. Furthermore, the PROSPER researchers' analysis did not include skin cancer. Considering the relatively short-term nature of statin trials, it is the incidence of such an easily detectable, superficial cancer that would provide the strongest clue as to the future cancer-causing potential of statins. Only two of the statin trials have reported skin cancer incidence; the 4S and HPS simvastatin trials. Increases in skin cancer were noted in both(9,91).

Also providing little reassurance was a report in early 2006 by Japanese researchers on the incidence of lymphoid malignancies (lymphoma and myeloma) among statin users. Knowing that immune-suppressing drugs increase the risk for these malignancies, and that statins may exert immune-suppressing effects(92), they examined the association between statin use and development of lymphoid malignancies in a case-control study. The cases were 221 consecutive patients with proven lymphoid malignancies hospitalized in the Department of Hematology of Toranomon Hospital in Tokyo, Japan between 1995 and 2001. The two control groups comprised 442 and 437 inpatients without malignancies from the Departments of Orthopedics and Otorhinolaryngology of the same hospital. The controls were matched individually with cases for age, sex and year of admission. A 224 percent higher frequency of statin use was found among patients with lymphoid malignancies compared to the control patients(93).

In the CARE trial, breast cancer, another readily detectable malignancy, developed in twelve women from the treatment group but in only one of the control individuals--a highly significant difference(6). Breast cancer was also the malignancy for which the greatest increase was noted in the PROSPER trial. The possibility that statins will lead to future increases in cancer incidence cannot be flippantly dismissed.

Statins and Birth Defects

It is estimated that one to three percent of statin prescriptions are for women of childbearing age. NIH researchers analyzed fifty-two cases of first-trimester statin exposure reported to the Food and Drug Administration (FDA) from 1987 through 2001, and observed a disproportionately high occurrence of severe central nervous system defects and limb deformities. The findings, reported in the April 8, 2004 issue of the *New England Journal of Medicine*, showed that twenty of fifty-two babies exposed to statins in the womb were born with malformations(94). *"We can't tell whether the defects were caused by the use of statin medications, but other birth defect studies suggest that these are the kinds of problems that occur if the embryo does not get enough cholesterol in early pregnancy to develop normally,"* said one of the authors, Dr. Maximilian Muenke, a senior investigator and chief of the medical genetics branch at the National Human Genome Research Institute in Bethesda, MD.

Of the twenty babies born with malformations, four had severe central nervous system defects, and five had malformed limbs. There was also a case of a very rare birth defect called holoprosencephaly, which occurs when the brain fails to divide properly. *"These are such very rare birth defects that one would not expect to find the number we found in a population this small,"* Muenke said(95).

The authors pointed out that all the adverse birth outcomes were associated with the use of 'lipohilic' statins (those that are attracted to lipids in the body), such as cerivastatin, lovastatin, atorvastatin, and simvastatin. The lipophilic statins achieve concentrations in the embryo/placenta similar to those seen in maternal plasma, and lipophilic statins have been shown to cause birth defects in animal studies. No malformations were reported among fourteen infants exposed to pravastatin, a hydrophilic drug that has low tissue penetration and has not caused reproductive abnormalities in animals.

Laboratory research conducted since Muenke's report suggests that statins may indeed be toxic to the developing fetus. When Israeli researchers exposed human first trimester placental explants to a medium containing simvastatin, they observed that the drug sharply inhibited normal migration and proliferation of cells in the explants, while increasing apoptosis (cell death)(96).

Pregnant women should avoid statins like the plague. The problem is, pregnancies are often unplanned and many women do not know they are pregnant until after four to six weeks of pregnancy. Fetal exposure to statin drugs can happen inadvertently before a woman is even aware she is pregnant. The biggest irony of all this is that there is absolutely no reason for females to be taking statins in the first place: As Chapter 23 clearly explains, clinical trials have repeatedly shown that statin drugs do not offer any mortality benefit whatsoever to women!

Statins and Impotence

As if rhabdomyolysis, cognitive dysfunction, potentially fatal kidney failure, and possible increases in the risk of birth defects, cancer and heart failure were not bad enough, researchers recently added another ailment to the ever-growing list of adverse statin side effects: Erectile dysfunction.

A systematic review by UK researchers of case reports, clinical trials and information from regulatory agencies, found that both statins and fibrates were associated with erectile dysfunction and impaired libido. In many cases, symptoms improved after drug withdrawal, but resumed once the lipid-lowering therapy was reinstated(97).

Investigators from the Netherlands Pharmacovigilance Centre have also reported a number of statin-associated sexual dysfunction cases. They described two cases in which dysfunction was accompanied by significant reductions in testosterone, providing a strong clue as to why statins can interfere with sexual capacity. The first patient was a forty-six-year-old male with initial serum cholesterol of 275 mg/dl. The patient started treatment with twenty milligrams of fluvastatin daily, which was then increased to forty milligrams daily. Shortly after initiation of statin therapy, the patient noticed a decrease in libido. His testosterone value was measured and determined at 207 ng/dl (normal range for adult men: 345-1008 ng/dl). At this time his cholesterol level had decreased to 228 mg/dl). Fluvastatin was withdrawn and five days later his testosterone had increased to 380 ng/dl. The patient's libido also returned to normal.

The second patient, a fifty-four-year-old male, started treatment with pravastatin to lower his cholesterol level of 236 mg/dl. Within days of commencing pravastatin, he experienced a decrease in his libido. His testosterone level was 167 ng/dl, while his total cholesterol level had decreased to 174 mg/dl. When pravastatin was discontinued seven months later, his libido returned to normal after a few days. Four months later, his testosterone level had risen to 657 ng/dl. The center received six more reports concerning decreased libido in association with the use of statins, one of them concerning a woman. In three cases the outcome is known: two patients recovered after withdrawal of the suspected drug and one recovered after switching to another statin(98).

More recently, researchers analyzed statin-associated impotence cases collected by the Spanish and French pharmacovigilance systems. Thirty-eight cases of impotence associated with statins were identified in the Spanish database, with impotence disappearing after drug withdrawal in 93 percent of the cases. In France, 37 cases were reported, and in 85% of these recovery was observed after drug withdrawal(99).

Statins versus Testosterone

While it may be hated by disgruntled feminists the world over, the hormone testosterone is extremely important for men *and* women alike. Libido, cognition, muscle and bone growth are just some of the vital functions positively influenced by healthy levels of testosterone in both sexes.

Statins inhibit the activity of an enzyme required for cholesterol production known as HMG-CoA reductase, and hence may potentially inhibit the synthesis of steroid hormones derived from cholesterol, including testosterone. Furthermore, high-dose simvastatin has been shown to directly suppress testosterone synthesis in lab studies by inhibiting the 17-ketosteroid-oxidoreductase catalyzed conversion of dehydroepiandrosterone and dehydroandrostenedione to androstenediol and testosterone, respectively. In susceptible individuals, these effects of cholesterol drugs may translate to a very real reduction in sexual capacity.

The adverse hormonal effects of statins don't just hit below the belt; the Australian Adverse Drug Reaction Advisory Committee also lists eleven reports of gynaecomastia (growth of breast tissue in males) associated with simvastatin use. The UK Committee on Safety of Medicines has also noted cases of gynaecomastia associated with cholesterol drug use(97).

Statins: Journey Into the Unknown

To maintain their lipid-lowering effects, statins must be administered on a life-long basis. The established ability of statins to promote rhabdomyolysis and cognitive dysfunction, a plausible connection with birth defects and heart failure, reports of carcinogenicity from rodent studies and increases in superficial cancers noted in human trials warrant extreme caution. Given the complete lack of data on the effects of decades of statin administration, users can consider themselves part of a mass experiment in progress, the outcome of which is largely unknown. Warnings for statin use to be limited to high-risk patients--where dramatically shortened life expectancies may override any concerns about long-term side effects--have been completely overshadowed by the relentless promotional efforts of drug companies. These efforts have been further bolstered by enthusiastic endorsements from health authorities who are besides themselves at finally having clinical data that, on the surface, appears to support the lipid hypothesis.

Are we witnessing the unfolding of another officially endorsed health disaster? Only time will tell. For those who do not want to find out the hard way, there are numerous non-drug measures that can help alleviate the risk of CHD. In Sections Two and Three, we will learn how increases in the intake of omega-3 fats, fruits, nuts, vegetables and certain dietary supplements, as well as exercise, stress reduction, sound sleep, and a low-to-moderate carbohydrate diet provide a far more judicious preventive alternative to toxic statin drugs for those with no clinical signs of CHD.

Chapter 10

"An almost endless number of observations and experiments have effectively falsified the hypothesis that dietary cholesterol and fats, and a high cholesterol level play a role in the causation of atherosclerosis and cardiovascular disease. The hypothesis is maintained because allegedly supportive, but insignificant findings, are inflated, and because most contradictory results are misinterpreted, misquoted or ignored."

Uffe Ravnskov, M.D., Ph.D.

Money, Politics and Cholesterol

An Unproven Theory Becomes Accepted Dogma

With such a flimsy scientific foundation, the lipid hypothesis should have been discarded a long, long time ago. Instead it has become one of the central tenets of modern day health care, thanks largely to the efforts of influential health organizations, powerful financial interests, government bureaucrats and researchers engaged in questionable scientific practices. Through clever manipulation of the media, the medical profession and public opinion, they succeeded in turning a theory riddled with inconsistencies into official health policy.

The Early Days

In 1957, the American Heart Association published a report evaluating the evidence for the newfound hypothesis that dietary fat was somehow involved in the causation of heart disease(1). When reading this report, it is hard to believe it was published by the same organization that just a few years later would be wholeheartedly endorsing the notion that animal fat and cholesterol increased the risk of CHD.

The authors of this report summarized the major arguments put forward in support of the lipid hypothesis, being careful to present evidence both for and against the fledgling theory. The report correctly noted that atherosclerosis produced in animal experiments was similar, but not identical, to that seen in humans, and cautioned that the results of animal experiments and clinical studies with patients were *"not necessarily applicable to healthy individuals."*

Addressing claims of an alleged upward spiral in CHD deaths, the authors wrote: *"Undoubtedly the wide use of the electrocardiogram...and the inclusion in 1949 of Arteriosclerotic Heart Disease in the International List of Causes of*

Death play a role in what is often believed to be an actual increased "prevalence" of this disease."

The report emphasized that regional statistics of CHD incidence were at best *"a crude index"* and that cross-country comparisons, which would later become a central pillar of the anti-cholesterol argument, were even less reliable. The validity of food consumption data was discussed, and evidence was presented suggesting that such data, frequently used to associate fat with CHD, often substantially overestimated the percentage of calories derived from fat. This was especially true of animal fat, of which significant proportions were often discarded during consumption and lost as a result of certain cooking methods.

The authors acknowledged that while elevated cholesterol levels and high fat intakes were associated with higher rates of CHD in certain populations, the exact opposite relationship was seen amongst others.

As far as changes in fat intake were concerned, the authors noted that total fat intake had changed little since the turn of the century, but that the use of hydrogenated fats had increased greatly. It was stressed that while polyunsaturated oils had been shown to lower cholesterol levels, there was no proof that they could lower the actual incidence of CHD. The authors concluded, *"the evidence at present does not convey any specific implications for drastic dietary changes, specifically in the quantity or type of fat in the diet...on the premise that such changes will definitely lessen the incidence of coronary or cerebral artery disease."*

Compare this cautious summary with the following recommendation to individuals at increased risk of CHD that was issued in an another AHA report just four years later: *"The reduction or control of fat consumption under medical supervision, with reasonable substitution of poly-unsaturated for saturated fats, is recommended as a possible means of preventing atherosclerosis and decreasing the risk of heart attacks and strokes. This recommendation is based on the best scientific information available at the present time."*(2)

Whereas the previous report had spanned twelve-and-a-half pages and cited eighty-seven references, the 'updated' version filled little over two pages and included a mere twenty-three references.

One has to wonder what happened in those four short years to markedly change the AHA committee members' attitude towards the role of dietary fats in CHD. It certainly wasn't the emergence of convincing new scientific research; the first randomized trial examining the substitution of polyunsaturated fat for saturated fats (which showed an increase of CHD deaths among subjects fed corn oil) was not published until 1965.

Something that did undergo marked change was the composition of the AHA's nutrition advisory committee. Only two of the five authors responsible for the cautious 1957 report returned to pen the 1961 guidelines; among the new arrivals were Ancel Keys and Jeremiah Stamler, another famous proponent of the lipid hypothesis. The remaining members of the committee were Irvine Page, Frederick Stare, Edgar Allen, and Francis Chamberlain.

The AHA's proposed link between cholesterol and CHD, coupled with experimental evidence that polyunsaturated fats lowered cholesterol, presented a huge opportunity to the vegetable oil industry, one that was seized upon immediately. An intensive promotional campaign aimed at increasing awareness of the 'heart-healthy' benefits of polyunsaturated oils was launched. Advertisements in both the popular media and medical journals alerted physicians and the public alike to these wondrous (and unproven) benefits, and a number of researchers who subscribed to the cholesterol theory became vocal supporters of polyunsaturated oils.

In 1963, Alan Blaketon and Jeremiah Stamler co-authored *Your Heart Has Nine Lives*, a self-help book advocating the Prudent Diet(3). The book encouraged readers to replace saturated fats from animal foods with polyunsaturated oils, and told readers to *"de-emphasize"* eggs, butter, full fat cheeses and untrimmed meats. The authors' support for polyunsaturated fats was not based in any way on sound evidence, but creative speculation that science would eventually, hopefully, validate. According to the book's 'Acknowledgements' section, Stamler had received *"significant research support"* (money) from the Corn Products Institute of Nutrition and from the Wesson Fund for Medical Research (Wesson are a manufacturer of vegetable oils). Stamler also thanked the American Oil Company for its *"invaluable cooperation"* with his research activities.

A quick read through *Your Heart Has Nine Lives* provides a revealing insight into the mindset of early cholesterol-theory proponents. According to Blaketon and Stamler: *"Beyond any doubt, the heart plague, especially among middle-age men, is a relatively recent development. There has never been an epidemic of this kind before in history."* The authors further claimed *"today we are on solid scientific ground in our knowledge of the risks and causes of heart attacks."* Obviously, the authors could not cite any controlled dietary intervention trials to help illustrate this *"solid scientific ground"*. All they could do was to emphasize that research was in progress, and mention the *"promising"* National Diet-Heart Project, a pilot study which went on to find no difference in CHD rates between control subjects and those eating a Prudent diet.

Despite the paucity of supportive evidence, the authors had little hesitation about deriding critics of the new guidelines: *"Those who argue against general application of present knowledge offer no hope for years to come against premature heart attacks. They should face this fact about their position, and consider whether they are being truly cautious and truly careful about human lives."*

While morally denigrating those who could not bring themselves to support dietary guidelines that were at best speculative, the authors had no qualms about expressing their care and caution towards human welfare by recommending consumption of unprecedented amounts of polyunsaturated oils, of which the health consequences were completely unknown at the time. They quoted none other than Ancel Keys as saying: *"The absence of final, positive proof of a hypothesis is not evidence that the hypothesis is wrong."* Of course not, but nor can it be used to justify the wholesale endorsement of guidelines that may one day harm millions of people.

Frederick Stare, through his syndicated column in the *Los Angeles Times*, became a prolific advocate of polyunsaturated oils. In a 1969 column he stated: *"To my knowledge, I've never heard of too much polyunsaturated fat for man..."*(4) Subsequent promotional campaigns for Procter and Gamble's Puritan Oil featured Framingham Director Dr.William Castelli and former AHA president Dr. Antonio Gotto, Jr. The latter's efforts included sending a letter promoting Puritan Oil printed on a DeBakey Heart Center letterhead to practicing physicians in 1988(5). The DeBakey Heart Center at Baylor College of Medicine was named after famous cardiac surgeon Michael DeBakey; Gotto's use of the Center's stationery was rather ironic considering DeBakey himself had conducted a study in the early sixties showing little relationship between cholesterol and CHD in 1,700 patients(6).

Throughout the 1960's, the AHA's efforts garnered increasing acceptance for the cholesterol theory, but many remained unconvinced. Even the American Medical Association at first opposed the lipid hypothesis, warning that *"the anti-fat, anti-cholesterol fad is not just foolish and futile. . . it also carries some risk."*

In 1959, the Food and Drug Administration (FDA) warned: *"The role of cholesterol in heart disease has not been established. A causal relationship between blood cholesterol levels and these diseases has not been proved. The advisability of making extensive changes in the nature of the dietary fat intake of the people of this country has not been demonstrated."*(7)

The FDA reaffirmed its stance on the lack of science behind the lipid hypothesis in 1965 when it wrote: *"...any claim, direct or implied, in the labeling of fats and oils or other fatty substances offered to the general public that they will prevent, mitigate, or cure diseases of the heart or arteries is false or misleading, and constitutes misbranding within the meaning of the federal Food, Drug and Cosmetic Act."*(8)

Back in 1965, the pharmaceutical companies had not yet developed cholesterol-lowering drugs. Today, these have become the largest-selling category of prescription drugs in the world; today, the FDA--infamous for its overly cozy relationship with the drug industry--is now an ardent supporter of the lipid hypothesis.

In a 1969 report, the Diet-Heart Review Panel of the National Heart Institute stated: *"It is not known whether dietary manipulation has any effect whatsoever on coronary heart disease."* Members of the panel worried that cutting total fat, and replacing saturated fats with polyunsaturated fats, could have an unforeseen adverse impact on health. The National Heart Institute went on to become the National Heart, Lung, and Blood Institute (NHLBI), which, along with the AHA, would become a major prime mover in the push to gain acceptance for the lipid hypothesis. However, the Diet-Heart-Review panelists at the time, to their credit, could not endorse speculative dietary recommendations whose safety and effectiveness was largely a mystery. Numerous future key players in the cholesterol saga would not be hampered by any such inhibitions.

Enter the Bureaucrats

Gary Taubes is an American science journalist whose articles, which focus primarily on exposing questionable scientific practices, have earned him numerous international awards. It is not surprising that he eventually turned his attention to investigating the anti-saturated fat, anti-cholesterol phenomenon, an area where shoddy science has run rife. Taubes is probably best known for his controversial article *What if it's all been a big FAT lie?,* which literally caused a sensation when it appeared in the *New York Times Magazine* in July 2002.

Just over a year before his *NYT* article was published, Taubes penned an article titled *The Soft Science of Dietary Fat*, which was featured in *Science* magazine(9). Taubes had written the article after interviewing scores of researchers and civil servants, poring through piles of government reports and congressional transcripts, and studying the scientific literature. The result was a revealing exposé on the behind-the-scenes political maneuvering that was instrumental in winning widespread acceptance for the cholesterol theory.

Taubes describes how one of the early catalysts for the eventual dominance of the cholesterol paradigm was Senator George McGovern's Select Committee on Nutrition and Human Needs, which had been founded in 1968 with the goal of eradicating malnutrition in America. By the mid seventies, after establishing a series of landmark food assistance programs, McGovern's committee had largely fulfilled its original mandate and should have called it a day.

It didn't. True bureaucracies don't willingly die, after all; instead they ask for more money to tackle 'pressing new issues'. In this case, the committee's general counsel, Marshall Matz, and staff director, Alan Stone, both young lawyers, decided that it would address 'overnutrition', the tendency for many Americans to eat too much of the wrong type of foods. It was a *"casual endeavor,"* Matz told Taubes. *"We really were totally naïve, a bunch of kids, who just thought, 'Hell, we should say something on this subject before we go out of business.' "* Marshall and Alan's *"casual endeavor"* was readily endorsed by McGovern and his fellow senators, many of whom were reportedly following the then-fashionable guidelines of famous low-fat author Nathan Pritikin.

The committee listened to two days of testimony on diet and disease in July 1976, then assigned Nick Mottern, a former labor reporter with no scientific background and no experience in writing about science, health or nutrition issues, to compile the first Dietary Goals for the United States. When gathering his information on fat, Mottern relied almost exclusively on Mark Hegsted, a Harvard School of Public Health nutritionist who believed unconditionally in the benefits of restricting dietary fat.

Under the influence of Hegsted, Mottern came to view dietary fat as the nutritional equivalent of cigarettes. Mottern's final report recommended that Americans trim fat to thirty percent of their daily calories and saturated fat to only ten percent, paralleling advice given by the AHA. When *Dietary Goals* was unveiled in 1977, it met with an avalanche of criticism from numerous researchers, health authorities, and the dairy, beef and egg industries. The criticism from those with considerable financial interests at stake proved advantageous to the report's authors, who were able to quickly dismiss critics of the report as food industry apologists.

McGovern's committee finally wound up in 1977, but at the USDA, former consumer-activist and recently appointed assistant secretary Carol Tucker Foreman felt it was imperative to convert McGovern's recommendations into official policy. Seeking scientific support, she consulted the National Academy of Sciences (NAS), but the academy's president Philip Handler, an expert on metabolism, told Foreman that Mottern's Dietary Goals were *"nonsense"*. Acting on advice from McGovern's staffers, Forman then hired Hegsted. Their collaboration led to the first edition of *Using the Dietary Guidelines for Americans*, which contained dietary fat recommendations virtually identical to those in *Dietary Goals*.

Shortly after this, the NAS Food and Nutrition Board released its own guidelines, *Toward Healthful Diets,* which advised Americans not to agonize over fat intake but simply to watch their weight, and let everything else take care of itself. The media in particular was highly critical of the board's recommendations, and criticized the NAS for offering advice that conflicted with that given by the USDA and McGovern's committee. The USDA then leaked a report to the press stating that two of the twelve NAS panelists consulted to the food industry, and that the board itself was funded by industry donations. When these connections were aired in the media, the credibility of the NAS took a beating, as did dietary fat and cholesterol. The low-fat argument received a significant boost, with the press, politicians and layman alike increasingly buying into that idea that fat consumption was harmful and should be restricted.

Putting the Cart Before the Horse

The low-fat theory was rapidly transforming from myth into accepted truth, but there was one small problem. Actually, for advocates of the lipid hypothesis, it was a potentially huge problem; despite all that had been written against cholesterol and animal fat, there was not a single well-designed trial that could be used to show any CHD or longevity benefits from low-saturated fat diets. As we saw in Chapter 8, it wasn't for lack of trying--numerous trials had been conducted, but all failed miserably to prove the validity of the lipid hypothesis. Researchers were now pinning their hopes on a series of multi-million dollar super-studies funded by the NHLBI that would, hopefully, finally prove the validity of the cholesterol-lowering argument.

The results of the first four of these were published between 1980 and 1984, and included the Framingham, Honolulu and Puerto Rico projects (see Chapter 6) as well as a Chicago study that failed to show any benefit from eating less fat. The fifth was the massive MRFIT clinical trial, where the only intervention of any benefit was smoking cessation. The NHLBI had spent hundreds of millions of dollars in an attempt to prove the lipid hypothesis, and had so far come up empty-handed.

The sixth study was the 140 million dollar Lipid Research Clinics Coronary Primary Prevention Trial (LRC-CPPT), which examined the effect of cholestyramine (a drug belonging to the fibrate family, the predecessors to statins) in middle-aged men with extremely high cholesterol levels. LRC-CPPT was in no way a dietary trial--both the treatment and control groups received the same dietary advice(10).

When the final results for the LRC-CPPT were tabulated, thirty patients (1.6 percent) in the treatment group suffered a fatal heart attack compared to thirty-eight (2.0 percent) in the control group, a miniscule absolute difference of only 0.04 percent. The researchers, of course, did not include these unimpressive figures in the study's summary. Instead they quoted the more striking, but misleading, 'relative risk' reduction figure of 24 percent. Relative risk (RR) is the percentage that 0.04 percent comprises of 2 percent (the death rate in the control group), and means little in the absence of absolute figures, which show the exact number of CHD deaths.

Quoting RR in the absence of absolute figures is a favorite tool of researchers looking to amplify the impact of otherwise uninspiring results. The mortality difference of eight deaths between the cholestyramine group and the control group occurred amongst 3,806 men over a period of 7.4 years. How do we know whether this piddling difference was due to the effect of cholestyramine or purely a chance occurrence?

In an attempt to answer such questions, researchers use mathematical formulations known as 'statistical tests'. The results of these tests will conclude that the results are either statistically significant--that is, they are probably real--or not statistically significant--meaning that they are probably not real. Statistical tests are by no means infallible, as there is always the possibility that they may conclude a difference is significant when in reality it is purely a chance occurrence. All said and done, statistical tests are a 'best guess' proposition; to know with full certainty whether small differences such as those seen in the LRC-CPPT were real or not would require omnipotence.

To improve the odds of achieving a correct guess, scientists can opt to use the strictest possible statistical tests. The two most widely used tests employ a 'probability' level of either 0.05 (meaning that the probability of error is five in 100, or 5 percent) or 0.01 (where the probability of error is one in 100, or 1 percent).

The greatest degree of accuracy in determining the statistical significance of study results is essential when those results may be used to encourage millions of people to begin expensive and life-long treatment with potentially toxic drugs. The authors of the LRC-CPPT appeared to be in full agreement with this notion--at least initially.

Cooking the Books

Upon the commencement of a major trial it is customary for the researchers involved to publish a protocol report in a medical journal outlining the study's goals and design. In their 1979 protocol report, the designers of the LRC-CPPT stated that *"... since the time, magnitude and cost of the study make it unlikely that it could ever be repeated, it was essential to be sure that any observed beneficial effect of cholesterol-lowering was a real one. Therefore,* [significance] *was set at .01 rather than the usual .05."* The 0.01 level *"was chosen as the standard for showing a convincing difference between treatment groups."*(11)

When the final results were published in 1984, the LRC-CPPT researchers appeared to have suffered a severe bout of collective amnesia. They had used, not the 0.01 level, but the 0.05 level in their statistical tests! This blatant abandonment of the earlier and more exacting published protocol was also accompanied by the use of what is known as a 'one-sided', or 'one-tailed', test. Those familiar with statistical tests know that opting for the one-tailed test instead of the more stringent 'two-tailed' test had the effect of lowering the significance level even further.

Even after adopting the use of statistical tests that were looser than the patrons of a singles bar after happy hour, the LRC-CPPT researchers had to combine fatal *and* non-fatal coronary events before they could only just barely obtain statistically significant supportive results! Neither the differences in fatal nor non-fatal coronary events reached significance when considered separately.

After greatly relaxing their pre-set standards of statistical significance, and selectively emphasizing the misleading RR figures, the LRC-CPPT researchers were ready to claim that they had found *"strong evidence for a causal role for* [total cholesterol and LDL] *in the pathogenesis of CHD."*

They further claimed that the shamelessly exaggerated results *"support the view that cholesterol-lowering by diet would also be beneficial"*, even though numerous clinical trials had already shown dietary cholesterol-lowering to be nothing but a complete failure.

The discrepancies with the LRC-CPPT did not stop there. When total mortality was calculated, death rates from non-CHD causes were higher amongst cholestyramine recipients compared to controls. In fact, overall death rates between the two groups were almost identical--sixty-eight (3.6 percent) died in the treatment group, compared to seventy-one (3.7 percent) in the control group.

In reality, the NHLBI had spent yet another outrageous sum of money on a study showing no mortality benefit whatsoever from cholesterol-lowering treatment. Of course, that was not how the results were reported--the researchers simply ignored the increase in death from other causes and hailed the miniscule reduction in CHD deaths as a breakthrough.

The study's authors claimed that the alleged benefits of cholesterol-lowering *"could and should be extended to other age groups and women and ... other more modest elevations of cholesterol levels."* This claim was made despite the fact that the trial participants were all middle-aged men with cholesterol levels higher than ninety-five percent of the population.

Armed with the 'supportive' results of the LRC trial, the NHLBI began a massive publicity campaign, enlisting the help of a willing media. *Time* magazine, for example, featured a report with the hyperbolic headline: *"Sorry, It's True. Cholesterol really is a killer."* The cover for an issue carrying a follow-up story, *"And Cholesterol and Now the Bad News ..."*, depicted a plate with two eggs and a strip of bacon arranged to look like a sad, frowning face. Such tomfoolery gave the impression that organizations like the AHA, NHLBI, and low-fat 'gurus' like Nathan Pritikin, had been right all along.

While the shenanigans surrounding the reporting of the LRC trial were enough to leave any sane observer shaking their head in disbelief, they were nothing compared to what was about to follow...

Chapter 11

"The alternative to scientific experiment is the expert committee. Unfortunately, just as one cannot be sure of the relationship between risk factors and disease, we cannot be sure of the relationship between the opinion of the committee and the truth: the opinion of the committee will depend on who is selected for it."
Dr. J.R.A. Mitchell

Creating a 'Consensus'

How scientists 'agreed' to let shady science validate the cholesterol hypothesis.

The greatly exaggerated results of the LRC-CPPT trial inspired the NHLBI to convene the Consensus Development Conference in Bethesda, Maryland, in December of 1984. The aim of the gathering was to determine how the wildly overblown results from this single trial could be transformed into dietary guidelines for the American public. Professor Basil Rifkind, the director of the trial, headed the conference and also decided who was invited to appear on the panel that devised the recommendations.

The title 'Consensus Conference' implies that the panel members reached a unanimous conclusion during the two and a half day gathering, but nothing could be farther from the truth. While many of the conference participants were eager to institute guidelines based on the LRC-CPPT trial, others were highly critical.

Biostatician Paul Meyer remarked: *"To call 'conclusive' a study which showed no difference in total mortality, and by the usual statistical criteria, an entirely nonsignificant difference in coronary incidents, seems to me a substantial misuse of the term."* Professor Michael Oliver from the U.K. also pointed to the increase in non-CHD mortality that negated the reduction in CHD deaths, and asked *"why explain these results away?"*

The failure of cholesterol-lowering treatments to lower overall death rates was flippantly dismissed by British epidemiologist Richard Peto, who explained that there had *"already been fifteen or twenty trials, but in every one something ridiculous happened."* Peto then went onto claim that, although no single trial was convincing, the sum of the trial results was impressive when considered together. How a series of failures could somehow appear successful when considered collectively is anyone's guess; after all, twenty zeros still add up to nothing.

Participants also disagreed on the dietary guidelines that were to be instituted, whilst others expressed concern over the rush to formulate recommendations based on such inconclusive evidence. These cautious commentators were simply ignored.

At the end of the second day, the chairperson shocked many of the attendees when he stood up and announced: *"It has been established beyond a reasonable doubt that lowering elevated blood cholesterol levels will reduce the risk of heart attack deaths due to coronary artery disease."* According to the Consensus report(1), the panel had *"agreed"* that:

- *"The blood cholesterol level of most Americans is undesirably high, in large part because of our high dietary intake of calories, saturated fat, and cholesterol."* The results of numerous clinical trials and epidemiological studies, including those sponsored by the NHLBI, showing that saturated fat was not in any way connected to CHD, were blatantly ignored.
- *"In countries with diets lower in these constituents, blood cholesterol levels are lower, and coronary heart disease is less common."* As we have seen, cross-country comparisons are without question the least reliable of all epidemiological evidence. Embarrassing 'paradoxes' like France, where high saturated fat consumption accompanied low rates of CHD, were not discussed, nor were the published reports of CHD-free East African nomads and Pacific Islanders who ate diets very high in saturated fat.
- *"There is no doubt that appropriate changes in our diet will reduce blood cholesterol levels. Epidemiologic data and over a dozen clinical trials allow us to predict with reasonable assurance that such a measure will afford significant protection against coronary heart disease."* The report's authors must have been looking at research conducted in some far away galaxy; here on planet Earth, over a dozen clinical trials have failed miserably in their attempt to show any benefit from dietary cholesterol-lowering.
- *"All Americans (except children under 2 years of age) be advised to adopt a diet that reduces total dietary fat intake from the current level of about 40 percent of total calories to 30 percent of total calories, reduces saturated fat intake to less than 10 percent of total calories, increases polyunsaturated fat intake but to no more than 10 percent of total calories, and reduces daily cholesterol intake to 250 to 300 mg or less."* The recommendations to reduce saturated fat were not supported by any clinical evidence, only highly selective interpretation of epidemiological data. The recommendation to increase polyunsaturated fat intake was given despite the complete failure of this fat source to favorably alter mortality outcomes in tightly controlled trials. Dietary cholesterol had shown almost no relationship with blood cholesterol levels, except in animal experiments of questionable relevance, but the panel evidently figured it would recommend dietary cholesterol restriction any old how. Even young children were not exempt from the new

guidelines, a truly appalling development. Growing bodies are dependent on adequate supplies of essential fatty acids and fat soluble vitamins, and the fact that the long term effects of fat restriction in children were unknown evidently mattered little. The report's authors also had no qualms about exposing children to the potentially dangerous effects of increased polyunsaturated fat consumption.

- *"Plans be developed that will permit assessment of the impact of the changes recommended here as implementation proceeds and provide the basis for changes when and where appropriate."* Unbeknownst to them, the American people were about to become participants in a huge dietary experiment. As they would be encouraged to adopt a lifelong dietary regimen of which the outcome was largely unknown, the authors figured it might be a good idea to monitor the results in case changes were required. How thoughtful.

Ulterior Motives

At the end of the second day of the conference it was also announced that the panel had recommended the establishment of a nationwide cholesterol education plan, *that printed copies of the plan would be available at 8.30 am the very next morning, and that a press conference had been scheduled three hours after that to announce the plan to the public.* Upon hearing this announcement, many observers believed the true agenda of the conference had finally been revealed; the consensus conference appeared to be little more than a pre-orchestrated event designed to accelerate acceptance of the cholesterol theory(2).

The NHLBI proceeded to launch the National Cholesterol Education Program (NCEP) in November 1985 with the goal of *"reducing illness and death from coronary heart disease (CHD) in the United States",* which it hoped to achieve by encouraging Americans to lower their cholesterol levels. National, state and local organizations were enlisted in a massive, ongoing campaign that continues to this day. The campaign was designed to raise awareness of the 'benefits' to be had from lowering blood cholesterol via the guidelines recommended in the consensus report, and explicitly targeted physicians, other health professionals, and the general public.

The Aftermath

One need not look far to see that the cholesterol propaganda campaign has been an absolutely astounding success. Fat-phobia has spread not just across America, but all over the globe. A hugely profitable industry has grown out of the public's 'need' for reduced fat foods, with food manufacturers tripping over themselves to develop and market all manner of highly-altered foodstuffs which typically bear little resemblance to their natural state, but are nonetheless considered healthy because of the *"low-fat, cholesterol-free!"* livery proudly emblazoned across their packaging.

The trend for sensationalist reporting remains alive and well, with popular media carrying stories on a daily basis warning of the dire consequences from eating allegedly dangerous, 'artery-clogging' saturated fats. According to NHLBI figures, millions more people have discovered the joys of fretting over their cholesterol levels, with the percentage of Americans getting their blood cholesterol checked increasing between 1983 and 1995 from thirty-five to seventy-five percent. The NHLBI is also proud of the fact that *"in 1995, physicians reported initiating diet and drug treatment at much lower cholesterol levels than in 1983, levels close to NCEP recommendations."*(3)

1984 will go down in history as the year of the 'cholesterol coup', the year that proponents of the lipid hypothesis finally succeeded in gaining official acceptance of their theory. The ease with which they did so was unprecedented, and a source of deep concern to those who believe in the scientific method. When someone proposes a new theory, especially one that appears to contradict all available evidence, the onus is on them to provide convincing evidence as to why their hypothesis should be considered. For a new theory to then be accepted as scientific fact, the supporting evidence should be overwhelming, consistent and repeatedly demonstrable, not riddled with inconsistencies and contradictions that must be evaded and distorted in order to make it appear valid.

The claim that saturated fat and cholesterol, natural constituents of our diet for millions of years, caused heart disease was indeed a radical proposition, especially in light of the fact that the so-called 'rise' in CHD correlated far more closely with the increased consumption of historically recent food items such as sugar, refined carbohydrates and polyunsaturated vegetable oils. The NHLBI consensus report unreservedly indicted cholesterol and saturated fat, based on the utterly insignificant results of a single drug trial. History abounds with examples of individuals who have presented theories with far more solid evidence than the NHLBI panel could ever dream of possessing, yet were greeted with ridicule and even violent opposition to their ideas.

This paradoxical scenario led many to ponder the true reasons for the remarkably swift acceptance of the Consensus recommendations. Some of these reasons shall be discussed in the next chapter.

Chapter 12

"What passes for knowledge is often no more than well-organised ignorance."
Dr. J.R.A. Mitchell

"If We Want Your Opinion, We'll Give it to You!"

How the food and drug industries actively perpetuate the wildly profitable cholesterol hypothesis.

By the time the NHLBI convened the Consensus Development Conference in 1984, the AHA and NHLBI had publicly committed themselves to the anti-saturated fat, anti-cholesterol concept, and had spent hundreds of millions of dollars trying to prove its validity. If these authorities were forced to admit that the lipid hypothesis was invalid, the consequences in terms of embarrassment, loss of prestige and financial status would have been quite severe. It would have been exceedingly difficult for organizations like the AHA and NHLBI to justify their exalted status, and to continue to attract hundreds of millions of dollars in funds every year, if they were to admit that their cholesterol theory was a bust. Millions of people cajoled into forsaking their favorite foods and pushed onto lipid-lowering drugs would not have taken kindly to the revelation that the anti-animal fat and anti-cholesterol paranoia they had been successfully indoctrinated with was wholly unnecessary.

The desire by health organizations to save face is by no means the only factor driving the continued perpetuation of the lipid hypothesis. Another huge motivator is the staggering sum of money to be made from cholesterol-free, low-fat foods and lipid-lowering drugs.

You Scratch My Back, and I'll Scratch Yours

Most members of the general public would not even begin to realize just how much money is lavished upon 'impartial' health authorities by food and drug manufacturers. With over 630 products bearing the 'heart-check' logo, it is estimated that the AHA earned over two million dollars from its certification program in 2002(1). Among the 'wholesome' foods that the AHA has deemed worthy of its heart-check are(2):

- General Mills Cheerios, Cocoa Puffs, Cookie Crisp, Corn Chex, and Count Chocula;
- Healthy Choice Low Fat Ice Creams,

- Chocolate Moose Milk Chocolate Drinks;
- Malt-O-Meal Frosted Mini Spooners, Honey Graham Squares, and Honey Nut Toasty O's;
- Kellogg's Frosted Mini-Wheats Big Bite;
- Kellogg's Nutri-Grain Cereal Bars;
- Pop-Secret 94% Fat Free Butter Microwave Premium Popcorn.

Official endorsement of such nutrient-depleted and refined carbohydrate-rich pap is no doubt a major reason why we are now burdened with unprecedented levels of obesity and diabetes, and why the incidence of heart disease has failed to decline despite a marked drop in smoking. In order to guard against heart disease, a truly healthy diet should possess the following two characteristics:

1) The ability to prevent the development of elevated blood sugar levels;
2) The maximum possible concentration of cardio-protective vitamins, minerals, trace elements, amino acids, and antioxidant phytochemicals per calorie.

The highly processed 'foods' listed above do not even begin to meet either of these criteria, but consumers are unlikely to be made aware of this so long as the giant health organization continues to receive up to $7,500 per product per year to endorse these same foods.

Pharmaceutical giant Merck, which manufactures the cholesterol-lowering statin drugs Mevacor and Zocor, has spent $400,000 financing an AHA program inculcating 40,000 doctors with cholesterol treatment guidelines (these guidelines, as we shall learn shortly, are written by researchers with financial ties to cholesterol-lowering drug manufacturers like Merck). Other lipid-lowering drug manufacturers that contribute funds to the AHA include Pfizer, Astra-Zeneca and Bristol-Myers-Squibb.

Another organization which just can't bring itself to say a bad word about highly processed low-fat foods is the American Dietetic Association (ADA). The official association for America's dietitians has received financial contributions from, among others, the National Soft Drink Association, ConAgra, Grocery Manufacturers of America, Monsanto, Procter and Gamble, Potato Board, National Pasta Association, American Soy Products, National Dairy Council and the National Cattleman's Beef Association. The ADA issues 'fact sheets' providing information on various nutrition and health topics; most of these are underwritten by companies whose products are discussed in the fact sheets. Manufacturers that have given at least $100,000 towards the production of these sheets include Coca-Cola, Kellogg, Kraft Foods, Weight Watchers International, Campbell Soup, National Dairy Council, Nestle USA, General Mills, Monsanto, Nabisco, Procter and Gamble, Ross Products, Wyeth-

Ayerst Labs and Uncle Ben's(1). The extensive food industry support given to organizations such as the ADA may explain why dietitians are so fond of claiming that *"there is no such thing as a bad food"* and that *"all foods consumed in moderation have a place in a varied, healthful and balanced diet"* (except of course, those containing all but miniscule amounts of saturated fat). Such pragmatic and non-offensive tripe ensures that these organizations and their members do not bite the numerous hands that feed them.

The American Diabetes Association is the nation's premiere diabetic organization. For some bizarre reason, it insists that the country's carbohydrate-intolerant diabetics should eat a carbohydrate-rich diet. Among the few parties that would benefit from such regrettable advice are drug companies and the manufacturers of low-fat, carbohydrate-rich foods. Lo and behold, these can be found in abundance on the Association's sponsor sheet. The following is only a partial list of the companies that each donated between $100,000-750,000 to the Association in 2002(1):

- $750,000: Abbott Laboratories; Aventis Pharmaceuticals; BD Consumer Healthcare; Bristol-Myers Squibb Company; Eli Lilly and Company; GlaxoSmithKline; Merck & Co., Inc.; Novartis Pharmaceuticals Corporation; Novo Nordisk Pharmaceuticals; Pfizer Inc; Takeda Pharmaceuticals North America, Inc.
- $500,000+: Bayer Corporation; Kraft Foods; Roche Diagnostics Corporation.
- $250,000+: Abbott Laboratories, Ross Product Division (Glucerna); AstraZeneca; Merisant U.S., Inc. (Equal Sweetener); Wyeth Pharmaceuticals.
- $100,000+: Archway Cookies, LLC; Coolbrands International, Inc. (Eskimo Pie); CVS/pharmacy; General Mills, Inc. (Fiber One); Good Neighbor Pharmacy; KOS Pharmaceuticals, Inc.; Murray Sugar Free Cookies; Ocean Spray Cranberries, Inc.; Ortho-McNeil Pharmaceutical, Inc.; Rite Aid Pharmacy; Roche Pharmaceuticals; Schering Plough Healthcare Products, Inc.; Specialty Brands of America (Cary's Sugar Free Cookies); The Procter & Gamble Company; Voortman Cookies Limited.

The ability of these authorities to remain impartial whilst being lavished with industry money is extremely suspect, especially when one considers some of the highly questionable advice these authorities spew forth.

Science For Sale

While both the food and pharmaceutical industries profit handsomely from the lipid hypothesis, the latter is arguably most dependant on the continued propagation of cholesterol paranoia. While the food industry could adapt to the abandonment of the cholesterol paradigm by reformulating many of its staple products, the drug giants would be faced with the prospect of losing their most lucrative line of revenue. As such, the pharmaceutical industry goes to great lengths to keep the current anti-cholesterol mania thriving. A cornerstone of their campaign is the cultivation of a supportive consensus in the scientific community.

Most of us would like to think that scientists are incorruptible individuals engaged in a single-minded pursuit of the truth. Many observers, however, have voiced alarm at the increasingly blurred boundaries between big business and science. Along with organizations like the NHLBI and the AHA, pharmaceutical companies are a major source of research grants, which are a scientist's bread and butter. Nowadays, seventy percent of all money channeled into CHD drug trials comes from the pharmaceutical companies themselves.

The financial ties between drug companies and clinical researchers are not merely limited to grant support. As former *New England Journal of Medicine* editor-in-chief, Marcia Angell, M.D., explained in a May, 2000 editorial: *"Researchers serve as consultants to companies whose products they are studying, join advisory boards and speakers' bureaus, enter into patent and royalty arrangements, agree to be listed authors of articles ghostwritten by interested companies, promote drugs and devices at company-sponsored symposiums, and allow themselves to be plied with expensive gifts and trips to luxurious settings. Many also have equity interest in the companies"*(3).

Needless to say, this 'goodwill' does not extend to those who rock the boat. Commenting on Angell's editorial, one M.D. wrote: *"As an academic psychiatrist and neurologist, I have been invited by pharmaceutical companies on a number of occasions to educate my colleagues on such topics as depression and dementia...Several months ago, however, I wrote a series of case reports reflecting my experience with the side-effect profile of a certain medication. The problem was that the profile was less favorable than that of medication made by a competitor of one of the companies for which I often spoke. My invitations to speak suddenly dropped from four to six times per month to essentially none."*(4)

In the same journal, Thomas Bodenheimer, M.D., cited a number of studies showing that researchers with ties to drug companies were indeed more likely to report favorably on the products of those companies than researchers without such ties(5). After interviewing pharmaceutical company executives, clinical researchers, medical writers and physicians from commercial research organizations, Bodenheimer uncovered some very disturbing findings.

The clinical investigators Bodenheimer spoke with relayed numerous instances where the drug giants used contracts forbidding publication of results without their prior approval to avoid the release of negative findings. Researchers who discovered that a drug had serious side effects or that it offered no advantage over existing drugs were threatened with legal action if they went public. When research on a particular drug yielded mixed results, manufacturers shelved the negative studies and ensured that only the positive results were submitted for publication. When one researcher found that a drug he was studying caused adverse side effects and sent a manuscript detailing these effects to the sponsoring company, it *"vowed never to fund his work again and published a competing article with scant mention of the adverse effects."*

A more recent and even more extensive analysis of the scientific literature bears out the findings of Bodenheimer. Researchers analyzed data from eight individual articles, encompassing a total of 1,140 original studies, that addressed the association between industry sponsorship and research outcome. When the results of all these studies were pooled, they showed that industry-sponsored research was 3.6 times more likely to produce favorable findings than studies with no financial ties to the industry. The study also found that: *"Approximately one fourth of investigators have industry affiliations, and roughly two thirds of academic institutions hold equity in start-ups that sponsor research performed at the same institutions."*(6)

Biased and coercive activity by drug companies is in no way confined to American shores; in June 2005, the *Medical Journal of Australia* published the results of a survey involving medical specialists. Twenty-one percent of those with an active research relationship with the pharmaceutical industry reported examples of potentially serious research misconduct, including: Delayed publication or outright suppression of key negative findings; editing of a report to make a drug look better; concealment of findings relevant to the study's conclusions; and alteration of patient data or statistics(7).

Drug Company Influence Goes All the Way to the Top

The cash-laden tentacles of the pharmaceutical industry have penetrated even into the highest levels of government bureaucracy. The NHLBI is a branch of the National Institutes of Health (NIH), the federal government's center for medical research on humans. The NIH's top scientists are among the highest paid employees in the government, and its studies can affect the commercial viability of new drugs and the stock prices of biomedical companies.

Dr. H. Bryan Brewer Jr., a high-ranking scientist at the NIH, was considered *"one of the nation's leading experts on cholesterol"* and part of a team that wrote the cholesterol guidelines that encouraged more aggressive prescription of cholesterol-lowering drugs. As the *Los Angeles Times* reports: *"What doctors were not told for years is this. While making recommendations in the name of the NIH, Brewer was working for the companies that sell the drugs.*

Government and company records show that from 2001 to 2003, he accepted about $114,000 in consulting fees from four companies making or developing cholesterol medications, including $31,000 from the maker of Crestor (AstraZeneca)"

In the August 21, 2003 issue of the *American Journal of Cardiology*, Brewer wrote that Crestor's *"benefit-risk profile ... appears to be very favorable"*. He assured doctors there was no basis for worry about rhabdomyolysis, claiming that, *"No cases of rhabdomyolysis occurred in patients receiving* [Crestor] *at 10 to 40 milligrams."*

But eight cases of rhabdomyolysis were reported during clinical trials of Crestor. One case involved a patient who took the drug in ten milligram doses, according to records filed with the Food and Drug Administration and reviewed by the *LA Times* under the Freedom of Information Act. FDA records also show that it received seventy-eight reports of rhabdomyolysis among patients taking Crestor during its first year on the market. Two of those patients died.

AstraZeneca sales representatives have routinely provided copies of Brewer's journal article about Crestor to doctors nationwide, the *LA Times* reported(8).

Brewer was hardly the only NIH employee writing recommendations for the public with one hand and receiving drug company money with the other. The *LA Times* revealed in late 2003 that hundreds of NIH employees had been accepting consulting fees from biotech and pharmaceutical companies at least since November 1995, when then-NIH Director Harold E. Varmus relaxed the Institute's conflict-of-interest rules. Current Director Dr. Elias A. Zerhouni told a congressional subcommittee in January 2004 that an internal review showed a total of 527 agency employees had engaged in paid consulting arrangements with 1,515 outside employers since 1999. Some of these contracts involved such major cholesterol-lowering drug manufacturers including Pfizer, Wyeth Pharmaceuticals, and AstraZeneca(9,10).

Zerhouni did not identify how much money had been paid to the NIH scientists in fees or stock options from these outside companies. In fact, in 2003, more than ninety-four percent of the NIH's top-paid employees were not required to publicly disclose consulting income. Nonetheless, an *LA Times* story from January 2005 indicated that there were some very sizable sums of money involved. The story reported on an NIH Alzheimer's researcher who was under investigation for accepting more than $500,000 of drug company money without seeking permission or reporting the income to the agency as required(11).

In response to the resultant uproar over the revelation that employees from the Government's foremost research agency were regularly engaging in potentially compromising financial relationships, Zerhouni announced that NIH directors had stopped accepting consulting fees and stock options from drug companies. In early 2005, the ban was finally extended to include all NIH staff(12). Rather than being relieved that their employer was finally acting to resolve the image-blackening conflict-of-interest issue, NIH employees quite literally greeted the decision with howls of protest(13). After being flooded with 1,300 comments by employees and threats of high-level defections, Zerhouni agreed in August 2005 to loosen the ethics rules he unveiled in February. Under the final regulations, about 200 senior staff members will be required to divest large stock holdings in drug and biotechnology companies, far fewer than the 6,000 employees who would have had to divest under the original proposal(14).

FDA: The Food and Drug *Alliance*?

The Food and Drug Administration (FDA) is the massive government agency that decides which new drugs will be allowed into the market, when a drug should be pulled from sale because of safety concerns, and whether specific health claims can be made for individual food products and supplements.

In September 2000, *USA Today* reported that fifty-four percent--more than half--of the experts hired to advise the FDA on the safety and effectiveness of medicines had financial relationships with drug manufacturers that would be helped or hurt by their decisions. Some of these advisors had helped a pharmaceutical company develop a medicine then served on an FDA advisory committee that judged the drug!

Financial conflicts typically included stock ownership, consulting fees, research grants, a spouse's employment and payments for speeches and travel. Federal law generally prohibits the FDA from using experts with financial conflicts of interest, but *USA Today* found that the FDA had waived the restriction *more than 800 times* since 1998!

When *USA Today* analyzed potential financial conflicts at 159 FDA advisory committee meetings between January 1998 and June 2000, it found that:

- At ninety-two percent of the meetings, at least one member had a financial conflict of interest.
- At fifty-five percent of meetings, half or more of the FDA advisers had conflicts of interest.
- At meetings where broader issues were discussed, ninety-two percent of members had conflicts.
- At the meetings dealing with the fate of a specific drug, thirty-three percent of the experts had a financial conflict.

As alarming as they are, the figures unearthed by *USA Today* actually underestimate the true percentage of researchers with financial conflicts; many of these conflicts are considered too small to require disclosure or a waiver and were therefore not counted in *USA Today's* study. According to FDA guidelines, a committee member can be paid up to $50,000 a year by a drug company without any financial conflict being disclosed if the work was on a topic other than what the committee is evaluating. Committee members can also own up to $5,000 in stock in the company appearing before the committee.

The FDA stopped making details of financial conflicts public in 1992, after controversies about whether the financial interests of committee members had biased decisions on breast implants, the controversial anti-depressant Prozac, and a drug to treat Alzheimer's disease(15). The FDA is not the only bureaucracy that appears to subscribe to a 'what they don't know won't hurt 'em' philosophy of public disclosure--according to the *Los Angeles Times,* the NIH issued a form instructing employees who reported their income confidentially not to reveal details of conflicting financial industry ties. Ah, good old government transparency…

Selective Science

In 1992, Swedish researcher Uffe Ravnskov, M.D., PhD, examined the frequency with which researchers cited successful and unsuccessful cholesterol-lowering trials in their published papers. He found that trials whose results were reported as supportive of the lipid hypothesis were cited almost six times as frequently as those that were not(16).

A few years later, Ravnskov examined a number of commonly cited scientific reviews supporting the lipid hypothesis, documenting numerous instances where the authors ignored contradictory findings, quoted studies incorrectly, inflated the importance of insignificant favorable results and cited non-supportive studies as if they were supportive. He even noted instances where authors cited other reviews as supporting evidence. Published scientific reviews are supposed to represent the conclusions of authors who have conducted a sweeping survey of the available clinical evidence, not the rehashed opinions of other review authors. What's more, after examining these cited reviews, Ravnskov found they often did not even support the argument presented in the original review(17).

It is easy to present a convincing case for just about any theory when one quotes only supporting research and conveniently ignores contradictory evidence. Such a practice should be utterly abhorred by any scientist whose primary mission is an impartial search for the truth, but selective citation is anything but rare amongst cholesterol researchers. When one's livelihood depends upon funds handed out by major purveyors of the lipid hypothesis, there exists substantial incentive to take the path of least resistance.

The potential for the pharmaceutical industry to influence public health policy is readily illustrated by the financial ties of the NCEP committee that sets America's cholesterol guidelines. These are the official blood cholesterol targets that the nation's doctors abide by when counseling their patients. Over the years, the upper recommended limits for ideal blood cholesterol levels have gradually sunk lower and lower, allowing doctors to place millions more on cholesterol-lowering medications.

In May 2001 the NCEP revised its guidelines, categorizing the entire population into one of three categories according to CHD risk. Each category was assigned an upper limit of LDL cholesterol. Individuals exceeding their assigned threshold were given three months to achieve their target LDL level, and if their efforts were unsuccessful, the initiation of drug therapy was recommended. Certain groups were advised not to even bother fussing with the initial drug-free period; those with diabetes and pre-existing CHD were encouraged to begin drug therapy right away. The only two side effects listed for statin use in the NCEP guidelines were the relatively benign-sounding terms *"myopathy"* and *"increased liver enzymes"*.

The financial disclosure information at the end of the article, required by the *Journal of the American Medical Association*, shows that six of the fourteen NCEP committee members had received financial support from multiple pharmaceutical companies. The resultant list read like a *Who's Who* of lipid lowering drug manufacturers(18).

In July 2004, the NCEP updated its guidelines yet again, recommending even lower target LDL levels in all but the lowest risk CHD category, again creating millions of new customers for cholesterol-lowering drug manufacturers(19). Again, the panel was comprised of individuals with conflicting financial ties. This time, all but one of the nine panelists had received grants or consulting or speakers' fees from the manufacturers of some of the most popular statin medications on the market, including Pfizer, Bristol-Myers Squibb, Merck and AstraZeneca(20).

Who's Your Pusher?

Clinical researchers are not the only group of professionals among whom the pharmaceutical industry endeavors to cultivate a compliant attitude. In an article titled *Physicians' Ties With the Pharmaceutical Industry: A Critical Element of a Wildly Successful Marketing Network,* Jerome P. Kassirer, MD, former editor-in-chief of the prestigious *New England Journal of Medicine*, gave numerous examples of how drug companies influence physicians' prescribing behavior, including:

- Free gifts to physicians and medical students;
- Paying respected medical figures to lend their name to articles that have been ghost-written by authors employed by drug companies;
- Sponsoring free continuing education courses for physicians that are biased in favor of the sponsoring company's products;
- Sponsoring the publication of literature containing diagnostic and treatment guidelines for doctors that favor the sponsoring company's products;
- Paying researchers and practitioners to deliver presentations at drug-company-sponsored symposia which, again, place a favorable slant on the sponsoring manufacturers' products;

Kassirer recalls how, during his tenure as editor-in-chief at the journal, it became increasingly difficult to obtain authors who did not have financial ties to the companies whose products were being discussed in submitted articles. In fact, Kassirer's successor found it so difficult to find authors without conflicting financial ties he abandoned the journal's conflict-of-interest policy in 2001! (21)

Buying Doctors' Allegiances

Many doctors on the receiving end of such drug company 'hospitality' would indignantly object to the suggestion that it influences their prescribing practices in any way. The available evidence, however, paints a very different picture.

Each year, drug companies spend billions of dollars maintaining an army of highly trained sales reps whose job is to convince doctors of the value and superiority of their products. Pfizer, for example, maintains a force of 13,000 salespeople who are continually trained and tested. According to a January, 2003 article in *Forbes* magazine, *"...trainees go through weeks of simulated sales calls in a mock physician's office, built like a movie set on one of Pfizer's upstate New York campuses. On the simulation stage, former sales reps play harried and irritable doctors. Trainees are timed and judged on their ability to deliver a pitch for a Pfizer drug."*(22)

Confidential documents obtained from drug giant Merck and presented at a hearing of the House Government Reform Committee on May 5, 2005, further illustrate just how meticulously drug company salespeople are groomed. Merck's sales staff were given instructions as detailed as how long to shake a physician's hand--three seconds--and how to eat bread when dining with doctors--*"one small bitesize piece at a time."* Sales representatives were offered $2,000 bonuses for meeting sales goals, and worked in campaigns with such code-names as 'Project Offense' to try and boost sales of the company's best-selling Vioxx, even as regulators were about to increase label warnings about the increased risk of cardiovascular disease that accompanied use of the drug. *"Don't bring up the heart risks",* warned a February 9, 2001, memo.

When doctors asked about those risks, Merck sales reps were to refer to a 'cardiovascular card' with data suggesting that Vioxx could be safer than other anti-inflammatory drugs. The card, however, did not include the very study raising the first warning signal that Vioxx could harm(23).

Drug companies bear the considerable expense needed to cultivate and maintain such highly skilled sales teams for one simple reason--they get results.

An extensive review by Ashley Wazana, M.D., published in a January 2000 issue of the *Journal of the American Medical Association,* examined the impact of drug company interactions on physicians' prescription-writing habits and found that:

- *"Meetings with pharmaceutical representatives were associated with requests by physicians for adding the drugs to the hospital formulary and changes in prescribing practice",* even when the requested drugs presented little or no therapeutic advantage over currently-used drugs.
- Interaction with pharmaceutical representatives was also found to increase the preference for new drugs, and the rapidity with which they were prescribed. The prescription of cheaper generic drugs, meanwhile, declined in conjunction with such interaction.
- Acceptance of samples, free meals, and funding for travel and lodging to attend 'educational symposia' were all associated with increased requests for addition of sponsors' drugs to hospital dispensaries and increased prescribing of these drugs.
- *"Drug company-sponsored continuing medical education (CME) preferentially highlighted the sponsor's drug(s) compared with other CME programs"* and also influenced prescription habits in favor of the sponsor's products.

Interestingly, one of the reviewed studies found that while eighty-five percent of medical students agreed it was improper for politicians to accept a gift, *"only 46% found it improper for themselves to accept a gift of similar value from a pharmaceutical company."*(24)

A recent study of physicians in northwest England underscores Wazana's findings. The study found that the number one source of drug information for physicians was the pharmaceutical industry itself. Physicians were most commonly introduced to new drugs through pharmaceutical sales representatives, and pharmaceutical companies were the greatest influence on their decisions of which drugs to prescribe. Almost three-quarters of the doctors regarded drug company representatives as an efficient way to obtain new drug information. While the doctors claimed to be generally wary of the drug industry's objectives, they tended to believe that its information would be selective but accurate. The physicians believed that they could generally spot misleading information, but only seventeen percent sought out evidence from peer-reviewed journals before making prescribing decisions. According to the researchers, physicians *"were largely reactive and opportunistic recipients of new drug information, rarely reporting an active information search."*(25)

To make matters worse, much of the drug company propaganda with which doctors are bombarded appears to have very little basis in reality. A recent study by independent researchers in Germany found that ninety-four percent of the information contained in advertising material and marketing brochures sent out by drug companies to GPs is not supported by available scientific evidence. They found around fifteen percent of the brochures did not contain any citations, while another twenty-two percent contained citations of studies that could not be found. Most of the remaining sixty-three percent contained information that was connected with the cited research articles but did not reflect their results. Only six percent of the brochures contained statements that were supported by identifiable scientific literature. The researchers found that medical guidelines from scientific societies were misquoted or changed, drug side effects and risks were downplayed, non-supportive study results were suppressed, treatment effects were exaggerated and beneficial drug effects were drawn from animal studies(26).

The Anti-Cholesterol Militia

While health agencies, drug companies and food manufacturers have without a doubt been the prime movers behind the great cholesterol hoax, they didn't do all the work. Any discussion about the perpetuation of the lipid hypothesis would be incomplete without mentioning the important role played by the huge army of independent anti-cholesterol commentators. These have included the swarm of low-fat diet authors that proliferated during the eighties and nineties, numerous well-meaning but highly misguided 'consumer advocacy' groups and, of course, the countless ratings-hungry media outlets that have run alarmist stories about saturated fats and cholesterol over the years.

While the list of published low-fat diet authors runs longer than the Mississippi, the most famous and influential is unquestionably the late Nathan Pritikin. It was in 1979 that he introduced the *Pritikin Program for Diet and Exercise*, which was followed by several other international bestsellers, including *Live Longer Now, The Pritikin Weight Loss Manual* and *Diet For Runners*. Pritikin was initially branded a quack by a hostile medical profession when he stated that heart disease was reversible through a combination of diet, exercise and stress management. When evidence accumulated to suggest that this multi-factorial approach could effectively treat diabetes and heart disease, the tide of opinion began to turn. Pritikin captured the attention of physicians, researchers, government leaders and millions of lay people around the world.

Unfortunately, many of these individuals swallowed Pritikin's anti-fat vitriol hook, line and sinker, not realizing that his multiple intervention program succeeded not because of, but in spite of his extreme dietary fat guidelines. Other influential authors who went on to win fame and fortune by fanatically preaching the low-fat gospel were Richard Simmons, Susan Powter and Dean Ornish (see Appendix B at the end of this book for a more complete discussion of Ornish and Pritikin).

A shining example of how the misguided angst of independent activists can be readily harnessed by vested financial interests was the vicious scare campaign targeting tropical oils that peaked in the late 1980's. In 1986, a consumer advocacy group known as the Center for Science in the Public Interest (CSPI) and the American Soybean Association launched an all-out attack on tropical oils. The CSPI's antagonism towards tropical fats arose not because they had been documented to cause any adverse health consequences--they hadn't, and still haven't--but simply because of their high saturated fat content.

As for the soybean industry's involvement, coconut and palm kernel oils had a long and safe history of use in the food industry, providing a major impediment to the growth of the vegetable oil industry. Soybean farmers and their families were encouraged to write to the media, government officials and food companies, expressing their 'concern' over the use of highly saturated tropical fats like palm and coconut oils in the American food industry.

In 1988, Nebraska billionaire Phil Sokolof, founder of the National Heart Savers Association, jumped on the bandwagon by launching full-page newspaper advertisements that contained scathing anti-tropical fat rhetoric. Sokolof, convinced that an elevated cholesterol level reading was the sole explanation for a heart attack he suffered at age forty-three, was, and remains, a highly vocal and active campaigner against saturated fat and cholesterol.

Sokolof's *Poisoning of America* campaign denounced companies for using tropical oils, with one newspaper advertisement featuring an illustration of a coconut with a burning fuse, likening the humble tropical nut to a bomb. Sokolof also took a swipe at food giant McDonald's for cooking its fries in beef tallow. Cowering to public pressure, McDonald's stopped using tallow and switched to using polyunsaturated vegetable oils. Food manufacturers and outlets using tropical oils followed suit, switching to supposedly 'healthier' polyunsaturated oils to avoid negative publicity. Until recently, the NHSA web site (now defunct) still boasted of these 'achievements'(27); what was not mentioned was that the campaign succeeded in replacing heat-resistant saturated fats with oxidation-prone vegetable oils that were riddled with trans and omega-6 fatty acids (see Chapter 17)--hardly a development worth celebrating!

Ironically, field studies of tropical populations that consumed high-fat coconut products on a daily basis, such as the Kitavans, Pukapukans and Tokelauans, found them all to possess outstanding cardiovascular health(28, 29). A recent comparison of two margarines, one containing predominantly coconut oil and the other mostly monounsaturated fats, tentatively suggests the former may have beneficial effects on the body's anti-clotting capabilities(30).

Although there was not a shred of sound scientific evidence to support this negative publicity blitz, the media readily picked up on the story, running alarmist articles on the tropical fat 'scandal'. The foreign-based tropical oil industry made attempts to counter these scare tactics, but was paid little attention. Scientists familiar with tropical oils also tried to set the record straight, but were similarly ignored. The campaign against tropical oils was yet another powerful testament to the ability of money and scare-mongering hype to successfully fan the flames of ignorance.

The Gravy Train Rolls On...

To keep the cholesterol bandwagon rolling merrily along, food and drug companies actively support scientists who perpetuate the cholesterol myth, spare no expense in molding a conformist mindset among doctors, and 'donate' large sums of money to the 'impartial' organizations that create and promote public health guidelines.

Readers could be forgiven for concluding that the diet-heart research arena contains about as much integrity as a room full of politicians. Fortunately for us, not all researchers have sold out to vested interests. The field of science contains many shining stars whose findings not only contradict the lipid hypothesis, but provide strong clues as to what really causes CHD.

In Section Two, we will look closely at their discoveries and find out just what we can do to avoid heart disease.

SECTION TWO
What *Really* Causes Heart Disease?

Chapter 13

"It is a dispiriting fact that, when faced with diseases of unknown cause, the medical profession unerringly manages to get cause and effect completely the wrong way round."
Malcolm Kendrick, M.D.

Beyond Cholesterol.

If not cholesterol, then what?

Thanks to years of incredibly effective propaganda, the average layperson's understanding of coronary heart disease runs something like this: Larry Lipid regularly eats foods that are high in fat, especially saturated fat, causing his blood to become filled with lots of nasty fat and cholesterol particles. These globules menacingly proceed through Larry's bloodstream, looking for a comfy spot on his artery walls where they can settle and begin to multiply. Once they have found a suitable location, these mischievous particles form a 'fatty deposit' that begins to grow larger and larger, just like the evil gelatinous mass from the old horror movie *The Blob.* This fatty deposit eventually grows to the point where it blocks the entire artery, halting blood flow to Larry's heart and triggering a potentially deadly heart attack. As a terrified Larry clutches his chest and waits for the paramedics to arrive, he finally sees the error of his ways and vows that, if he survives, he will never eat another turkey thigh or chicken wing again.

Although subscribed to by much of the lay public and, evidently, many health professionals, the above version of events is about as realistic as the Flat Earth Theory. The 'cholesterol-clogs-arteries' scenario might be acceptable in a children's storybook, but individuals who are serious about avoiding heart disease need to know what *really* occurs in the run-up to a life-threatening coronary event.

The Long and Short of CHD

Coronary heart disease is a complex malady that, in the simplest of terms, can be considered as consisting of two phases; a *chronic* and an *acute* phase. The chronic phase involves the development of atherosclerosis, a process in which plaque forms inside our arteries over many years.

In the human cardiovascular system, atherosclerosis occurs most severely, not in the veins or capillaries, but in the larger arteries where blood volume and pressure is greatest. Inside these large arteries, atherosclerosis strikes most prominently in the areas where they curve and divide(1). These susceptible areas experience the greatest 'shear stress', a term used to describe the pressure and friction exerted against blood vessel walls as blood pulsates through them. This observation alone should alert readers to the illogical nature of the cholesterol theory; after all, if simple elevations in blood cholesterol were responsible for atherosclerosis, then plaque formation should occur uniformly throughout the entire cardiovascular system, rather than primarily in the areas of large arteries where the greatest shear stress is experienced.

Because of the inevitability of shear stress, even the healthiest among us will possess at least a small degree of atherosclerosis by the time we reach our seventies(2). In healthy, well-nourished arteries, the effect of shear stress is minimal, and atherosclerotic build-up does not reach potentially dangerous levels. In many individuals however, the formation of atherosclerosis occurs at an accelerated pace, impairing proper arterial function and dramatically increasing the likelihood of a coronary event.

Fatty Streaks

Fatty streaks, which are irregular yellow discolorations near the surface of the artery, are considered to be the earliest visible manifestations of what eventually becomes advanced atherosclerotic plaque. Repeatedly cited as evidence that blood lipids are initiators of atherosclerosis, fatty streaks in fact are not layers of fat but congregations of mainly macrophage white blood cells located under the endothelial cells that line the surface of arteries. Fatty streaks may also contain lymphocytes, leukocytes, platelets, and smooth muscle cells(3). The macrophages have a foamy appearance due to high concentrations of cholesterol and phospholipids in their cytoplasm, but a high cellular lipid content does not in any way prove that cholesterol is the causative factor. In fact, it is most disingenuous to claim that elevated serum cholesterol causes fatty streaks or promotes the transformation of fatty streaks into advanced atherosclerosis when careful investigations repeatedly show no relationship between serum cholesterol levels and extent of atherosclerosis. The extensive involvement of white blood cells merely reinforces the contention that atherosclerosis is not the product of simple blood cholesterol elevations, but an inflammatory immune response to arterial injury. The latter concept will be discussed in more detail shortly.

The continued development of arterial plaque involves the thickening and calcification of the artery wall, which leads to a loss of elasticity. Advanced atherosclerosis involves the additional accumulation of fatty and fibrous deposits within arterial plaque. This atherosclerotic plaque build-up can accumulate to the point where it prominently bulges underneath the inner wall into the bloodstream, forming what is known as an *atheroma*. This tumor-like formation is a mixture of collagen, calcium, arterial muscle cells, white blood cells, blood platelets, and yes, fatty acids and cholesterol. This protruding mass is often covered by a fibrous cap, not unlike the scar tissue that forms on your skin after you cut yourself.

Clearly, atheromas are not mere blobs of fat that randomly stick to artery walls. As Figure 13b shows, growth of an atheroma takes place *inside* the artery wall, not on the surface as commonly depicted in the popular media.

Arterial Injury

Advanced atherosclerosis is essentially the manifestation of arterial injury. This injury may be caused by a variety of factors, as we shall discuss shortly. For now, it is important to remember that when the body is injured, it inevitably attempts to repair itself.

Cholesterol is likely found in the atheroma for the same reason that all the other components of an atheroma are present: as part of the body's attempt to repair a damaged section of artery. Cholesterol is used by every cell in the body to supply all-important structural integrity to the cell membrane. This important quality may be why the body channels cholesterol into atherosclerotic plaques, which are essentially areas of the artery containing a high proportion of damaged cells. If arteries are not damaged, cholesterol will not accumulate within them. Blaming cholesterol for atherosclerosis makes about as much sense as blaming paramedics for the carnage they face after arriving at a road accident scene.

The Acute Phase

The mere presence of advanced atherosclerosis in the coronary arteries is no guarantee that one will succumb to a coronary event. For a heart attack to occur, there has to be some sort of trigger, some kind of stimulus that suddenly brings coronary blood flow to a grinding halt.

Enter the acute phase of CHD.

The majority of life-threatening coronary events are believed to occur either when a narrowed section of artery undergoes spasm and blocks blood flow to the heart, or when the fibrous scar tissue covering an atheroma ruptures. In the latter instance, the contents of the atheroma spill into the bloodstream, causing the blood to rapidly clot. These blood clots, or *thrombi*, may completely block the artery at the site of rupture or may break away and travel through the bloodstream, eventually becoming 'jammed' in another area narrowed by plaque build-up. Once a coronary artery is completely blocked, the heart is denied the oxygen and nutrient-rich blood that it requires to keep pumping, and the terrifying sequelae of myocardial infarction ensue.

130

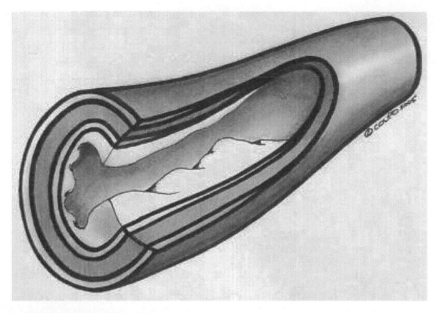

Figure 13a (above) depicts the popular but erroneous 'fatty deposit' scenario of atherosclerosis as typically portrayed to the public. In this scenario, particles of fat and cholesterol allegedly stick to the arteries walls like mud inside a pipe. **Figure 13b (below)** is a far more accurate representation of atherosclerotic plaque build-up. Plaques develop, not on the surface of the artery, but between the inner and outer walls. They are not comprised simply of fat and cholesterol, but also arterial muscle tissue, white blood cells, collagen, calcium, and blood platelets.

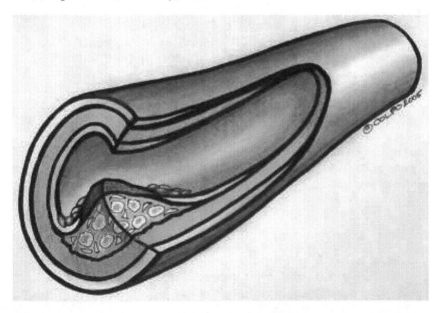

In the case of *ischemic* stroke, the same process is enacted, but it occurs in the arteries that lead to the brain instead of those adjacent to the heart (*hemorrhagic* stroke involves a different procession of events; it occurs when blood vessels in the brain rupture, flooding surrounding tissues with blood).

In order to maximize our chances of avoiding CHD and ischemic stroke, we must abandon the untenable belief that mindlessly lowering blood cholesterol levels to meet some arbitrary guideline will produce beneficial results. We must instead concentrate on preventing advanced atherosclerosis, arterial spasm, plaque rupture and thrombi formation.

The Causes of Arterial Injury

What exactly causes our arteries to become weakened, damaged and, ultimately, blocked? The following is by no means an exhaustive list, but it covers most of the major known contributors:

Chronic stress. Psychological stress arouses the activity of hormones that cause our arteries to spasm and our blood to clot. It also lowers the levels of important anabolic hormones that we need for tissue growth and repair. Poor sleep habits can also exert effects similar to those of chronic stress.

Increased free radical activity. Smoking, high bodily iron levels, environmental pollution, excessive alcohol consumption, a high unsaturated fat intake, and a diet deficient in antioxidants all act to significantly increase the production of free radicals inside our bodies. This excess of free radicals directly damages our arteries.

High blood sugar levels. When we consume diets excessively high in carbohydrates--especially those rich in refined carbohydrates--or when we become overweight, or when we are chronically stressed or sleeping poorly, our blood sugar levels rise. High blood sugar levels increase free radical activity, deplete our bodies of vitamin C, and cause increased *glycation,* a phenomenon that is extremely deleterious to both cardiovascular and overall health.

Poor nutrient intake, especially of key vitamins, minerals, amino acids, plant phenols, and long-chain omega-3 fatty acids. Science has clearly illustrated that eating inadequate amounts of these nutrients--as a great many of us do--is an open invitation to arterial degradation and subsequent cardiovascular disease.

Lack of physical activity. A lack of physical activity results in declining blood sugar control, impaired arterial function, body fat gain, and greater susceptibility to the effects of chronic stress--all of which impart a greatly increased risk of heart disease.

Impaired nitric oxide (NO) release. If you're wondering what on earth a highly reactive gas like NO has to do with heart disease, the answer is everything. As you will learn in Chapter 20, healthy NO levels within arteries are absolutely essential for proper cardiovascular function. Unfortunately, many of us stubbornly persist with dietary and lifestyle habits that are extremely effective in suppressing NO activity.

The factors I have listed above are not merely 'associated' with CHD--they serve as direct catalysts for the disease process itself. Interestingly, the majority of these factors also possess the ability to raise total and/or LDL cholesterol levels. Unfortunately, hordes of researchers continue to confuse cause with effect, assuming that cholesterol is the guilty party.

Cholesterol is an essential substance that our cells cannot live without. The notion that it causes heart disease--or any other disease--would be downright hilarious if not for the shameful fact that it has been accepted as a pivotal precept of contemporary medicine.

Arteries On Fire: CHD as an Inflammatory Disease

Like many injuries, the body's response to arterial damage involves inflammation. When an ankle is badly sprained and it subsequently becomes swollen and painful, that is inflammation in action. The heat, redness and swelling are a result of extra blood being channeled to the area, which brings with it immune cells that break down injured tissue. As these damaged cells are being removed, the body begins creating healthy new ones to take their place. If an injured ankle is given sufficient rest and exposed to an abundant supply of the nutrients it needs to repair itself, its owner will usually be back up and running around at full speed within a week or two.

As many stubborn athletes have found out the hard way, when one tries to 'work through' an injury it often becomes worse instead of better. The injured area never gets a chance to repair itself, but instead sustains greater damage with each passing day. Inflammation quickly transforms from a helpful short-term process into an escalating cascade of muscle and connective tissue damage. Serious injury eventually forces the driven athlete to stop and listen to their body. What should have been a minor interruption to one's training schedule becomes a major, and often career-ending, setback.

Now imagine the same scenario occurring inside your arteries. Because of poor nutrition, excessive stress, insufficient sound sleep, infectious disease, cigarette smoking, excessive alcohol consumption--or perhaps because of a combination of some or all of these factors--the structural integrity of your coronary arteries becomes compromised and a particularly susceptible portion becomes damaged. Your body will immediately begin to repair the wounded area, activating the inflammatory mechanisms of the immune system in the process(1).

If, like a stubborn athlete working though an injury, you continue the activity/s that initially caused this arterial damage, you can bet your last dollar that the inflammatory process will follow suit. Inflammatory proteins and enzymes and white blood cells of the immune system will accumulate at the site of injury, along with arterial muscle cells, blood platelets, collagen, calcium, and cholesterol. All of these agents become players in a self-perpetuating cycle of continued inflammation that, if not curtailed, leads to ever-worsening atherosclerotic build-up.

Sometimes a struggling cardiovascular system will send out warnings to its owner, perhaps in the form of angina pains, that something is not quite right under the surface. At other times, when the cardiovascular system has already sustained damage so severe that it simply cannot continue to function properly, it will let its owner know in no uncertain terms. For many CHD victims, the immense crushing chest pain that heralds the onset of a heart attack is the first-- and often last--warning that something is amiss.

The idea that atherosclerosis is an inflammatory 'repair-to-injury' process is not a controversial one. In fact, it enjoys almost unanimous acceptance among cardiovascular researchers. The major bone of contention among these scientists is what initiates damage to the arteries, what keeps the whole process going, and of course, what should be done to stop it.

Modern medicine searches frantically for the single magic bullet that will 'cure' heart disease, but all the available evidence indicates that CHD is a multi-faceted disease influenced by a wide variety of factors. The following chapters present evidence showing that CHD is largely a disease arising from, and aggravated by, nutritional deficiencies and imbalances, infectious agents, and modifiable lifestyle factors such as physical inactivity and chronic stress. To myopically focus on only one or two of these factors while neglecting the rest will yield sub-optimal results at best, and prove totally ineffective at worst.

In the next chapter we will begin our CHD-fighting mission by learning about one of the greatest--yet most underrated--enemies of cardiovascular health known to mankind.

134

Chapter 14

"We are, perhaps uniquely among the earth's creatures, the worrying animal.
We worry away our lives, fearing the future, discontent with the present, unable
to take in the idea of dying, unable to sit still."
Lewis Thomas.

Don't Stress!

Your heart will be forever thankful.

CHD prevention campaigns have long centered around dietary factors. Every day, all over the world, researchers, health authorities, politicians, health writers, doctors, nutritionists and internet forum participants heatedly debate the cardiovascular merits of animal fats, fish, red meat, milk, vegetable oils, *trans* fatty acids, sugar, whole-grains, soy foods, low- versus high-carbohydrate diets, vitamin supplements--the list goes on and on. While mind-boggling sums of money, scientific manpower and media exposure have been devoted to the link between diet and CHD, a woefully inadequate amount of attention has been awarded to what is easily one of the greatest CHD instigators of all--psychological stress.

Stress and CHD

Exponents of the diet-heart theory frequently cite the increase in CHD that often awaits those who migrate from less developed regions of the world to modernized countries like America. Almost unanimously, these exponents point to the so-called 'fatty' Western diet as the cause. But is it really? Could it be that the increase in CHD that commonly afflicts migrant populations often has little to do with diet and everything to do with the act of migrating itself? If you think this sounds far-fetched, please read on. The connection between migration and increased CHD provides valuable clues about the causation of heart disease that can benefit all of us--even if we've never ventured more than a hundred miles from home!

Stress and the Japanese

In Chapter 3, we discussed the work of Dr. Michael Marmot, a British researcher who examined the incidence of CHD among Japanese men who migrated to America. Marmot noted that, overall, Japanese-Americans had a much higher rate of CHD than men who remained in Japan. Marmot also observed that the increased risk was totally unrelated to blood cholesterol levels(1). What he instead found was that those men who retained their traditional cultural practices continued to enjoy the same low rate of CHD as

135

their compatriots back home. Those men who abandoned traditional Japanese cultural practices, on the other hand, suffered a dramatic increase in CHD risk(2).

Traditional Japanese culture places great emphasis on family and community cohesion. Marmot believed that Japanese-American men who abided by these traditional social customs were protected from the detrimental cardiovascular effects of stress. In contrast, those who embraced Western culture, with its emphasis on competition and material acquisition, were afforded no such protection.

Italian-Americans, Stress and CHD

In 1962, researchers began paying close attention to the people of Roseto, a picturesque town located in the northeastern corner of Northampton County, Pennsylvania. Roseto was founded by Italian stoneworkers who had begun migrating to the area in the 1880's. Up until the mid-sixties, the residents of this town were a tight-knit community who lived almost as if they were still back in Italy, retaining a strong emphasis on family and community relationships. Roseto's loyalty to traditional Italian customs was accompanied by a very low rate of CHD, one that could not be explained by traditional risk factors. In the nearby town of Bangor, the death rate from heart attack was twice that of Roseto, despite similar smoking and dietary habits.

Beginning around 1965, the winds of change started to blow through Roseto. The social structure became less and less orientated towards family and community cohesion and instead began to revolve around individual goals and more materialistic values. During this period of stark social change, the prevalence of and mortality from CHD increased sharply, eventually matching the rate seen in nearby Bangor(3). Again, the rise in CHD could not be explained by a change in the classic risk factors, such as cholesterol, smoking, hypertension, diabetes, or obesity.

Psychological Upheaval and its Impact on Health

Two-and-a-half-thousand years ago, the Greek physician Hippocrates wrote that *"those things which one has been accustomed to for a long time, although worse than things to which one is not accustomed, usually give less disturbance"*. The 'Father of Medicine' knew that life events resulting in major psychological upheaval could have a very real and harmful impact on physical health.

It goes without saying that migrating to a new country involves major upheaval. The monumental migration that characterized the twentieth century arose not because people got bored and casually decided they could benefit from a change of scenery; it occurred because people sought to escape poverty, war, and even persecution. Leaving one's homeland often meant saying goodbye to family members and lifelong friends, with no guarantee they would ever be seen again.

Few of us who have grown up in our country of birth could even begin to imagine what it must have felt like to arrive in a new land equipped with little more than a suitcase and the clothes we were wearing; to be faced with the daunting task of establishing a whole new life in a completely unfamiliar environment; to be confronted with the urgent need to find work in a country where we could hardly speak the language, of obtaining accommodation, dealing with racism, and establishing a new social network--all at once! To say that migration would have been a stressful endeavor for many of its participants would be one of the great understatements of all time.

Migrants who formed closely-knit social networks with those who migrated from the same country or region would have been able to obtain solace, support and camaraderie from people who truly understood what they were going through. Such social solidarity would have gone a long way towards cushioning the difficulties and uncertainties inherent in forging a new life in a strange land. By reducing feelings of fear, uncertainty, helplessness and social isolation, it would have protected their cardiovascular systems against the destructive effects of stress.

Migrants are hardly the only people who experience chronic stress. Anyone who faces uncertainty about their future, relationship difficulties, financial problems, substance abuse, family rifts, difficulties at work or school, bereavement, social isolation, or chronic health problems is susceptible to the effects of stress. Almost all of us are likely to experience at least one of these adversities at various points throughout our lifetimes, which means a good deal of us are potential candidates for stress-induced illnesses--including CHD.

How Stress Can Break Your Heart

When we become acutely stressed, our internal environments undergo a striking transformation; our bodies, in effect, go into red alert. Blood is diverted away from organs and tissues participating in 'non-essential' activities--such as digestion, immune function, growth and repair--and re-routed towards those involved in dealing with imminent danger, such as the muscles and heart. Our reflexes sharpen, our muscles tighten, and our hearts start beating faster in anticipation of intense physical effort. This is the famous 'fight-or-flight' response, which is triggered when the body releases substances known as *catecholamines*. The two most abundant catecholamines released during stressful times are *norepinephrine and epinephrine* (adrenaline). Stressful situations also cause the body to secrete abundant amounts of the catabolic hormone *cortisol*.

Norepinephrine and epinephrine exert pronounced effects on the cardiovascular system: they increase heart rate and dilate blood vessels in muscles, allowing for increased blood flow to support muscular effort. High levels of catecholamines also increase blood viscosity and encourage blood clotting, a development that serves to minimize blood loss from any injury that may occur while frantically fighting or fleeing danger. Meanwhile, cortisol raises our blood sugar levels, ensuring a ready supply of fuel for the brain. In order to achieve these elevated blood sugar levels, cortisol overrides the action of insulin. In other words, during brief periods of stress we become temporarily insulin resistant.

In an emergency situation, these are all highly beneficial changes that effectively prepare us to do battle with imminent threats, or to run like crazy in order to save our very lives. It is when the sympathetic nervous system--which is responsible for kick-starting the fight-or-flight response--becomes activated on a regular basis that stress itself becomes a life-threatening danger.

The right amount of catecholamines and cortisol, released at the right time, is essential to good health. In contrast, excessive catecholamine levels released at inappropriate times are anathema to good health. When an unhappy marriage, unfulfilling job, or financial difficulties cause us to become chronically stressed on a long-term basis, our bodies enter a state where they become increasingly susceptible to elevated blood sugar levels (see next chapter) immune dysfunction, arterial constriction and spasm, and blood-clotting.

Work and Stress

Relatively few of us will ever experience the hardship of migrating to another country. However, the majority of us will spend a significant portion of our lives participating in another common source of stress--work. As the majority of the adult population spends the greatest part of its waking hours engaged in the process of making a living, the potential for work-derived stress to negatively impact upon public health is huge.

Stereotypical images of highly-stressed and heart attack-prone executives notwithstanding, researchers have found that it is those at the bottom of the corporate ladder who in fact suffer the highest incidence of work stress and heart disease.

In 1978, Professor Marmot published the first of many papers reporting on the Whitehall studies, possibly the largest long-term investigations of health within an organization ever conducted. Marmot and his team initially followed over

17,000 British civil servants for seven-and-a-half years, observing a stepwise increase in CHD incidence from the highest to the lowest grades of employment. Men in the lowest grade, who were employed as messengers, had 3.6 times the CHD mortality of men in the highest employment grade (administrators)(4).

In the subsequent Whitehall II study, which examined a much broader array of mental and physical health correlates, the researchers found that civil servants with the highest work demands and the lowest decision latitude suffered the highest incidence of CHD(5). Those with low job control had nearly double the risk of being diagnosed with CHD than those enjoying high job control(6). Numerous other groups have since confirmed the Whitehall findings(7-10).

Closely related to the issue of low job control is what researchers call 'effort-reward imbalance'--that is, expending high effort and reaping relatively little reward. The feeling that one is working hard, or long, or both, but getting nowhere, or that's one's future career prospects give little cause for optimism, is an all-too-common cause of anguish. So too is the perception that one's work efforts are not being justly rewarded. A recent literature review found that effort-reward imbalance at work was associated with increases in CHD risk that ranged from 1.5-fold to a whopping 6.1-fold!(11)

The same review also found that job strain was associated with up to five-fold increases in CHD risk. The wave of corporate downsizing that gained increasing momentum during the late nineties has left more and more individuals working ever-longer hours, struggling to keep up with workloads that were previously tackled by two, three, and sometimes more, people. The majority of studies that have examined health outcomes in survivors of downsized workplaces have reported significant increases in health problems and medically certified sickness leave(12).

The most recent of these, a 7.5-year follow-up study of over 22,000 municipal employees in Finland, found that cardiovascular mortality was twice as high among employees who had survived major workplace downsizing compared to those who had experienced no downsizing. The increased risk was most marked during the first four years after downsizing, during which time survivors of trimmed-down workforces were more than five times as likely to succumb to a fatal cardiovascular event!(13)

A twenty-five-year follow-up of Finnish metal industry workers--all initially free of cardiovascular disease--found that those with high job strain, manifested by high demands at work and low job control, had a 2.2-fold cardiovascular mortality risk compared to colleagues with low job strain. Employees with effort-reward imbalance (reflected by low salary, lack of social approval and few career opportunities relative to efforts required at work) suffered a 250 percent increased risk of cardiovascular death(14).

All Work and No Play...

A 2001 survey found that, on average, employed American adults work forty-six hours per week, with around forty percent now working fifty or more hours per week. The survey also found that an increasing number of Americans are working longer hours than five years previously; they are also spending less time participating in organized social activities, having sex, enjoying leisure activities, or sleeping(15,16). This is a worrying trend, because research shows that increasing one's workload at the expense of exercise, sleep, and other restorative activities bodes poorly for future health.

In the early nineties, Japanese researchers found that men who worked eleven hours a day had 2.5 times the risk of suffering a heart attack than those who worked seven to nine hours per day. A similar increase in heart attack risk was seen in those who had extended their daily work time by three or more hours in the recent past(17). A more recent study found that men who worked over sixty hours per week were twice as likely to have suffered a heart attack than those working forty or less hours per week. Longer working hours were related to fewer days off, shorter hours of sleep, and more days per week with less than five hours of sleep(18). Numerous other studies confirm that prolonged working time is associated with an increased risk of heart attack(19-22).

More than Just a Statistical Association

When presented with epidemiological studies linking stress to CHD, are we looking at a causal or merely secondary association?

Abundant experimental evidence indicates that we are observing a direct association. When psychological stress is induced in volunteers through such activities as frustrating tasks, recalling angry experiences, or public speaking, researchers have observed the following(23-27):

- Dilation (widening) of healthy arteries, but constriction of atherosclerotic arteries;
- Arterial spasm, leading to reduced blood flow to the heart;
- Increased blood platelet aggregation;
- Increased production of fibrinogen, a protein that assists in the formation of blood clots;
- Abnormalities in ventricular function;
- A reduced ability of the heart to refill with blood (researchers have observed reductions of around fifty percent!);

- Reduced cardiac output;
- ECG changes indicating ischemia (oxygen deprivation of the heart) at lower blood pressure and heart rates than that seen with exercise-induced ischemia!

In support of these results, numerous investigators have found that individuals with low job control, high job strain and more pronounced effort/reward imbalance tend to have higher levels of fibrinogen, higher blood pressure readings, and a greater predisposition to heartbeat irregularities(28-32).

Marriage and Stress

Despite being the butt of many jokes, across-the-board research findings show that, overall, marriage is associated with better health. In contrast to their married counterparts, unmarried women have fifty percent higher mortality and unmarried men have a 250 percent higher death rate(33). Unmarried people are also far less likely to report being happy with life than married people.

These findings apply only to those in stable marriages; unmarried people are happier, on average, than those in troubled marriages(34). Those who remain in stable marriages enjoy greater overall longevity than both those who have never been married and those who have experienced divorce(34,35).

The scientific literature is replete with studies linking marital discord to a wide range of health disorders, most notably heart disease(36,37). In the massive MRFIT trial, in which 10,904 of the participating men were married at baseline, a nine-year follow-up revealed that those who subsequently divorced suffered an increased risk of cardiovascular and overall mortality(38).

As part of the Stockholm Female Coronary Risk Study, researchers examined and interviewed hundreds of Swedish women aged thirty to sixty-five who had been hospitalized for heart attack, then monitored them over the next five years. Among the 187 women who were married or cohabiting with a male partner, marital stress was associated with a three-fold increased risk of a recurring coronary event--even after adjustment for such factors as age, estrogen status, education, smoking, diabetes, blood pressure, blood triglycerides and left ventricular dysfunction(39).

In the Healthy Women Study, the marital status and quality of 393 premenopausal women was assessed, along with a number of cardiovascular risk factors. More than a decade later, the investigators assessed the extent of atherosclerosis in the women's arteries using a technique known as electron beam computed tomography. They found that women in satisfying marriages had the least atherosclerosis in the carotid arteries and aorta, and less rapid progression of carotid atherosclerosis when compared to those trapped in the least-satisfying marriages. Women who did not have a partner had intermediate levels of atherosclerosis(40).

Experimental findings show that marital conflicts can instigate a variety of harmful biochemical changes within the body. When researchers from Johns Hopkins University asked couples to discuss a topic on which they heatedly disagreed for ten minutes, blood pressure increases were observed in both sexes(41).

In another revealing series of experiments, both newlywed and older couples were studied whilst staying in a hospital research unit. Subjects who displayed more negative or hostile behaviors during a thirty minute discussion of marital problems showed larger and more sustained increases in blood pressure, epinephrine, norepinephrine and adrenocorticotropic hormone (which stimulates the release of cortisol) and greater declines in immune function compared to less negative subjects(42,43).

When researchers conducted similar experiments but encouraged husbands and wives to try and actively influence their partners' opinions during the discussions or to simply disagree, some rather interesting findings emerged. Among husbands attempting to influence their wives' opinions, those exhibiting hostile behavior experienced marked rises in blood pressure. Such blood pressure increases were not seen among husbands who merely disagreed with their wives. Hostile husbands also displayed an increase in heart rate, regardless of whether they were simply disagreeing or actively trying to change their wives' minds(44,45). Marital discord does not just drain one's spirit, but directly assaults the cardiovascular system itself.

Depression and Heart Disease

Scientific evidence for a link between depression and heart disease dates back at least to the 1930's, when published studies first reported a higher incidence of heart disease deaths among depressed psychiatric patients(46,47). Since these early seminal reports, a vast and remarkably consistent body of evidence has accumulated showing that depression, be it mild or severe, significantly increases the risk of cardiovascular mortality(48).

Researchers from the University of Cincinnati recently published a thorough, methodical review of published prospective studies in which individuals initially free of heart disease were followed for periods ranging from four to forty years. Some of the studies detected up to 3.5-fold increased risks of developing coronary heart disease for individuals suffering depressive symptoms. When the results of all these studies were pooled together, the researchers found that subjects with symptoms of depression were two-thirds more likely to develop CHD(49).

Another recent pooled analysis, incorporating data from 35,0000 study participants, found a fifty percent increased risk of fatal or non-fatal heart attacks in those who had depressed mood. Among those who suffered from more severe depression, the likelihood of heart attack was increased 2.7-fold(50). To help put these figures into perspective, a similar analysis by the Surgeon General found that smoking a pack a day or more conferred a 2.5-fold risk of developing CHD(47). In other words, major depression is every bit as bad for your heart as regular cigarette smoking, a habit that the Surgeon General in 1983 described as "... *the most important of the known modifiable risk factors for coronary heart disease in the United States."*(51)

As for stroke, studies conducted so far have established a 1.7- to 2.6-fold risk for folks with a history of depression, after adjusting for such predisposing factors as age, blood pressure, smoking, and heart disease(52,53).

In addition to predicting heart disease among healthy subjects, depression also increases the risk of mortality among those with existing CHD. One study found that the risk of death during the first six months after a heart attack was almost six times higher in depressed than non-depressed patients(54). Compounding the problem is the fact that depression is very common in CHD patients--around twenty to forty-five percent of post-heart attack patients exhibit symptoms of depression(55).

Lighten Up!

While Hollywood and MTV continue to glorify the hotheaded 'bad boy' stereotype, a large volume of research shows that a hostile and impatient manner effectively primes one for increased sickness and an early death. Controlled experiments show that hostile individuals respond to provocation, conflict and disagreement with larger increases in blood pressure and heart rate than more agreeable folks(56-58). It is perhaps not so surprising then, that:

- A study of almost 13,000 middle-aged men and women followed for up to six years found that, among people with normal blood pressure, a strong, angry temperament (defined as a tendency toward quick, minimally provoked, or unprovoked anger) was associated with a 128 percent increase in the risk of fatal and non-fatal heart attack(59).
- In the sixteen years following the conclusion of the MRFIT trial, participants who were rated as highly hostile were far more likely to die of cardiovascular causes than men with low hostility scores; the most hostile men had a 240 percent greater risk of cardiovascular death than those exhibiting the least hostility. High-hostile men who had a non-fatal event during the trial were especially susceptible to cardiovascular death after the trial; with a greater than eight-fold risk increase for those in the highest category of hostility!(60)

- A nine-year follow-up of nearly 3,000 men from South Wales found that suppressed anger resulted in a seventy percent increase in heart attack risk(61).

Losing a Loved One

Bereavement is something that virtually all of us will encounter at some point in our lives. Those who have lost a loved one will need little reminder of just how devastating this experience can be. When someone you have known for decades is suddenly gone, the subsequent emotional shellshock can readily bring forth feelings of intense sadness, despair, anger, and guilt. A significant volume of research shows that how well we cope with the loss of loved ones can have a sizable impact on our own future survival prospects.

Numerous studies have examined the impact of losing a spouse on subsequent mortality in the widowed. With few exceptions, these studies have found that after the death of a partner, mortality among surviving spouses increases in comparison to those who remain married. This excess mortality risk is most pronounced in the first six months of bereavement, after which time it returns to baseline levels--usually within the following six months. While suicide, accidents, and homicide deaths are far more common among the recently widowed, the bulk of their early excess mortality is due to coronary events(62).

Cholesterol and Stress

In Chapter 2, we learnt how the association between elevated cholesterol and CHD mortality begins to dissipate from age fifty onwards. Thus, the entire anti-cholesterol charade has been built upon epidemiological associations detected in individuals under this age, who comprise only a tiny percentage of all CHD victims.

Orthodoxy has never provided a feasible explanation as to why high cholesterol should be a risk factor for CHD in younger folks, but not in seniors. Are we really supposed to believe that cholesterol is a highly dangerous cardiovascular toxin for younger folks, but suddenly becomes harmless after the fifth decade of life? Such a claim is nothing short of a physiological absurdity.

There exists a far more realistic proposition, and I'll try and lay it out as simply as possible:

1. Work is a major source of psychological stress;
2. Psychological stress raises cholesterol (as demonstrated in numerous controlled experiments(63-65));
3. Most people retire from work during the fifth and sixth decades of life;

4. Cholesterol elevations therefore accompany stress-related coronary disease in younger patients, but lose their statistical association with CHD as people retire and leave the stress of the workforce behind them.

When researchers present us with data showing an epidemiological relationship between cholesterol and heart disease in younger folks, what we may really be looking at is the destructive effect of work stress. For the last forty-plus years, medicine has been blaming cholesterol for crimes that were in all likelihood committed by chronic psychological stressors!

Stress and Food: A Deadly Mix?

One cardiovascular researcher who has distanced himself from the great unthinking mass of cholesterol-obsessed investigators is Dr. Malcolm Kendrick, from Cheshire in the UK. In 2002, Kendrick published a paper in the innovative journal *Medical Hypotheses* that placed the CHD spotlight on the critical postprandial period(66). For those wondering what on earth a 'postprandial period' is, it's those several hours following a meal in which blood levels of various nutrients and hormones are elevated.

Among these elevated nutrients and hormones are blood glucose and insulin. As Chapter 18 will further elucidate, elevated blood glucose is a major contributor to cardiovascular morbidity and mortality. Elevated insulin has also been implicated as a direct antagonist of cardiovascular health.

Both blood glucose and insulin are elevated after a meal, due to the digestion of food and the subsequent transport of glucose and amino acids into the bloodstream. If there are factors present which significantly amplify this post-meal rise in blood glucose and insulin, then the postprandial period may present a critical phase in the development of CHD.

Kendrick is by no means the first cardiovascular researcher to focus on the postprandial period, but he is the first to hypothesize the potentially atherogenic connection between the post-meal period and psychological stress. According to Kendrick, the presence of psychological stress in the postprandial period--a phenomenon that can significantly amplify the usual post-meal rise insulin and blood glucose--may dramatically accelerate the progression of heart disease. This widely overlooked phenomenon may even help explain the famous 'French Paradox'!

The Beginning Of The End: Declining Blood Sugar Control

Eating too many calories and/or carbohydrates, and engaging in too little physical activity promotes high blood glucose levels, which must be brought back into the normal range via the actions of insulin. One important mechanism by which insulin helps clear glucose from the blood stream is to shuttle it into the muscles where it is stored as glycogen.

If elevated spikes in blood glucose occur on a regular basis, then the muscle cells eventually become desensitized to the effects of insulin. Instead of welcoming in glucose from the bloodstream, the insulin receptors on the outer membranes of the muscle cell begin to increasingly ignore insulin's signals. The muscle cells, in effect, have become *insulin resistant.*

The body initially attempts to overcome this lack of response by getting the pancreas to secrete even more insulin. The pancreas, however, eventually becomes burnt out from the task of continually producing and releasing large amounts of insulin. As insulin secretion from the tiring pancreas begins to wane, blood sugar levels continue to rise. If this scenario progresses far enough, we will develop Type 2 diabetes and require oral medication or even insulin injections to keep our blood sugar levels under control.

Stress and Blood Sugar

A further cause of insulin resistance, as discussed earlier, is psychological stress. In controlled experiments, infusion of stress hormones produces an immediate but temporary insulin resistant state in healthy human subjects(67,68). If excessive catecholamine and cortisol levels occur during the post-meal period as a result of psychosocial stresses, then even greater rises in blood glucose and insulin release can be expected.

Hyperinsulinemia

We now know that elevated blood glucose is a potent enemy of cardiovascular health, but a high output of insulin brings its own can of worms. Hyperinsulinemia may cause impaired arterial function, increased free radical production, inhibition of blood clot breakdown, and the proliferation of arterial muscle cells--all integral features of atherosclerotic plaque build-up(69,70). When combined with the ability of high blood sugar to increase glycation, free radical activity, arterial dysfunction and blood clotting, these effects of hyperinsulinemia may provide a highly destructive double-whammy to cardiac health.

The Pima Paradox

The Pima Indians of North America are well known for their extreme susceptibility to insulin resistance and Type 2 diabetes, with up to seventy percent of the male population suffering from the latter! Given that the Pima population suffers one of the highest rates of insulin resistance and diabetes in the world, one would also expect them to exhibit frighteningly high rates of cardiovascular mortality.

Whilst Pima Indians with diabetes do indeed suffer 2-3 times the rate of diabetes as non-diabetic Pima Indians, they still suffer less than half the CHD rate of that seen in typical Caucasian populations!(71,72)

Remember that stress, along with diet and physical inactivity, is an important promoter of insulin resistance and type 2 diabetes. The body's hypothalamic-pituitary-adrenal axis (HPA axis) is a major part of the neuroendocrine system that controls reactions to stress. Chronic stress can damage the HPA axis, leading to abnormal patterns of cortisol and catecholamine release.

Insulin resistant Pima Indians, however, show little evidence of central or sympathetic nervous abnormality(73). This suggests that the influence of diabetes and insulin resistance on the development of CHD in this population is limited to dietary mechanisms; modern Western populations in contrast, not only consume excessive calories/carbohydrates but also experience high levels of recurrent psychosocial stress. The absence of such stress patterns in the diabetic Pima population may explain why they still enjoy relatively low rates of CHD.

The French Paradox

Kendrick also cites the example of the French, who enjoy one of the lowest national CHD rates in the world. As Kendrick points out, the French have a similar rate of diabetes and obesity, and obtain a similar amount of exercise as the British. The Brits and French also share similar rates of smoking, obtain a similar percentage of calories from animal fats and fruits/vegetables, and possess similar average body mass index, cholesterol and blood pressure readings. In addition, the French have one of the highest rates of anti-depressant use in Europe, so a lack of stress cannot account for the low rate of CHD(74). Then again, maybe it can: that is, if there is a lack of stress in the critical postprandial period among this population.

What's Your Hurry?

Anyone who has spent time in Southern Europe will have observed how meals tend to be consumed in a much more relaxed manner than in most other Western nations. Whilst Southern Europeans traditionally take a three hour break in the middle of the day, workers in countries like the U.S. barely have time to let their lunch settle before having to head back to the office or factory floor.

Could the convivial mealtime approach of the French and their Mediterranean neighbors help explain why they enjoy rates of CHD lower than those seen in other modernized countries, where alarm clocks abruptly cut short the natural sleep cycle, where highly-refined, high-carbohydrate breakfasts are followed by a mad rush to arrive at work on time, where lunch is often eaten consumed whilst hunched over an office desk, and where dinner is often gulped down in a hurry so that the kids can be taken to rehearsals/sports/scouts/etc?

The Australian Migrant Paradox

I remember from a young age that, despite being extremely hard-working individuals, my Italian grandparents never rushed a meal. Lunches and dinners at my grandparents' house were unhurried, jovial events that seemed to last forever. Perhaps the retention of mealtime behavior akin to that of my grandparents explains why Greek and Italian migrants to Australia enjoy significantly lower rates of CHD than their Australian-born counterparts, despite having a far higher susceptibility to diabetes and overweight(75-78). In the families of their Italian-Australian/Greek-Australian offspring, where a faster-paced lifestyle with more emphasis on material achievement is commonplace, heart disease has occurred with increasing frequency and at a younger age.

Mom Was Right--Don't Gulp Down Your Food!

If necessary, unhook the phone while you eat and turn off the TV news if the nightly parade of corruption and injustice consistently presses your hot buttons. Eat in an unhurried manner, chew your food thoroughly, and savor its taste and aroma. Eating is unquestionably one of life's greatest pleasures, so why rush it? After your meal is finished, don't jump up from the table and plunge yourself back into the day's activities; instead, make it a regular habit to sit contentedly in a relaxed, quiet environment for at least thirty minutes after eating.

Don't forget the benefits of carbohydrate-controlled nutrition--consuming low to moderate carbohydrate meals comprised primarily of low or 'No' glycemic index foods (see Chapter 16) will go a long way towards limiting the extent of postprandial blood glucose elevations.

If you can regularly avail yourself of upbeat, jovial company or some funny movies/shows/literature, so much the better--a study with type 2 diabetics showed that the postprandial rise in blood glucose was significantly lower on a day in which the subjects attended a comedy show, as compared to a day in which they attended a monotonous lecture(79).

Another Piece of the CHD Puzzle Falls Into Place?

Kendrick may have stumbled across a major piece of the CHD puzzle. A number of studies have shown that measurement of post load glucose, which more closely resembles the postprandial state, is a stronger predictor of CVD than fasting glucose in both non-diabetic and diabetic patients(80-82). Avoiding stress during and after a meal may help alleviate post-meal insulin resistance, and the resultant exaggerated blood levels of glucose and insulin. This in turn, may reduce the formation of atherosclerotic plaque and blood clots during the post-meal period; a period which occurs for most people at least three times each and every day.

Don't Underestimate Stress

Every year, countless lives are lost due to CHD that is induced and aggravated by chronic psychological stress. Authorities have traditionally underestimated the true impact of psychosocial factors like stress, preferring instead to focus on simplistic and often useless health measures, such as lowering cholesterol and minimizing saturated fat intake. A recent National Institutes of Health editorial acknowledged that: *"To date, psychosocial factors have not been the target of sustained public health efforts for the reduction of CVD risk in either primary or secondary prevention strategies."*(83)

Strategies for reducing stress are so important that I have devoted an entire chapter to them in Section Three. In the meantime, let's find out just what is wrong with the modern diet, and why it dramatically increases the risk of CHD.

Chapter 15

"Food is an important part of a balanced diet."
Fran Lebowitz

It's the Food, Stupid!

Real health requires real food.

Human beings, like virtually every other species on the planet, rely on the food they eat to deliver the nutrients needed for optimal health. We need food, not only for calories to meet our energy requirements, but also for the hundreds of *vitamins, minerals, trace elements, amino acids* and *fatty acids* necessary for growth, repair and resistance to disease. When our bodies receive inadequate amounts of these *micronutrients*, then our organs and tissues can malfunction and we become increasingly susceptible to disease and premature death.

If health authorities are serious about discovering the true role of diet in CHD, then they desperately need to rid themselves of their current anti-cholesterol, anti-saturated fat obsession and instead become acquainted with the fundamental influence exerted by dietary-derived micronutrients upon coronary health. They must begin acknowledging that the modern Western diet delivers woefully inadequate amounts of many nutrients, and far too many of certain others. This distorted pattern of intake is a direct consequence of humankind's shift from its natural diet of fresh meats, vegetables, fruits and nuts, to the current modern diet which is dominated by cereal grain products and heavily processed and refined foods.

Micronutrients and Heart Health

The interaction between food-derived micronutrients and the cardiovascular system is extensive and complex. Below are just a few examples of how the mighty micronutrients exert a profound effect upon our cardiovascular health:

- *Vitamin C, copper,* and key amino acids such as *proline* and *lysine* are needed for healthy formation of collagen, the 'mortar' which quite literally holds our arteries together;
- The amino acid *arginine* is necessary for the production of nitric oxide, a substance that allows our arteries to expand and contract properly;
- *L-carnitine, co-enzyme Q10, taurine,* and *magnesium* all play key roles in energy production and muscular contraction, and are therefore absolutely essential for healthy cardiac function;

- *Omega-3 fatty acids* help prevent inflammation, the formation of blood clots and the occurrence of potentially fatal irregularities in heartbeat;
- *Selenium* and *vitamins A, C* and *E* directly act as antioxidants, preventing free radical-induced damage to the heart and arteries.

A deficiency in even one of these heart-healthy nutrients poses a direct threat to our cardiovascular health. Given that the modern Western diet is deficient in many of the above nutrients, it shouldn't take a rocket scientist to work out why Western nations are plagued by epidemic levels of heart disease and stroke…

Designer Foods Versus the Foods We Were Designed to Eat

When all is said and done, the ultimate diet for any animal--human or otherwise--is the one they were designed by nature to eat. Any competent veterinarian could readily tell you this, but most 'human veterinarians' (doctors) and the authorities they look up to for guidance appear to be totally blind to this simple fact.

For almost their entire 2.4 million-year history, humans lived as hunter-gatherers, subsisting on freshly killed meats and plant foods that could be eaten either raw or with a minimum of preparation, such as wild vegetables, fruits, berries, and nuts(1). Around 10,000 years ago, human history changed irrevocably with the dawn of the Agricultural Revolution(2). The exact reason for humankind's switch to agriculture is still a source of much debate, but a combination of accelerating population growth and diminishing wild game availability due to climatic changes and prolific hunting appears to be the most likely cause(3).

With the adoption of farming, the human diet underwent a massive and fundamental change in a relatively brief space of time, from a high-protein regimen based on meats and wild vegetation to a high-carbohydrate pattern based on cereal grains--a food source that was essentially alien to the human digestive tract (unlike the meats and wild plants that humans evolved on, cereal grains are virtually inedible in their raw state(4-6)). It is no coincidence that the emergence of pottery, which would have allowed humans to soak and cook grains and thus make them edible in significant quantity, occurred around the same time as the onset of agriculture(7).

If cereal grains were a far healthier food than meat, as health authorities and dietitians repeatedly tell us, then the shift from a meat-based diet to a grain-based diet during the onset of the Agricultural Revolution should have been accompanied by a significant improvement in health and longevity. The archeological record shows just the opposite; societies that abandoned the meat-based hunter-gatherer diet and adopted cereal grains as their new staple experienced a characteristic reduction in stature, a decrease in life span, an increase in infant mortality, an increased incidence of infectious diseases, an increased prevalence of iron deficiency anemia, an increased incidence of bone disorders, and a jump in the number of dental caries and tooth enamel defects. Rather than constitute a boon to health, the shift from a hunter-gatherer diet to a grain-based diet was accompanied by an overall decline in the quantity and quality of life(8).

The Industrial Revolution

After the dawn of agriculture, some ten millennia would pass before the human diet would again undergo such dramatic and fundamental changes. Eventually, the first in a series of high-impact shocks to human health occurred around 150 years ago with the onset of the Industrial Revolution, where newly emerging technologies allowed for the wide-scale production of sugar, refined flours and refined vegetable fats. This was followed by the twentieth century's rabid proliferation of highly processed, colorfully packaged, calorie-rich but nutrient-poor 'convenience' foods. During the latter half of the last century, the consumption of these nutrient-depleted man-made foods underwent exponential growth after health authorities launched the 'Cholesterol Revolution'. Healthy animal foods such as meats and eggs became the subject of fanatical denunciation due to their 'harmful' saturated fat content, while authority-endorsed low-fat and cholesterol-free junk foods flooded the market. The consumption of these pseudo-health foods, along with increasing physical inactivity, not only prevented the decline in CHD incidence that should have resulted from the widespread reduction in smoking--it also produced the greatest number of obese and diabetic individuals that the world has ever seen.

Modern Diets, Modern Diseases

As a result of the Agricultural, Industrial, and Cholesterol Revolutions, we humans now derive the bulk of our calories from foods that were alien to the human digestive tract for 99.7 percent of its evolutionary history. Incredibly, Americans now obtain over three-quarters of their calories from staples that were non-existent during the Paleolithic, including cereal grains (twenty-two percent of calories), potatoes (three percent), sugar and other sweeteners (eighteen percent), vegetable oils (seventeen percent), dairy products (eleven percent), and alcoholic beverages (four percent). While nutrient-dense staples like meats, eggs, nuts, fruits, vegetables and seafood once furnished virtually all of our calories, they now provide a mere twenty percent of our daily energy intake!(9)

Hey, Who Took My Nutrients?

Health officials appear to have convinced themselves that the path to nutritional utopia involves swapping refined cereal grains for whole grains, and are now hell-bent on convincing us of the same. An objective analysis of the facts shows that they are sadly misguided.

Cereal grains--whole or refined--are nutritional weaklings. They contain no vitamin C, no vitamin D, no B12, no vitamin A and (with the sole of exception of yellow maize) no beta-carotene. While important nutrients like carnitine, creatine, carnosine, conjugated linoleic acid (CLA), vitamin B12, and the omega-3 fatty acids EPA and DHA can only be found in animal foods, there is not a single vitamin, mineral or trace element found in cereal grains that cannot be supplied either by animal products or non-cereal plant foods like vegetables, fruits and nuts.

Cereal grains and legumes also contain high concentrations of substances that researchers collectively classify as *anti-nutrients*. Among these are *inositol hexaphosphate,* more commonly known as *phytate*. This substance binds to minerals such as iron, calcium, magnesium, and zinc in the gastrointestinal tract, significantly reducing their absorption by the body(10-12). The last thing most people need is to impair the assimilation of such nutrients, all of which are essential for healthy cardiovascular function, and many of which are already woefully inadequate in the average American diet(13-15).

In cereal grains, anti-nutrient content is highest in the outer husk, which means that 'healthy' whole-grains actually have a far higher phytate content than refined grain products. Attempting to improve one's mineral status by eating more whole-grains is, at best, a 'two-steps-forward, two-steps-backward' proposition. While such a strategy does indeed increase the intake of zinc, iron, magnesium and calcium, it also promptly increases their excretion from the body! The end result is that overall mineral status improves only marginally, remains unchanged, or even worsens!(16-20)

A substance known as *pyridoxine glucoside*, which has been shown to reduce the availability of vitamin B6 by seventy-five to eighty percent, occurs widely in plant foods, including cereal grains(21). As a result, B6 from cereal grain products is absorbed with far less efficiency than that from animal foods(22). Researchers who fed young men different foods containing pyridoxine glucoside found that as dietary glucoside levels increased, the vitamin B6 status of the subjects decreased(23). Again, increased wheat fiber consumption merely worsens the situation; B6 from whole wheat bread is five to ten percent less available than that from white bread, and the addition of wheat bran to the diets of young men reduced the availability of B6 by seventeen percent(24,25).

Given the importance of vitamin B6 for efficient homocysteine metabolism (see Appendix E), and that low B6 and high homocysteine levels are associated with increased CHD risk, the cardiovascular implications of a diet high in cereal grains and low in meat are worrying. Following the edicts of health officials, who urge us to eat just such a diet (one needs to look no farther than the USDA's abominable food pyramid to see how deeply entrenched this line of thinking has become) will significantly worsen one's B6 status and increase one's risk of CHD. An analysis of menus specifically designed by dietitians to meet these anti-meat guidelines found that half of them failed to deliver the recommended dietary allowance for B6--an allowance that some researchers believe has been set too low(26,27).

Cereal grains not only contain no detectable vitamin D, but also actively encourage deficiency of this important vitamin by impairing its absorption. It has long been recognized that high cereal grain consumption induces vitamin D deficiency in various animal species, including primates, our closest animal relatives(28,29). By studying the fate of radiolabeled vitamin D, researchers observed significantly increased excretion of vitamin D in healthy human volunteers fed sixty grams of wheat fiber daily(30).

Vitamin D deficiency is surprisingly common among Americans, especially during the winter months. Professor Michael Hollick and his colleagues from the Boston University School of Medicine observed that a third of healthy Boston adults aged 18-29 were vitamin D deficient by the end of winter. The risk of deficiency rises in the elderly and among dark-skinned individuals; forty-two percent of African American women and eighty-four percent of black elderly folks throughout the U.S. were vitamin D deficient by the end of winter(31).

Poor vitamin D status has been linked to increased risk of breast, prostate and colon cancers, osteoporosis and other bone disorders, Type 1 diabetes, arthritis, infertility, PMS, chronic fatigue and depression, Seasonal Affective Disorder, multiple sclerosis, musculoskeletal pain, and heart disease(31-45). Ironically, the few foods that contain vitamin D are mostly items that have fallen out of favor thanks to orthodoxy's fanatical anti-fat and cholesterol campaign, such as cod liver oil, butter, whole milk, liver and egg yolks. Exposure to the most efficient vitamin D source of all--sunlight--has also decreased dramatically thanks to the efforts of health authorities who mistakenly believe avoiding the sun is the best way to prevent skin cancer.

The numerous nutritional shortcomings of whole-grains may help explain why the only randomized clinical trial to have ever examined the hypothesis that wheat fiber can reduce CHD actually found a small increase in coronary and overall mortality(46). Lowered antioxidant defenses may have been a possible contributor to this 'surprising' result: when type 2 diabetics consumed a low-wheat fiber diet and a high-wheat fiber diet containing bran-rich bread and breakfast cereal for three months each, LDL cholesterol oxidation was increased during the high-wheat fiber phase(47).

The Nutritional Magic of Meat

Let us now contrast the distinctly uninspiring nutritional profile of cereal grains with that of meat. Admonitions to restrict the consumption of animal flesh are issued beyond counting, despite the indisputable fact that it is *the most nutritious food known to humankind.*

Meat contains high quality protein, which is essential for growth and repair of the body's tissues and organs, including those of the cardiovascular system. In the Nurses Health Study, fourteen years' follow-up of over 80,000 initially healthy women revealed that higher protein intakes were associated with a lower risk of CHD(48).

Cereal grains have a very low protein content. One would need to consume seven to eight slices of wholemeal bread, or four to five cups of cooked brown rice, to equal the amount of protein contained in one three ounce serving of porterhouse steak. Furthermore, cereal protein is of very low quality. While animal products contain high levels of all the essential amino acids, cereal grains are deficient in the essential amino acid lysine. In fact, all protein-containing plant foods possess distinctly inferior amino acid profiles when compared to meat, eggs, and dairy products. Legumes, for example, are low in important sulfur-containing amino acids such as methionine, tryptophan, threonine and cysteine(49). Vegetarian proponents claim that this shortcoming of plant foods can be overcome by eating cereal grains together with legumes, as each will supposedly compensate for the amino acid deficiencies of the other. It sounds good in theory, but legumes also have a very low total protein content; four ounces of boiled lentils contains less than eight grams of protein, while the same amount of untrimmed porterhouse steak contains twenty-one grams. No matter how creative you get with your cereal/legume combinations, you will still be faced with the task of consuming copious amounts of these bulky, gas-forming foods in order to achieve an optimal protein intake. In addition to sending your intake of anti-nutrients through the roof, such a dietary pattern will likely exert some rather, uh, anti-social effects upon your intestinal canal. For those who still believe they can satisfy their protein requirements entirely from plant foods, good luck, but please, don't ever sit next to me on the bus…

Meat is the richest source of the all-important B-vitamins. This includes vitamin B12, which is found in small amounts in eggs and milk and whose bio-available form is non-existent in plant foods. Abstinence from meat is a major reason why vegetarians are far more likely to suffer from B12 deficiencies than omnivores(50).

Meat, especially chicken, pork and red meat, is the only appreciable source of *carnosine*(51). Emerging research suggests this novel amino acid may accelerate wound healing, boost the immune system, rid the body of toxic metals, and even help fight against cancer(52). Carnosine is a potent antioxidant and is shaping up as an especially effective agent against *glycation*, a harmful process that is accelerated by high blood sugar levels (see chapter 18). In laboratory studies, carnosine exhibits a far stronger ability to prevent glycative damage than the more widely studied anti-glycation compound, aminoguanidine(53).

The potent anti-glycation effects of carnosine may explain why a comparison of vegetarians, vegans and meat-eating omnivores revealed the latter to have significantly lower levels of nasty glycation end-products circulating in their bloodstreams. The difference could not be explained by total carbohydrate intake, blood sugar, age or kidney function, as all these variables were similar between the vegetarian and omnivorous groups(55).

Meat is also the only noteworthy source of *L-carnitine,* with lamb constituting the richest source of all. In Chapter 24, we will learn how heart attack patients receiving supplements of this remarkable amino acid had a significantly improved survival outlook compared to control subjects(54). Heart failure patients have also been shown to benefit from supplemental L-carnitine(56,57).

Meat, together with fish, is by far the best source of *creatine,* an amino acid used by the body to form adenosine tri-phosphate (ATP), the chemical source of energy that powers our cells. Over the last decade, creatine supplements have become extremely popular with strength athletes(58), but research has also shown creatine to improve exercise tolerance in patients suffering from congestive heart failure(59,60).

When healthy young men who normally consumed an omnivorous diet were switched to a lacto-ovo vegetarian diet for twenty-six days, significant decreases in muscle creatine content were observed(61). Another study showed that whilst higher peak blood levels of creatine could be achieved through supplementation, the same amount obtained via red meat consumption caused more prolonged and consistent blood levels(62).

Meat, along with certain species of fish and seafood, is a rich source of *taurine*, an important amino acid whose concentration in eggs, milk, and plant foods ranges from negligible to none(63,64). Taurine is found in high concentrations in the heart, brain and central nervous system, where it helps stabilize the cellular response to nervous stimulation. Taurine possesses antioxidant capabilities, and has been shown in double-blind clinical trials to improve cardiac function in patients with congestive heart failure(65-67). While taurine cannot be found in plant foods, herbivorous animals are able to synthesize it from other dietary amino acids. Humans are also able to manufacture their own taurine, but with far less efficiency than herbivorous animals, as evidenced by significantly lower blood taurine levels in vegans and among rural Mexican women reporting low meat intakes(68,69).

Fruits, Nuts, and Vegetables: The Plant Kingdom's True Nutrient Superstars!

Similar to meat, the nutritional quality of fruits, vegetables and nuts is far superior to that of cereal grains. Fruits and veggies provide such valuable nutrients as folic acid, vitamin C, and the various *carotenoids*, including *alpha-carotene, beta-carotene, lycopene, cryptoxanthin* and *lutein*. Nuts and seeds, meanwhile, are excellent sources of many otherwise hard-to-get nutrients; magnesium, for example, is found in abundance in Brazil nuts, almonds, sesame seeds, sunflower seeds, pumpkin seeds and cashews; the crucial mineral selenium is found in abundance in Brazil nuts; high concentrations of an important form of vitamin E known as *gamma-tocopherol* can be found in sesame seeds, pecans, walnuts, pistachios, pumpkin seeds, pine nuts, Brazils and cashews; gram for gram, the richest dietary source of the vital amino acid *arginine* is peanuts. While nuts and seeds truly are nutritional powerhouses, it must be mentioned that they also contain anti-nutrients such as phytates. In fact, on a per gram basis, the average phytate content of nuts and seeds is similar to that of grains and legumes. Of course, few people eat nuts and seeds in anywhere near the quantities that grains are typically consumed. Furthermore, soaking nuts and seeds for around six hours, and then roasting them, can significantly reduce their anti-nutrient content.

Scientists have also discovered a mind-boggling array of compounds in plant foods that they have collectively classified as *phytonutrients.* So far, tens of thousands of these phytonutrients have been identified, many possessing remarkable antioxidant and disease-fighting effects. In head-to-head comparisons, phytonutrient compounds known as *polyphenols* have been shown to possess many times the free-radical fighting power of more commonly known antioxidants such as vitamins C and E(70).

Another important group of phytonutrients are the *anthocyanins*, the compounds that impart color to fruits, vegetables and plants. Anthocyanins are considered a major contributor to the outstanding antioxidant activity often exhibited by red and blue plant foods(71). A recent study which compared the antioxidant power of various phytonutrient classes found anthocyanins to be the most potent of all(72).

In lab experiments, anthocyanins have been shown to exert potent artery-widening effects(73). When administered to hamsters, anthocyanins from bilberry significantly reduce inflammation and subsequent blood vessel injury in capillaries that have been deliberately exposed to free-radical promoting damage(74). When these anthcyanins are fed to diabetic rats, they maintain normal capillary function, while untreated rats experience the marked deterioration of capillaries characteristic of diabetes(75). Oxidation of blood lipids in rats fed anthocyanins is reduced dramatically compared to control rats not receiving anthocyanins(76). In humans, supplementation with chokeberry anthocyanins also produces marked reductions in oxidized LDL cholesterol levels(77,78).

When one considers the powerful and highly favorable anti-oxidant, anti-inflammatory and artery-dilating effects of anthocyanins, it is of little surprise that diets rich in berries have been associated with significantly reduced CVD and all-cause mortality(79). As well as protecting against cardiovascular disease, anthocyanins may also protect against DNA damage and cancer, peptic ulcers, cataracts, diabetic retinopathy, and allergic reactions(80-89).

Sadly Neglected

Needless to say, the potent antioxidant phytonutrients found in plants won't help you if you don't eat them. Sadly, consumption of fresh fruits and vegetables in America is pitifully low. A USDA food intake survey published in 1996 found that the average American consumed a miniscule eighteen grams of dark green and deep yellow vegetables per day--the equivalent of half of a small carrot!(90)

According to a 2004 AC Nielsen poll, more than eighty-five percent of consumers are not eating the federally recommended minimum of five servings of fruits and vegetables a day, with only twelve percent reporting daily consumption of five or more servings(91). Nearly half of those questioned ate just one or two servings of produce a day. To make matters worse, the produce most commonly eaten by Americans is not particularly high in antioxidants; iceberg lettuce, tomatoes, French fried potatoes, bananas and orange juice are the most commonly consumed fruits and vegetables, accounting for nearly thirty percent of all fruit and vegetables consumed(92).

Which are the most antioxidant-rich plant foods? Tables 15a and 15b display the antioxidant activity evident in various commonly eaten foods. The results in Table 15a were compiled as part of a joint effort by Norwegian and U.S. researchers, while those in 15b were derived by USDA researchers(93,94). Each group used different analytical methods, which helps explain why some of the antioxidant ratings vary markedly for the same foods between the two tables.

In Table 15a, the Neolithic-style food grouping of "cereals" and "pulses" features very few foods with an antioxidant content higher than 1mmol/100g. In fact, white flour from wheat and rice, the two most commonly eaten staples in the world, possess some of the poorest antioxidant values on the chart. In

Table 15b, cereal products fare a little better, while some of the pulses--namely navy, pinto and red kidney beans--actually show very high antioxidant values. It should be kept in mind that, for some reason, the values for pulses were determined per-gram of *dry* weight; humans, however, cannot safely eat navy, pinto or red kidney beans in their dry state. Cooking, which results in a wet weight two-three times greater than the dry weight of raw beans, would obviously dilute the per-gram antioxidant values figures significantly.

Irrespective of the differences evident in the two different charts, both indicate that the most antioxidant-rich plant foods in edible form are derived from the fruit, nut, and vegetable categories. Berries are especially well represented at the top end of the spectrum, providing more high-antioxidant items overall than any other group of plants. Pomegranates, plums, walnuts, sunflower seeds, pecans, hazelnuts, pistachios, ginger, dried fruits, and artichokes are some of the other foods that rated particularly high on the charts.

As you glance through Tables 15a and 15b, avoid the temptation of selecting a handful of antioxidant-rich foods from the charts, then consuming these items day in and day out in the hope of obtaining their health-promoting effects. Continually consuming the same foods every day is an extremely effective way of developing immune food sensitivities. Eating a wider selection of foods-- with their widely-differing nutrient profiles--exposes one to a much wider array of protective vitamins, minerals and phytochemicals, and decreases the likelihood of developing nutrient deficiencies. As researchers from Cornell University, NY recently wrote, *"...the additive and synergistic effects of phytochemicals in fruit and vegetables are responsible for their potent antioxidant and anticancer activities ... the benefit of a diet rich in fruit and vegetables is attributed to the complex mixture of phytochemicals present in whole foods."*(95)

It is also worth remembering that the antioxidant values in Tables 15a and 15b were obtained in the laboratory setting, but petri dishes and test tubes present a vastly different environment to that encountered inside the human body. Inside the human body, abundant consumption of carbohydrate-rich items like potatoes and grains can quickly raise blood sugar levels, which in turn can dramatically boost free radical activity. For this reason, dried fruits, which are high in antioxidants *and* carbohydrates, should also be eaten judiciously; consume smaller amounts regularly as opposed to large servings in a single sitting to avoid excessive spikes in blood sugar.

When considering not only antioxidant content, but also important qualities such as low carbohydrate content, relatively low allergenicity, and a consistent association with reduced levels of various diseases, the 'ultimate' plant foods may well be those sporting the color green; artichokes, asparagus, broccoli, Brussels sprouts, cabbage, cauliflower, endives, green beans, and romaine

Table 15a. Antioxidant Capacity of Various Plant Foods, Halvorsen et al.
(mmol of total antioxidants/100 g)

Berries		Vegetables	
Blueberry/bilberry,wild	8.23	Chilipepper	2.46
Blackcurrant	7.35	Kale	2.34
Sour cherry	5.53	Red cabbage	1.88
Blackberry	5.07	Red/green pepper Capsicum	1.64
Raspberry	3.97	Brussels sprout	1.14
Blueberry	3.64	Spinach	0.98
Raspberry	3.06	Asparagus	0.85
Strawberry	2.17	Celery	0.80
Redcurrant	1.78	Onion	0.67
Sweet cherry	1.02	Broccoli	0.58
		Avocado	0.41
Fruits		Lettuce	0.34
Pomegranate	11.33	Tomato	0.31
Orange	1.14	Garlic	0.24
Pineapple	1.04	Cauliflower	0.23
Kiwi fruit	0.91	eggplant	0.17
Papaya	0.62	Cabbage	0.09
Apricot	0.52	Squash	0.08
Mango	0.35		
Apple	0.29	**Cereals**	
		Buckwheat, wholemeal flour**	1.99
Nuts and seeds		Millet, wholemeal flour	0.82
Walnut	20.97	Maize, white flour	0.60
Sunflower	5.39	Oats, rough oatmeal	0.59
Hazelnut	0.49	Rye, wholemeal flour	0.47
Almond	0.30	Wheat, wholemeal flour	0.33
		Millet, white flour	0.25
Dried fruits		Rye, white flour	0.23
Apricot	3.24	Wheat, white flour	0.13
Prune	2.60	Rice, white flour	0.04
Raisins	0.80		
Figs	0.76	**Pulses**	
		Broad bean	1.86
Roots and tubers		Pinto bean	1.14
Ginger	3.76	Soya beans	0.82
Red beet	1.98	Lentils	0.49
Turnip	0.29	Kidney beans	0.38
Sweet potato	0.22	Chickpeas	0.23
Potato	0.09	Garden pea	0.12
Parsnip	0.09		
Carrot	0.04		

Table 15b. Antioxidant Capacity of Various Plant Foods, Xu et al.
(mmol of Trolox Equivalents/100 g)

Berries		Vegetables	
Blueberry, wild	92.60	Artichokes	94.09
Blueberry	62.20	Red cabbage	31.46
Blackberry	53.48	Spinach	26.40
Raspberry	49.25	Eggplant	25.33
Strawberry	35.77	Asparagus	16.44
Sweet cherry	33.61	Broccoli	12.59
		Onions, yellow	12.20
Fruits	73.39	Lettuce, romaine	9.89
Plums, black	62.39	Cauliflower	6.47
Plums	42.75	Celery	5.74
Apples, Red delicious	38.99	Pumpkin	4.83
Apples, Granny Smith	26.70	Tomato, raw	4.60
Apples, Golden Delicious	19.11	Lettuce, iceberg	4.51
Pears, green	18.63	Cucumbers	1.23
Peaches	18.14		
Orange	15.48	**Cereal grain products**	
Grapefruit, red	13.41	Corn flakes	23.59
Apricots	12.60	Bread, pumpernickel	19.63
Grapes, red	8.79	Oats, old-fashioned	17.08
Bananas	7.93	Bread, whole grain	14.21
Pineapple	7.49		
Nectarines	3.12	**Roots and tubers**	
Cantaloupes	1.42	Red beet	27.74
Watermelons		Potato	10.81-13.26
		Carrots, cooked	12.15
Nuts and seeds		Radishes	9.54
Pecans	179.40	Sweet potato	7.66
Walnuts	135.41	Carrots, raw	3.71
Hazelnut	96.45		
Pistachios	79.83	**Pulses**	
Almonds	44.54	Beans, small red	149.21
Peanuts	31.66	Beans, red kidney	144.13
Cashew nuts	19.97	Beans, pinto	123.59
Macadamias	16.95	Beans, black (dried)	80.40
Dried fruits		Black-eyed peas	43.43
Prune	85.78	Beans, navy	24.74
Dates	38.95	Green peas, (canned)	3.84
Figs	33.83	Snap beans (canned)	2.90
Raisins	30.37	Lima beans (canned)	2.43

lettuce, to name but a few.

Going Against the Grain

Clearly, cereal grains should *not* form the foundation of a healthy diet--that role should be relegated to the foods that the human species has been eating for its entire evolutionary history: namely meats, fruits, berries, vegetables, nuts and seeds. Cereal grains and legumes were not consumed by humans in any meaningful amount until the onset of the Agricultural Revolution some 10,000 years ago. While consumption of small amounts of these Neolithic staples may not produce untoward effects in most individuals, they should *never* be consumed at the expense of the aforementioned Paleolithic foods.

OK, enough about cereal grains; what about the modern-day plethora of highly-processed, colorfully packaged and aggressively advertised packaged foods?

These are the subject of the next chapter.

Chapter 16

"Rich western nations do not lack calories. They do lack true nourishment."
Dr. Bernard Jensen.

The Pseudo-Foods

You are what you eat--so don't eat junk!

When people think of junk food, they usually think of items like donuts, chocolate bars, hot dogs, soft drinks, cheeseburgers, fries and so on. Most folks do not realize that some of the less infamous staples they commonly eat, and often believe to be healthy and nourishing, are every bit as deserving of the 'junk' title as the aforementioned foods. Breads, bagels, soup mixes, 'health' bars, breakfast cereals, 'cholesterol-free' vegetable oils, and 'low-fat' biscuits and crackers are just a few of the many 'pseudo-foods' that fall into this very category.

If you stroll down your local supermarket isle, select a trolley full of items from the enormous array of colorfully-packaged processed foods, and carefully examine their labels, you will find almost universally that a significant portion of their calories will be derived from one or more of the following ingredients:

- Cereal flour (usually refined wheat flour)
- Sugar--most commonly corn syrup, but also sucrose, fructose, maltodextrin, dextrose (glucose), brown rice syrup, maple syrup, date sugar, cane sugar, corn sugar, beet sugar, etc, etc.
- Refined vegetable oils
- Hydrogenated vegetable fats

Why is this bad news for the average person's nutritional status? Let's find out…

The Great White Hoax

White flour is ubiquitous in today's food supply, found not only in breads, burger buns, bagels, pastas, donuts and pastries, but also as an ingredient in confectionery, many packaged foods, burgers, sausages, and even delicatessen meats.

One cup (125g) of white flour delivers ninety-five grams of carbohydrate, thirteen grams of protein, one gram of fat, and 455 calories. These calories come complete with a pathetically low micronutrient content; while white flour contains relatively high amounts of potassium and phosphorus, it contains miniscule amounts of calcium, iron, magnesium, zinc, copper, folate, and vitamins B1, B2, B5, B6, E and K. White flour contains no vitamin A, D or B12(1). Enrichment of flour significantly boosts the iron, folate and vitamin B3 content, and also produces small increases in vitamins B1 and B2, but does nothing to counter the numerous other nutritional shortcomings of this ubiquitous staple.

In addition, white flour and finely ground wholemeal flours rate very high on the *glycemic index* (GI), producing sharp and rapid rises in blood glucose levels. As we shall discuss further in Chapter 18, high blood glucose levels are a cardiovascular disaster waiting to happen. For those not yet familiar with the glycemic index concept, this is a measure of how high a given portion of a food item will raise blood sugar levels; foods that cause large, rapid spikes in blood glucose levels possess a high GI, while those that produce less pronounced, gentler rises in blood sugar have a low GI. Indeed, some GI tables use white bread as the reference food!(2)

Per gram of carbohydrate, foods with a high GI produce a higher peak in post-meal blood glucose and greater overall blood glucose levels during the first two hours after consumption than do foods with a low GI. Table 16a presents the GI values for various foods, derived from healthy, non-diabetic individuals and using glucose, with a GI of 100, as the reference standard.

The greatest benefit to be derived from GI charts is by taking careful note of the foods *not* included in them. Readers will notice that Table 16a does not list GI values for nutrient-dense foods like meat, poultry, eggs, and green vegetables. That's because these foods contain little or no carbohydrate, making it extremely difficult for research subjects to consume enough of them to cause noteworthy rises in blood glucose. Even when consumed in large amounts, these foods have little effect on blood sugar levels. Carb-centric nutritionists and researchers heatedly debate the merits of high-GI versus low-GI foods, but truly smart folks know it is 'No-GI' foods that should form the foundation of a healthy diet!

Thanks to their concentrated carbohydrate content and the high GI of these carbohydrates, products made from white flours and other refined carbohydrates possess what is known as a high *glycemic load* (GL). While the GI reflects the blood sugar-raising potential of equal amounts of carbohydrates from various foods, the glycemic load measures the effect upon blood sugar elicited by typical serving sizes of foods. When we look at watermelon, for example, we see that it has a very high glycemic index similar to that of white bread. However, to ingest the twenty-five gram amount of carbohydrate used to determine the GI of watermelon, one would need to eat almost 500 grams of raw melon, a considerable quantity of food to be consumed in one sitting. In stark contrast, a mere forty-five grams of white bread, or 1.5 slices, supplies the same amount of carbohydrate. In real life, white bread is far more likely to lead to the over-consumption of carbohydrates--and subsequent development of high blood glucose levels--than bulky foods like watermelon. This is why the former possesses a GL of 10, while the latter sports a GL of 4.

Sugar--It Ain't So Sweet

If you thought the nutritional profile of white flour was bad, wait until you get a load of sugars such as sucrose and high fructose corn syrup, the latter being the most widely used sweetener in the American food supply today. These sweeteners, which tie with vegetable oils as the second major source of calories in the American diet after cereal grains, have virtually no micronutrient content whatsoever--*none!* They provide nothing but pure calories, thereby constituting the worst value-for-calories proposition in the entire food supply! Like processed flour, these refined high glycemic sweeteners send blood sugar levels soaring.

Along with their lack of nutritional value, blood sugar-spiking sweeteners and flours cause the body to excrete increased amounts of chromium, a mineral that is vital for proper blood glucose and insulin metabolism(3). In one study, consumption of a diet high in sugar increased the loss of chromium in the urine from 10 percent to 300 percent, when compared to a diet in which the majority of carbohydrates were obtained from complex sources(4). In other words, refined carbohydrate foods create an increased need for chromium while at the same time causing the body to become depleted of it!

Vegetable Fat Foolishness

The overwhelming majority of vegetable oil consumed in the U.S. is in the form of soybean oil. This is added to a staggering array of processed foods during the manufacturing process, employed in restaurants and convenience food outlets for cooking and frying, and used in homes during cooking and in salad dressings. Soybean oil contains an abundance of omega-6 fat in the form of linoleic acid, which, as we shall discuss more fully in Chapter 19, is in no way a virtue; high linoleic acid intakes destroy the body's crucial balance between omega-6 and omega-3 fatty acids, dramatically increasing the risk of heart disease and cancer in the process.

Aside from excessive linoleic acid and modest amounts of vitamin E and K, soybean oil contains virtually no other vitamins, minerals or trace elements. Hydrogenated soybean oil does contain vitamin A and sodium but otherwise is almost as nutritionally depleted as its liquid cousin. Furthermore, animal and human studies show that linoleic-rich oils like soybean worsen one's nutritional status by decreasing the absorption of iron, zinc and copper(5-9).

Table 16a. Glycemic Index and Glycemic Load of Various Foods

	GI	GL		GI	GL
Beverages			**Fruit and Fruit Products**		
Apple juice, unsweetened	39-53	12	Apple, raw, golden delicious	39	6
Carrot juice, freshly made	43	10	Apricots, dried	30	8
Coca Cola	63	16	Banana	67	16
Cranberry juice cocktail (Ocean Spray)	68	24	Dates, dried	103	42
			Grapes, black	59	111
Fruit-flavored drink mix, orange	66	13	Kiwi fruit	58	7
Gatorade	78	12	Mango, raw	57	9
Grapefruit juice, unsweetened	48	11	Oranges, raw	37	4
Orange juice	50	13	Papaya, raw	59	13
Tomato juice, canned, unsweetened	38	4	Pineapple, raw	66	6
			Prunes, pitted	29	10
Breakfast Cereals			Raisins	64	28
All-Bran (Kellogg's)	38	9	Cantaloupe, raw	65	4
Cornflakes (Kellogg's)	75	19	Strawberries, fresh, raw	40	1
Grapenuts (Kraft Foods Inc)	75	16	Watermelon, raw	72	4
Muesli, assorted varieties	39-66	7-17	**Legumes**		
Porridge, whole rolled oats	52	111	Black-eyed beans	33	10
Porridge, quick, wholemeal oat flour	74	24	Butter beans	32	6
			Garbanzo beans	36	11
Raisin Bran (Kellogg's)	61	12	Haricot and navy beans	35	11
Shredded Wheat	67	13	Kidney beans	21	7
Special K (Kellogg's)	69	114	Lentils	29	5
Cereal Grains			Mung bean	31	5
Pearl barley, boiled	25	11	Peanuts	13	1
Corn, sweet	54	17	Soya beans, boiled	18	1
Millet, boiled	71	25	**Miscellaneous**		
Rice, white, boiled, assorted varieties	48-139	18-60	Chocolate	43	12
			Ironman PR bar, chocolate	39	10
Rice, brown, boiled	50-87	16-33	Jelly beans	78	22
Cereal grains-pasta			Mars Bar	65	26
Spaghetti, white	50	24	Pizza, various styles	30-80	7-22
Spaghetti, whole meal	42	17	Pop Tarts, double chocolate	70	25
Ravioli, meat-filled	39	15	Potato crisps, plain, salted	54	20
Cereal grains--bread			Power Bar, chocolate	56	24
Rye-kernel (pumpernickel) bread	41	5	Pretzels	83	16
Rye bread, sourdough	48	6	Pure-Protein bars, various flavors	22-43	2-6
Rye bread, dark, whole-meal flour	55	7	Sausages	28	1
Wheat bread, coarse whole-grain	52	10	Snickers Bar	68	23
Wheat bread, sourdough	54	8	Sushi	52	19
Wheat bread, whole-meal flour	75	9	**Nuts**		
White bread	70	10	Cashews	22	3
Dairy Products			**Vegetables**		
Ice cream, full-fat, vanilla	38	3	Beetroot	64	5
Ice cream, low-fat, vanilla	50	3	Carrots, boiled	40	1.5
Milk, full-fat	40	3	Green peas	53	4
Milk, skim	32	4	Pumpkin	75	3
Yogurt, regular	36	3	Parsnips	97	1
Yogurt, reduced-fat	27	7	Potato, various, boiled or baked	56-101	14-18
Yogurt, non-fat	24	3	Rutabaga	72	7
Dairy Alternatives			Sweet potato	46	13
Soy milk, full-fat (3%)	40	7	Yam	37	13
Soy milk, reduced-fat (1.5%)	44	8			
Soy yogurt, 2% fat, w/ sugar	50	13			
Tofu-based frozen dessert, choc. w/ high fructose corn syrup	115	10			

Adapted from: Foster-Powell K, et al. International table of glycemic index and glycemic load values: 2002. *American Journal of Clinical Nutrition*, Jul, 2002; 76: 5-56.

The bottom line is that soybean and other omega-6-rich vegetable fats do more than just skimp on the micronutrients; as an added bonus, liberal consumption of these fats decreases mineral absorption, worsens one's essential fatty acid balance, and increases the risk of disabling illness.

Cereal grains, sweeteners and vegetable oils account for a staggering fifty-seven percent of calories consumed in the U.S.! With more than half of all calories coming from these nutritionally anemic 'anti-foods', it's little wonder that chronic degenerative disease is rife in modernized nations like America!

The Great Nutrient Swindle

OK, so you don't eat a lot of cereal products, wouldn't even think of eating such pap as donuts or candy, rarely venture inside a McDonald's, and have long since banished soda from your diet. That's terrific, but don't breathe easy just yet.

Recent research shows that, by choosing the wrong cooking method, using commercially frozen produce and eating canned foods, even the most well-meaning and health-conscious individuals may be unwittingly depriving themselves of many of the beneficial nutrients found in fresh foods.

Commercially frozen foods are often soaked in hot water before freezing, a process known as 'blanching'. After studying twenty different types of commonly eaten vegetables, Finnish scientists discovered blanching destroyed up to one-third of the vitamin C content of vegetables, with a further slight loss during frozen storage. Folic acid proved to be particularly sensitive to blanching, with more than fifty percent being lost, although levels remained stable during freezing. While mineral contents remained stable, substantial losses (twenty to thirty percent) of antioxidant activity and phenol content (plant compounds with antioxidant properties) were detected in many vegetables. Carotenoids (such as beta-carotene and lycopene) were not affected by blanching or freezer storage(10).

In Spain, food scientists measured the levels of flavonoids remaining in fresh broccoli after cooking by four popular methods: steaming, pressure cooking, boiling or microwaving. The four treatments showed large differences in their influence upon broccoli's flavonoid content. Conventional boiling led to significant flavonoid loss (sixty-six percent), while high-pressure boiling caused considerable leaching (forty-seven percent) of one of the studied flavonoid derivatives into cooking water. The real shocker came when broccoli was microwaved; this method of cooking led to a whopping ninety-seven percent flavonoid loss! Steaming, on the other hand, had minimal effects on both total and individual flavonoid content(11).

What this basically means is that when you buy frozen vegetables and microwave them before eating, there's a good chance you will ingest *none* of the antioxidant flavonoids originally found in the plant!

When Japanese scientists examined the effect of different cooking methods on mineral losses in food, they found average reductions of around sixty to seventy percent in cooked foods as compared to raw or uncooked foods. Mineral losses from cooking were particularly high in vegetables. Among the various cooking methods they studied, mineral loss was greatest after boiling, followed by parching, frying and stewing. Slicing vegetables thinly then soaking them in water also caused large mineral losses. To prevent mineral loss, the authors suggested eating boiled food with the broth, adding a *small* amount of salt when boiling, and selecting a cooking method that produces less mineral loss; these include stewing, frying, parching, and steaming(12). Wherever possible, buy your vegetables fresh and adopt steaming as your main cooking method.

Canning also leads to large nutrient losses in food; fish and other seafoods lose an average forty-nine percent of vitamin B6 and twenty percent of vitamin B5. In canned meats, average losses of B6 and B5 are forty-three and twenty-three percent, respectively. In vegetables, canning causes B6 losses of fifty-seven to seventy-seven percent and B5 losses of forty-six to seventy-eight percent. Fruit and fruit juices, meanwhile, lose thirty-eight and fifty-one percent of B6 and B5, respectively. Large losses of manganese, cobalt, zinc and folate have also been documented in canned vegetables, as compared to their raw counterparts(13).

Food Fortification: No Substitute For the Real Thing

In response to concerns over the substantial nutrient losses resulting from processing, food manufacturers now routinely fortify their products with synthetic vitamins and minerals. The labels of these products then proudly boast about this 'enhancement', as if adding one or two isolated vitamins somehow makes up for the wide-ranging nutrient losses that occurred during manufacture.

We live in a world where the medical establishment is afflicted with a 'single bullet' mindset, where scientists desperately seek out the one magic pill that will once and for all conquer heart disease, another that will cure cancer, yet another that will eradicate diabetes, and so on. It is perhaps not so surprising, then, that food fortification with isolated vitamins and minerals has found such widespread acceptance. While food enrichment does offer some benefits, it is in no way a substitute for a hunter-gatherer-style diet of fresh foods.
To further understand this phenomenon, let's take a closer look at perhaps the most famous vitamin of all, vitamin C (ascorbic acid).

To C or Not to C

Around fifty million years ago, our earliest primate predecessors began evolving from an insect-based diet to one that revolved around fruits and other vitamin C-rich plant foods. After making this dietary switch, the ability to produce ascorbic acid inside the body was no longer necessary, and was subsequently relinquished during the course of evolution. As such, humans are among the small handful of species whose bodies cannot create their own vitamin C. While most other species can synthesize ascorbic acid from glucose, we humans must obtain our vitamin C from the food we eat.

Among its many functions, ascorbic acid helps an enzyme known as *prolyl hydroxylase* convert collagen's precursor, *procollagen,* into collagen itself. This collagen is then used to help provide structural integrity to skin, bone, tendons, ligaments, teeth, and blood vessels. Because efficient collagen formation is a must for healthy arteries, it is easy to envisage how inadequate intakes of vitamin C could pose a serious threat to our cardiovascular status.

By inactivating the gene for *L-gulonolactone-gamma-oxidase* (GLO)--the enzyme required to convert glucose into ascorbic acid--researchers have successfully bred mice that, like humans, cannot produce their own ascorbic acid. Supplementary ascorbic acid must be added to the drinking water of these mutant mice in order to prevent them from becoming vitamin C-deficient. When the vitamin is withdrawn from the rodents' diets, their blood and tissue ascorbic acid levels quickly plummet and after several weeks they become anemic, lose weight, and die.

Upon post-mortem examination of these GLO-deficient mice, researchers have observed arterial lesions in the thoracic aortic arch, at the point in the aorta where the carotid artery branches off--a point where blood flow-related shear-stress is especially high, and where atherosclerosis commonly occurs in humans. Microscopic examination of these lesions has revealed marked abnormalities in the portions of the arterial wall that are responsible for imparting elasticity and flexibility. This, the researchers conclude, arises from the lack of vitamin C required to generate the raw materials required for collagen formation and repair(14).

In GLO-deficient mice, vitamin C deficiency also produces significant reductions in the collagen content of atherosclerotic plaques. As a result, the fibrous caps covering the atheromas of mice receiving inadequate vitamin C are significantly thinner and more fragile than those seen in GLO-deficient mice receiving adequate vitamin C(15).

Similar to GLO-deficient mice, humans suffering from severe vitamin C deficiency--a condition known as scurvy--will die from its emaciating complications long before they will ever have the chance to experience a heart attack. However, numerous researchers have raised the possibility that milder vitamin C deficiencies may, over a longer period of time, contribute to coronary artery disease. Epidemiological evidence strongly supports this contention, with numerous studies finding higher blood levels and/or dietary intakes of vitamin C to be associated with lower incidences of CHD and stroke(16-20).

Modern Day Vitamin C Intakes

Our Paleolithic ancestors are believed to have averaged anywhere from a few hundred to a few thousand milligrams of vitamin C each day (depending on their geographical location)(21). In contrast, the average vitamin C content of the highly-processed, grain-based American diet is a mere 110-125 milligrams per day for men and 91-107 milligrams per day for women. Around twenty-five percent of U.S. adults consume less than sixty milligrams of vitamin C per day, while ten percent fail to ingest even thirty milligrams per day(22). When over 15,000 U.S. adults had their blood levels of vitamin C measured as part of NHANES, fourteen percent of males and ten percent of females met the official criteria for deficiency, while over twenty percent exhibited vitamin C 'depletion'(23).

Given these observations, one may readily conclude that widespread fortification or supplementation with ascorbic acid could help significantly lower the incidence of heart disease and stroke. Randomized, placebo-controlled clinical trials, however, have failed to show any reduction in CHD or stroke from vitamin C supplementation in amounts ranging from 120-500 milligrams daily(24-26). What could possibly explain this failure?

Real Food to the Rescue

Fruits and vegetables are by far the richest sources of vitamin C. As such, high dietary and/or high blood levels of vitamin C detected in epidemiological studies are strongly suggestive of greater fruit and vegetable intake (see Table 16b for the vitamin C content of various foods). Indeed, clinical experiments show that when subjects are fed fruit and vegetable-rich diets, their blood levels of ascorbic acid increase markedly(27-29). A comparison of middle-aged subjects randomized to consume either 100 grams or 500 grams of fruits and vegetables daily found that blood vitamin C levels decreased by thirteen percent in the former, but rose by fifty percent in the latter(30).

Along with vitamin C, fruits and vegetables also tend to be high in other important micronutrients such as folic acid and the various *carotenoids*, including *alpha-carotene, beta-carotene, lycopene, cryptoxanthin* and *lutein*. As we learnt in the previous chapter, fruits, vegetables and nuts contain a

Table 16b. Vitamin C content of various food items

Fruits and vegetables	Weight	Common measure	Vitamin C (mg)
Red peppers, sweet, raw	149g	1 cup	283mg
Broccoli, boiled, drained	156g	1 cup	101mg
Strawberries, raw	166g	1 cup	98mg
Brussels sprouts	156g	1 cup	97mg
Papaya, raw	140g	1 cup	87mg
Peas, boiled, drained	160g	1 cup	77mg
Kiwi fruit, fresh, raw	76g	1 medium	71mg
Oranges, raw	131g	1 orange	70mg
Hot chilli peppers, red, raw	45g	1 pepper	65mg
Cantaloupe, raw	160g	1 cup	59mg
Mangos, raw	207g	1 mango	57mg
Cauliflower, boiled, drained	124g	1 cup	55mg
Grapefruit	118g	1/2 g/fruit	39mg
Chestnuts, roasted	143g	1 cup	37mg
Raspberries, raw	123g	1 cup	32mg
Lemons, raw	58g	1 lemon	31mg
Blackberries, raw	144g	1 cup	30mg
Sweet potato, baked in skin	146g	1 potato	29mg
Tomato, raw, ripe	180g	1 cup	23mg
Blueberries, raw	145g	1 cup	14mg
Lettuce, cos or romaine, raw	56g	1 cup	13mg
Watermelon, raw	152g	1 cup	12mg
Pumpkin, boiled	245g	1 cup	12mg
Onions, boiled	210g	1 cup	11mg
Bananas, raw	118g	1 banana	10mg
Pears, raw	166g	1 pear	7mg
Peaches, raw	98g	1 peach	7mg
Apple, raw, with skin	138g	1 apple	6mg
Plums, raw	66g	1 plum	6mg
Cherries, sweet, raw	68g	10 cherries	5mg
Carrots, raw	72g	1 carrot	4mg
Celery, raw	120g	1 cup	4mg
Apricots, raw	35g	1 apricot	4mg
Cucumber, raw	104g	1 cup	3mg
Avocados, raw, California	29g	1 oz	5mg
Hazelnuts	29g	1oz	2mg
Animal foods			
Lamb brain	100g	3.5oz	16mg
Chicken/Turkey giblets	100g	3.5oz	13-14mg
Clam, raw	100g	3.5oz	13mg
Beef kidney	100g	3.5oz	9.4mg
Crab, cooked	85g	3.5oz	4-8mg
Tuna, Yellowfin, cooked	100g	3.5oz	1mg
Pork, center-loin, cooked	100g	3.5oz	1mg
Dairy Products			
Yogurt, plain, whole milk	227g	8oz	1mg
Cheese	29g	1oz	0mg
Cow milk, pasteurized, 3.25%	244g	1 cup	0mg
Grain and soy products			
Breakfast cereals, fortified, various	30g	1 cup	6mg
Rolled Oats	234g	1 cup	0mg
Rice (brown or white)	185g	1 cup	0mg
Bread (wheat, rye, corn, etc)	24g	1 slice	0mg
Muffins, oat bran	57g	1 muffin	0mg
Doughnuts	14g	1 donut	0mg
Soy milk	245g	1 cup	0mg

Source: USDA National Nutrient Database, Release 16.

veritable cornucopia of substances known as *phytochemicals*. Not surprisingly, controlled experiments not only show increased blood vitamin C levels among volunteers fed fruit and vegetable-rich diets, but also increases in blood levels of folate, carotenoids and phytochemicals.

Among the many phytochemicals found in fruits and vegetables are the *bioflavonoids*. In epidemiological studies, researchers have found a consistent association between high dietary bioflavonoid intakes and reduced risk of CHD (as well as cancer, diabetes, and even asthma(31,32)). Bioflavonoids exert a favorable influence on connective tissue formation and repair(33-35). In animal studies, bioflavonoids have been shown to slow the development of atherosclerosis, and to reduce the severity of vascular damage in animals who already have advanced atherosclerotic lesions(36-39).

Here's the important point; phytochemical compounds like bioflavonoids help vitamin C to do its job better, which is no doubt why the two occur alongside each other in the plant kingdom! In human subjects, consumption of a citrus fruit extract, rich in bioflavonoids, results in greater absorption of ascorbic acid than when the vitamin is administered alone(40). Furthermore, laboratory research shows that the bioflavonoid *rutin* amplifies the antioxidant effects of ascorbic acid(41).

In a study with healthy human volunteers, researchers compared the effect of taking 150 milligrams of supplemental vitamin C daily or consuming 250 grams of cactus pear each day, the latter providing a similar amount of vitamin C as the supplement. In addition to containing vitamin C, cactus pear also contains antioxidant phytochemicals known as *betalains*. During the two-week period of cactus pear consumption, blood test results indicated significant reductions in free radical damage to cellular lipids, increased concentrations of the powerful antioxidant glutathione and reduced LDL oxidation. Vitamin C supplementation produced none of these effects(42).

Relying solely on ascorbic acid supplements in an attempt to prevent CHD is a little like bringing a wooden club to a gunfight. Because the ascorbic acid in plant foods is accompanied by a vast array of artery-friendly bioflavonoids, good old-fashioned fruits and vegetables possess far greater disease-fighting firepower than isolated vitamin C. That is why, as we saw in Chapter 8, clinical interventions involving increased fruit and vegetable consumption have succeeded where trials using vitamin C supplements have so far failed in lowering CHD mortality.

There's No Substitute For Real Food

Despite its many truly wondrous achievements, science has not even come close to formulating a compound that can do what real food does; namely, provide optimal nourishment for the amazingly complex metabolic machine known as the human body.

What modern technology *has* delivered to us is a staggering array of pseudo-foods whose nutrient profiles are vastly inferior to those of the fresh foods from which they were derived. The average modern-day citizen's intake of many important vitamins, minerals, trace elements, fatty acids, phytochemicals and amino acids dramatically pales in comparison to that of his hunter-gatherer ancestors. The next several chapters will elucidate the unfortunate cardiovascular consequences of this regrettable development.

Chapter 17

"Nature must be obeyed, not orthodoxy."
Weston A. Price.

Revenge of the Radicals

How free radicals can wreck your health.

We cannot live without oxygen. Every single cell in our bodies needs it to survive and thrive, to fuel the amazingly complex metabolic symphony our bodies perform each and every day. While most of us can last days without water and even months without food, a lack of oxygen will kill us within minutes.

While oxygen is absolutely essential to life, it also has a dark side. As cells go about utilizing oxygen, they inevitably create incompletely burned particles of oxygen known as *free radicals*. A free radical is an atom that has been robbed of its electron, making it a highly reactive and unstable entity with the ability to cause major damage to our tissues and organs.

Free radical activity isn't all bad--a small amount is actually crucial to our well-being. Free radicals are utilized by the immune system to attack harmful viruses and bacteria, and they may even play a role in the growth of blood vessels and skin during wound healing(1,2).

It is when free radical production becomes excessive that problems occur. Remember all those peaceful protests you've seen on the television news that quickly degenerated into all-out riots? A similar scene occurs inside your body when free-radical production gets out of hand. Free radicals rapidly multiply, and as they scurry about looking for replacement electrons, they behave like angry vandals hell-bent on damaging our cells. The more free radicals produced, the greater the damage caused.

Excessive free radical activity can ravage the proteins and fats that make up our most vital tissues and organs. It can also attack the DNA inside our cells, where the genetic blueprint for healthy growth and repair can be found. Cardiovascular disease, cancer, diabetes, neurological disorders, and liver and kidney diseases are but a few of the many ailments promoted by heightened free radical production. In fact, free radical damage is believed to be a significant contributor to the aging process itself.

What increases free radical production? Radiation, cigarette smoking, excessive alcohol, polluted air, exposure to toxic chemicals, tissue injury, nutrient deficiencies, high blood sugar levels, and polyunsaturated vegetable oils can all increase the free radical burden in our bodies. It is not surprising, then, that many of these same factors have been shown to increase the risk of CHD.

Whodunit: Free Radicals, LDL, and CHD

The interaction between free radicals and LDL cholesterol is a perfect example of just how misleading and counterproductive the current obsession with blood lipids can be. LDL cholesterol, we are told, is the demonic lipoprotein that dumps big wads of cholesterol onto the walls of our blood vessels. To avoid this potentially deadly scenario, we must be sure to reduce our LDL levels by eating a low-fat diet and taking 'miracle' cholesterol-lowering drugs like statins.

During the eighties, some researchers began to realize that LDL cholesterol itself was not a reliable independent risk factor for CHD--half of those who suffer CHD have LDL levels within the normal limit. Among the 28,000-plus participants of the Women's Health Study, for example, forty-six percent of first cardiovascular events occurred in women with LDL cholesterol levels under 130 mg/dL--the 'desirable' target for primary prevention set by the NCEP(3). Even Daniel Steinberg, a leading scientific supporter of the lipid hypothesis, had to acknowledge that *"We have all seen myocardial infarction in patients with cholesterol levels <200; we have also seen patients with heterozygous familial hypercholesterolemia and cholesterol levels >300 who somehow survive into their 70s with no clinically evident CHD...patients with very different LDL concentrations can come to the catheterization laboratory with similar degrees of atherosclerosis."(4)*

In experimental studies, researchers found that LDL did not accumulate in atherosclerotic cells if it had not first undergone some form of degradation-- such as that caused by oxidative free radical damage(5,6). Proponents of the lipid hypothesis promptly modified their pet theory, embracing oxidized LDL as an additional 'cause' of atherosclerosis. The discovery of oxidized LDL cholesterol, they claimed, only further supported the value of lowering LDL cholesterol.

They were wrong.

The amount of LDL oxidation that takes place in the body is *not* dependent upon blood levels of LDL cholesterol. In animal studies, administration of antioxidant drugs like probucol retards LDL oxidation and arterial plaque formation, even when there is no change in blood cholesterol levels(7-11). In fact, administration of the antioxidant butylated hydroxytoluene significantly reduces the degree of atherosclerosis on the aortic surface of rabbits even though it *raises* LDL cholesterol levels!(10)

A similar dissociation is observed in humans. Among elderly Belgians, higher levels of oxidized LDL cholesterol were accompanied by a significantly increased risk of heart attack, regardless of overall LDL levels(12,13).

In Japanese patients undergoing surgery to remove plaque from their carotid arteries, blood levels of oxidized LDL cholesterol were significantly higher than those measured in healthy controls. Advanced carotid plaques extracted from the patients showed far higher levels of oxidized LDL than neighboring sections of artery that were disease-free. Elevated oxidized LDL was also associated with an increased susceptibility of plaque rupture. However, there was no association between oxidized LDL concentrations and overall LDL levels(14).

In 1997, Swedish researchers published the results of a comparison of CHD risk factors among men from Vilnius in Lithuania and Linkoping in Sweden. These two populations were chosen because men in the former town had a four-fold higher mortality rate from CHD than those in the latter. The researchers found very little difference in traditional risk factors between the two groups, except that the men from CHD-prone Vilnius had lower total and LDL cholesterol levels, which according to common wisdom should have placed them at lower risk of heart disease. When the researchers subsequently looked at some of the less commonly cited risk factors, they discovered that the men from Vilnius had significantly higher concentrations of oxidized LDL(15).

Further underscoring the irrelevance of total LDL cholesterol levels was a comparison of patients given aggressive LDL cholesterol lowering treatment (statins plus niacin) with those receiving less aggressive treatment (statins only). Despite greater LDL reductions in the former group, after 1.2 years of treatment there were no differences in calcified plaque progression as detected by electron beam tomography(16).

Oxidized LDL: Cause or Effect?

At present, researchers do not know for sure whether oxidized LDL cholesterol actually causes CHD, or is simply a consequence of the atherosclerotic process. Free radical damage is a contagious phenomenon, rapidly multiplying as incomplete atoms engage in an ever-escalating cycle of electron snatching. As such, it is not unreasonable to postulate that once LDL cholesterol becomes oxidized, it may spark heightened free radical activity in the tissues it comes into contact with. Whether this is in fact the case remains to be proven.

What is clear is that oxidized LDL concentrations are increased, not by elevated LDL levels, but by an increased free radical load in the body. This increased free radical burden, in turn, can arise when we eat too much of the wrong foods and not enough of the right ones. Regardless of whether oxidized LDL cholesterol is a culprit or innocent bystander, there is little doubt that increased free radical activity in the body will increase one's susceptibility to cardiovascular disease. So regardless of its exact role in the development of atherosclerosis, oxidized LDL can nevertheless serve as a helpful gauge of the body's antioxidant status.

If we wish to avoid CHD--along with cancer and numerous other lethal ailments--we must make every effort to boost our bodies' antioxidant defense systems. Luckily, this is not a difficult task.

Oil Change

Polyunsaturated fatty acids--which are found predominantly in vegetable oils and are unwittingly consumed in excessive amounts by a large percentage of the population--are highly susceptible to free radical damage. So too are the unfortunate folks who consume them, especially when the ingested oils have been used in high temperature cooking. Numerous studies show that consumption of heated vegetable oils dramatically increases harmful free radical activity in both animals and human volunteers(17-24).

In healthy male subjects, consumption of a diet containing fifteen percent polyunsaturated fatty acids--an amount not at all difficult to achieve in today's vegetable oil-laden food supply--resulted in significant increases in peroxidation, which refers to oxidative damage incurred by lipids inside our bodies. When the same volunteers proceeded to consume a diet in which the PUFA content was restricted to only five percent, peroxidation decreased notably(23).

In another study, volunteers consumed a diet rich in saturated dairy fats for four weeks and were then switched to either a high linoleic acid diet or a high oleic acid diet for another four weeks. Linoleic acid is an omega-6 fatty acid found in abundance in most polyunsaturated vegetable oils, while oleic acid is the dominant fatty acid in olive oil. An additional control group consumed their habitual diet throughout the study.

At the end of the each diet period, the researchers measured levels of *8-iso-Prostaglandin F2 {alpha}*, a byproduct of lipid peroxidation that causes blood vessels to constrict at high concentrations. They also measured levels of nitric oxide (NO), the all-important gas that allows our arteries to relax as blood passes through them. This amazing gas also exerts anti-inflammatory, anti-clotting and antioxidant actions.

After four weeks of the high linoleic acid diet, 8-iso-Prostaglandin F2 {alpha} was significantly increased whereas nitric oxide levels showed a marked decrease. In only one short month, the high linoleic acid intake had effectively created a pro-oxidative, vasoconstrictive environment. Continued on a long-term basis, this type of environment encourages deteriorating arterial function and, ultimately, cardiovascular disease. Interestingly, free radical and NO status were most favorable after the four-week saturated fat-rich diet and in the controls eating their habitual diet!(24)

Not surprisingly, LDL particles carrying a high proportion of polyunsaturated fatty acids are far more susceptible to oxidative damage than those enriched with saturated or monounsaturated fatty acids(25). Consumption of polyunsaturated vegetable oils has repeatedly been shown to increase LDL oxidation, even though it lowers LDL and total cholesterol levels!(26)

Because of their propensity to sustain and promote oxidative damage, polyunsaturated vegetable fats are no longer a prominent feature of mainstream dietary guidelines. Instead, researchers who are increasingly concerned about the harmful effects of low-fat, high-carbohydrate diets, but unable to discard their phobic attitude towards saturated fats, are now recommending diets high in monounsaturated fats. On the back of such recommendations and the publicity given to the Mediterranean diet concept, sales of monounsaturated fat-rich oils such as olive and canola have boomed during the last decade. After strolling down the aisle of my local supermarket the other day, I was stunned by the dozens of different olive oil brands and varieties now available, a stark contrast to the lonely handful sitting on store shelves some fifteen years ago.

Before people rush off to embrace monounsaturated oils as the next cardiovascular elixir, they should know that the claimed heart-healthy benefits of these oils have never been demonstrated. Their rapid rise to stardom has been fueled almost entirely by tales of low CHD rates among southern European countries where olive oil often forms a staple of the diet. Ironically, the country with the lowest rates of CHD in southern Europe is the one with the greatest intake of highly saturated animal fats--France!

Furthermore, the only group of researchers to ever put olive oil to the clinical test found it to be anything but a coronary liquid gold. Rose and colleagues randomized men with existing CHD to consume diets high in either corn oil, olive oil or animal fats for a period of two years, reporting their results in a 1965 issue of the *British Medical Journal*. By the end of the trial, only fifty-two percent of the corn oil group and fifty-seven percent of the olive oil group remained alive and free of heart attack. In contrast, a full seventy-five percent of the control subjects who kept eating their high animal fat diet remained free of either fatal or non-fatal heart attack(27).

In other words, the likelihood of an adverse outcome decreased as the saturation of the main fat source increased. To understand why this occurred, we need to take a quick look at the structure of fats. I'm going to delve into a little biochemistry here, but stay with me--this is extremely important!

The fats we eat are comprised of *fatty acids*. Every fatty acid contains a chain of carbon atoms. With the exception of the carbon atoms at either end of the fatty acid chain, each of these carbon atoms has two hydrogen atoms attached to it (the carbon atom at one end has one hydrogen and two oxygen atoms attached, while the carbon atom at the other end has three hydrogens attached). When all of the carbon atoms in a fatty acid, excepting the carbon atoms at each end, are bearing two hydrogen atoms, that fatty acid is referred to as *saturated*. Animal fats and tropical fats typically contain the greatest proportion of their fat as saturated fatty acids.

When a fatty acid contains one or more carbon atoms that happen to be missing one of its hydrogen atoms, then the fatty acid in question is termed an *unsaturated* fatty acid. Those carbon atoms possessing a solo hydrogen atom are referred to as *double bonds*. It is these double bonds that attract free radicals and render unsaturated fatty acids far more vulnerable to oxidative damage than saturated fatty acids. Polyunsaturated fatty acids, which contain two or more double bonds, are the most susceptible of all fats to free radical damage. Because monounsaturated fatty acids each contain only one double bond, they are much less prone to oxidative damage than polyunsaturated fats. By the same token, they are more susceptible to free radical attack than saturated fats, which are completely free of vulnerable double bonds.

Nature has accounted for the above by providing those who eat an evolutionary-correct diet of range-fed meats, eggs, fruits, vegetables, and nuts with just enough polyunsaturated fats to meet their essential fatty acid requirements--and no more. As for monounsaturated fats, nature presents them to us, not in oxidation prone oils, but as a part of whole foods that simultaneously contain a variety of potent antioxidants--foods such as meats, nuts, olives and avocados. When it comes to healthy fat intake, nature--not confused researchers, biased food manufacturers, nor the health organizations that receive royalties from these same manufacturers--knows best!

Antioxidants--Nature's Free Radical Fighters

In the comparison between Swedish and Lithuanian men we talked about earlier, higher LDL cholesterol oxidation in the latter was accompanied not only by lower overall LDL levels, but significantly poorer blood levels of important diet-derived antioxidants such as beta carotene, lycopene, and gamma tocopherol (a form of vitamin E)(28,29). Blood levels of these nutrients are largely determined by dietary intake, especially from the consumption of antioxidant-rich fruits, nuts and vegetables. Thus, while the Lithuanian men had lower LDL levels, they had a greater susceptibility to oxidized LDL due to what appeared to be a deficient intake of antioxidant-rich foods.

One of the major mechanisms by which fruits, nuts, seeds and vegetables prevent us from heart disease is not by lowering cholesterol, but by supplying our bodies with a powerful arsenal of free radical-fighting antioxidant nutrients. When healthy volunteers were given supplements of garlic--a herb with potent antioxidant properties--or a placebo, the former reduced lipoprotein oxidation by a third, even though blood cholesterol levels remained unchanged!(30)

In fact, numerous studies have demonstrated that the increased consumption of various fruit and vegetable products improves blood levels of antioxidants and concomitantly lowers the susceptibility of LDL cholesterol to oxidation(31-36). This effect of increased fruit and vegetable intake does not merely reflect the superfluous modification of yet another meaningless 'risk factor'; as we learnt in Chapter Four, increased fruit and vegetable intake has been shown in randomized, controlled clinical trials to reduce the most important CHD outcome of all--death.

Hopefully by know, I have well and truly convinced readers that fortifying their diet with non-cereal plant foods is a winning CHD prevention strategy. Let me now begin to tell you why abandoning the nonsensical low-fat paradigm may also be one of the best things you can do for your health.

Lowering Fat Lowers Antioxidant Defenses

Many of the important antioxidants found in plant foods, such as carotenoids, vitamin K, and the various forms of vitamin E, are fat soluble, and therefore require dietary fat for proper absorption. Boosting dietary fat intake has repeatedly been shown to increase the absorption of these vital nutrients(37-39).

A study published in the August 2004 issue of the *American Journal of Clinical Nutrition* illustrates why the fat-free food craze cannot end a moment too soon. Healthy volunteers were assigned to consume a salad meal on three separate occasions, with the same amount of spinach, romaine lettuce, cherry tomatoes and carrots being ingested each time. The meals differed only in their fat content, being alternately laced with salad dressings containing zero, six or twenty-eight grams of fat. The researchers then measured the amount of alpha-carotene, beta-carotene, and lycopene appearing in the bloodstream for up to twelve hours after the meal. After ingestion of the salad with fat-free dressing, there was essentially no increase in blood levels of these important antioxidants! Absorption of these fat-soluble antioxidants did increase with the reduced-fat salad dressing, but was by far the highest after consumption of the salad containing full-fat dressing(40).

A study appearing in a 2001 issue of the same journal showed that the absorption of lutein, a carotenoid that may protect against optical disorders, cardiovascular disease and cancer(41,42), was 235 percent higher when consumed with a high-fat spread as compared to a low-fat spread(43).

In the U.S., twenty percent of men and thirty-three percent of women report that they always choose low-fat instead of regular salad dressings, a choice that dramatically reduces their absorption of vital fat-soluble antioxidants in the vegetables they eat(44). This reduced absorption in turn, seriously retards their ability to neutralize highly damaging free radicals(45).

The current trend of substituting full-fat animal foods with low-fat varieties is also a big mistake; the fatty portion of these foods is where crucial fat-soluble vitamins A, D and E, are found. Cutting the fat from these items also cuts their valuable fat-soluble vitamin content, which is why low-fat dairy products are routinely fortified with synthetic vitamins A and D. No such fortification program exists for low-fat meats and, for some reason, vitamin E is not added to dairy foods. So when you throw out egg yolks, use non- or low-fat dairy products, and eat only lean varieties of meat and fish, you are effectively cutting your intake of essential fat-soluble vitamins(46).

Fighting Free Radicals

To reduce your body's susceptibility to free radical-induced damage:

- Avoid the consumption of polyunsaturated vegetable oils and foods that contain them;
- Avoid low-fat diets;
- Eat fresh meats and antioxidant-rich fruits and vegetables;
- Engage in regular physical activity;
- Use antioxidant supplements (see Chapter 27).

Lowering blood sugar levels lowers free radical activity, while eating fresh meats, fruits, nuts and vegetables provides potent antioxidants such as carnosine, selenium, carotenes, vitamins E, C and A, and a vast array of potent plant-based antioxidant phytochemicals.

Moderate exercise, meanwhile, improves the body's own antioxidant defense system. It does this in much the same way it improves your fitness: by imposing physical stress which forces your body to favorably adapt. In this case, exercise stimulates the activity of free radical fighting enzymes like superoxide dismutase and glutathione peroxidase, and increases cellular concentrations of powerful antioxidants such as glutathione(47,48). Be careful not to overdo it, as overly strenuous exercise can increase free radical activity, especially if it is being fuelled by a poor diet low in antioxidants. Be sure to read chapter 28 to learn how to sensibly embark on an exercise routine(49,50).

Focus on What's Important

Fussing over blood cholesterol levels whilst ignoring your antioxidant status-- as much of the population presently does--is a little like standing in the path of an oncoming truck and worrying about how your hair looks. Stop wasting your time, money and health on useless distractions like blood lipids, and start attending to the things that truly matter.

To this end, the next chapter will expand on another highly destructive but vastly underrated cause of heart disease; one that is aggravated by the low-fat, high-carbohydrate diets that orthodoxy has been enthusiastically recommending for the past thirty years.

Chapter 18

"Man may be the captain of his fate, but he is also the victim of his blood sugar"
Wilfrid Oakley

High Blood Sugar

Your Arteries' Worst Nightmare?

When people enthusiastically recite their blood cholesterol readings to me and ask how they can be lowered even further, my response is usually a disinterested *"who cares?"* When they then ask me what the ideal level of blood cholesterol is, I tell them, *"one you don't know and don't worry about"*. As they stand there scratching their head, I then ask them what their fasting blood glucose level is. Unless the respondent is a diagnosed diabetic, most will not have the foggiest idea.

Cholesterol does not in any way cause heart disease, but elevated blood sugar levels sure as hell do. It is no coincidence that adults with diabetes suffer up to five-fold increases in heart disease and stroke mortality than non-diabetics! Nor is it happenstance that men diagnosed with diabetes at forty years of age are estimated to die, on average, around twelve years earlier than those without diabetes. Diabetic women, meanwhile, can expect to lose around fourteen years of life(1).

Thanks to decades of anti-cholesterol paranoia, millions of people now keep a hawk-like watch on their cholesterol levels. High blood sugar, meanwhile, waltzes into their lives with no resistance whatsoever, stealing health from right under their noses like a seasoned thief in the night.

The Vital Role of Blood Glucose

Sufficient blood glucose is vitally important for proper brain and nervous system function. If blood sugar drops too low--a state known as *hypoglycemia*--the brain is unable to function optimally. Hypoglycemia produces a variety of symptoms, including mental 'fogginess', fatigue, depression, mood swings, tremors, excessive sweating, palpitations, dizziness, and sugar cravings. Severe episodes of hypoglycemia, sometimes experienced by insulin-using diabetics, can even be fatal if not quickly attended to.

Depending on the textbook one consults, hypoglycemia is usually defined as a blood glucose concentration below 60-70mg/dl, with symptoms usually kicking in around 50 mg/dl. One of the most common causes of low blood sugar is *reactive hypoglycemia*, which occurs after the consumption of too many carbohydrates, especially of the refined variety. Epidemiological studies indicate that chronic hypoglycemia is a state best avoided, for it is associated with an increased risk of cardiovascular and all-cause mortality.

A far more pressing problem in modernized nations characterized by abundant food availability and physical inactivity is high blood sugar, or *hyperglycemia*, which can eventually lead to diabetes. The incidence of diabetes has experienced runaway growth in modernized nations over the last thirty years and is rising rapidly in developing countries, where diets rich in highly refined carbohydrates and sedentary lifestyles are becoming the norm.

Determining Safe Blood Glucose Levels

Throughout the course of evolution, our bodies have developed finely tuned mechanisms for keeping blood sugar levels in a tight range. Unfortunately, such factors as stress, excessive carbohydrate intake, physical inactivity, obesity, poor sleep and drug use can easily derail our bodies' attempts to maintain normal blood sugar concentrations.

The two best-known measures of blood glucose are *fasting blood glucose* and *the 2-hour post-challenge* blood glucose test. Fasting blood glucose is an easily administered test that simply measures the amount of glucose contained in a sample of blood drawn after an overnight fast. The 2-hour post-load test is a little more time-consuming; it involves consuming a mixture containing seventy-five grams of glucose, then having your blood glucose concentrations measured two hours later. Both of these tests have been shown to strongly predict the future occurrence of cardiovascular events. The 2-hour test appears to be superior in this regard than fasting blood glucose--at least in older subjects--while the deployment of both these tests appears to be the best strategy of all(2-7). However, because it is obviously much more convenient to administer, fasting glucose is by far the most common measure of blood sugar used by doctors.

While the increased cardiovascular mortality risks associated with diabetes are well known, few people are aware of the risks posed by 'pre-diabetic' levels of blood-glucose. Pre-diabetes is currently defined as a fasting glucose level of between 100-125 mg/dl or a 2-hour post-challenge blood glucose level of between 140-199mg/dl (see Table 18a). A vast array of epidemiological studies have confirmed that individuals in these pre-diabetic categories suffer a significantly higher cardiovascular and all-cause mortality rate than those in the normal categories(8-21).

Using data from the third National Health and Nutrition Examination survey (NHANES III), researchers estimate that the current prevalence of diabetes in

Table 18a. Diagnostic thresholds for diabetes and lesser degrees of impaired glucose regulation		
	Test	
Category	Fasting Plasma Glucose	2-hour Plasma Glucose
Normal	<100 mg/dl (<5.6 mmol/l)	<140 mg/dl (<7.8 mmol/l)
Impaired fasting glucose (Pre-diabetes)	100–125 mg/dl (5.6–6.9 mmol/l)	-
Impaired glucose tolerance (Pre-diabetes)	-	140–199 mg/dl (7.8–11.0 mmol/l)
Diabetes	126 mg/dl (7.0 mmol/l)	200 mg/dl (11.1 mmol/l)

Source: The Expert Committee on the Diagnosis and Classification of Diabetes Mellitus: Follow-up Report on the Diagnosis of Diabetes Mellitus *Diabetes Care*, 2003; 26: 3160-3167.

the U.S. is 8.3 percent, affecting around 16.7 million people over the age of twenty years. Of these, twenty-nine percent, or 4.9 million people, are undiagnosed! To make matters worse, an estimated 6.1 percent of the population has impaired fasting glucose, representing 12.3 million people over twenty years old. All up, some twenty-nine million American adults are estimated to have either diabetes or impaired fasting glucose! These figures, by the way, do not include the rapidly growing army of diabetic and pre-diabetic children and teens(22).

To complicate matters even further, several large prospective studies have found that blood glucose levels at the upper end of what is currently considered to be the normal range also raise the risk of cardiovascular and all-cause mortality!

The bottom line is that a significant portion of Americans suffer from elevated blood glucose levels that greatly increase their risk of cardiovascular and all-cause mortality, but do not even know it. By raising awareness amongst this group of their increased susceptibility, and educating them about safe and effective methods for lowering their blood sugar, there exists an opportunity to make huge advances in the battle against cardiovascular disease.

The Deadly Legacy of Elevated Blood Sugar

The longest follow-up study to have ever examined the relationship between fasting blood glucose and cardiovascular mortality in non-diabetic individuals involved 1,973 Norwegian men. All had fasting blood glucose measurements below 110 mg/dl at the start of the study. They were allocated to one of four categories depending on their fasting blood glucose level; 1) 52-73 mg/dl; 2) 74-79 mg/dl; 3) 80-85 mg/dl, or; 4) 86-109 mg/dl.

After twenty-two years, 453 of the men had died, with just over half of these deaths stemming from cardiovascular causes. After adjusting for potential confounding influences, the lowest cardiovascular and overall mortality risks were observed in the 74-79 and 80-85 mg/dl categories. Compared to those whose initial fasting blood glucose levels were less than 89 mg/dl, men with a fasting blood glucose concentration of 89 mg/dl or greater suffered a fifty percent greater risk of cardiovascular death throughout the study!(23)

While the Norwegian study was the longest-running examination of fasting blood glucose levels and mortality, the largest was a project conducted in Texas. It involved over 40,000 men and women from Dallas and San Antonio, who were aged 20 to 82 years and who had their fasting blood sugar levels measured at the start of the study. After an average follow-up of eight years, the cardiovascular and all-cause death rate was lowest in those whose fasting blood glucose was between 80-89 mg/dl. After the researchers adjusted for age, sex and population, however, there was little difference in mortality risk across the 80-109mg/dl range, although the risk was still markedly higher both below and above this range(24).

Among 30,000 European subjects aged 30–89 years and followed-up for eleven years, the lowest cardiovascular mortality risk was observed in subjects with fasting blood glucose levels between 89-98 mg/dl (5.0–5.5 mmol/l), while the lowest risk for overall mortality belonged to subjects with fasting glucose concentrations between 80-89 mg/dl (4.5–5.0 mmol/l). Considering the results of all three studies, the lowest all-cause mortality risk seems to lie with a fasting blood glucose range of 80-89 mg/dl(25).

In contrast to the U-shaped mortality pattern seen with fasting blood glucose, numerous large prospective studies have found that increasing post-load glucose values are accompanied by a linear increase in both cardiovascular and all-cause death rates. All of these studies detected significant increases in CHD, stroke and all-cause mortality at the upper end of what is currently considered the 'normal' range(26).

Why is Elevated Blood Sugar So Dangerous?

High blood sugar promotes CHD in numerous ways; it stimulates free radical activity, reduces vitamin C uptake by our cells, impairs the immune system, decreases levels of nitric oxide in our arteries, inhibits the breakdown of blood clots, and dramatically increases *glycation*, a process in which glucose molecules irreversibly attach themselves to protein and lipid molecules inside the body. Among other things, glycation stimulates further free radical production and results in the formation of *advanced glycosylation end-products* (AGEs), also known as *glycoxidation* products(30).

In normal individuals, there is a gradual and linear accumulation of glycoxidative damage with aging, but this process is greatly accelerated in diabetics, a direct result of their chronically elevated blood sugar levels. Elevated blood sugar levels increase the glycoxidation of collagen in our artery walls, causing them to become increasingly rigid and reducing their ability to properly relax and contract as blood passes through them.

Scientists also believe that when collagen is glycoxidized, any constituent of the bloodstream that enters the vessel wall--such as white blood cells or cholesterol--may bind to this damaged collagen to a greater extent than would normally occur. If these constituents are themselves glycated, then this effect may be amplified even further. Macrophages, which are white blood cells that can enter tissues and engulf foreign invaders, have been shown to bind with AGEs; if transported into the artery wall by macrophages, these AGEs may further increase oxidative damage and inflammatory activity. The end result is dramatically accelerated formation of atherosclerotic plaque. To make matters worse, glycation slows the replication of vascular cells, impeding the body's attempts to repair damage to blood vessel walls.

Those who maintain constantly high levels of blood sugar are thrown into a vicious cycle of escalating cardiovascular damage. Even acute bouts of hyperglycemia produce ominous changes in cardiovascular function. In healthy male volunteers, deliberately induced high blood sugar levels, similar to those observed in poorly controlled diabetics, quickly produce a substantial rise in blood pressure, heart rate, and blood levels of artery-constricting catecholamines(31). Under these circumstances, the ability of arteries to relax and maintain optimal blood flow is impaired(32).

When normal and diabetic subjects are given seventy-five grams of glucose, subsequent blood tests indicate significantly increased formation of thrombin, an enzyme that promotes blood clotting(33). Significant increases in blood free radical activity and decreases in vitamins C and E concentrations are also observed(34-36). When subjects are given water instead, no such change in free radical activity or vitamin status is observed.

In a 1973 study, healthy subjects were fed 100 grams of carbohydrates in the form of glucose, fructose, sucrose, honey or orange juice. When blood was drawn from the subjects and incubated with *Staphylococcus epidermis* bacteria, a significant decrease in the ability of white blood cells to engulf the bacteria was observed. This effect was not seen when subjects ingested starch, which produced a lesser rise in blood glucose than all of the aforementioned sugars (excepting fructose, which has a minimal effect on blood glucose but still causes significant increases in free radical activity and glycation). The suppressive effect of simple sugars upon immune function was still evident five hours after their ingestion!

When another group of subjects fasted for up to sixty hours, causing a progressive decline in blood sugar concentrations, their white blood cells showed a significantly increased ability to devour the bacteria(37).

Those who insist on 'topping up their tank' throughout the day with sugar-rich foods, soft drinks and juices are, in effect, waging a continual assault on their cardiovascular and immune systems.

Blood Sugar Versus Vitamin C

In Chapter 16, we learnt how vitamin C (ascorbic acid) promotes the healthy formation of collagen, which forms the 'backbone' of our arteries. Glucose transporters are proteins found in our cell membranes that, as their name suggests, facilitate the transport of glucose from the bloodstream into the cell. Glucose transporters also perform another extremely important function; they move ascorbic acid from the blood into cells. As such, ascorbic acid and glucose compete with each other for entry into our cells, and when blood sugar levels are high, ascorbic acid is the loser(38). Compared to healthy individuals, concentrations of vitamin C inside cells are reduced by almost a third in diabetics(39). Within two hours of ingesting a solution containing one hundred grams of glucose, both diabetics and healthy folks show significant decreases in intracellular levels of ascorbic acid(40). High blood sugar levels, in effect, starve our cells of vitamin C!

Don't Overlook the Real Enemy

It's a pity so few of us would even have a clue what our fasting blood glucose is, because monitoring one's glucose levels is a far more useful and widely applicable predictor of one's future mortality risk than one's blood cholesterol levels. In elderly subjects, who comprise the bulk of CHD victims, elevated cholesterol levels either have no effect or are in fact associated with *increased* survival and longevity, whereas elevated blood glucose levels are associated with higher death rates in young *and* old alike.

Unlike cholesterol, elevated blood glucose levels are a causal, not secondary, factor in the development of cardiovascular disease. In the Diabetes Control and Complications Trial, early and intensive treatment to keep blood sugar levels close to normal in type 1 diabetics slashed the risk of cardiovascular disease by forty-two percent, and cut the risk of heart attack and stroke by fifty-seven percent--far better results than those achieved by any cholesterol or blood pressure drug!(41)

The administration of a fasting blood glucose test is every bit as quick and simple as obtaining one's blood cholesterol, but the information it yields is infinitely more valuable. Individuals over forty-five should also consider taking the 2-hour blood glucose test, especially if they are overweight. The NHANES III data shows that the 2-hour test will pick up a significant portion of individuals in this group who would otherwise come up clean if they relied only on fasting blood glucose measurements(42).

Achieving Optimal Blood Sugar Levels

The best way to reduce elevated blood glucose is to reduce the excess consumption of its dietary equivalent: carbohydrates. The sad reality is that a major portion of Americans--along with the residents of most other industrialized nations--simply eat and drink too many calories. When a substantial portion of these excess calories are in the form of carbohydrates-- especially of the refined variety--then the likelihood of developing disturbed blood glucose metabolism and subsequent CHD increases sharply.

Back in 1957, it was Professor John Yudkin who first called attention to the fact that national sugar consumption displayed a far stronger epidemiological association with coronary mortality than dietary fat intake(43). More recently, Harvard researchers found that glycemic load--a combined measurement of both the total carbohydrate content of a diet and the glycemic index of the foods in that diet--was a strong predictor of CHD risk. After monitoring over 75,000 women in the Nurses Health Study for ten years, they observed that as dietary glycemic load increased, so too did the incidence of fatal and non-fatal CHD. After adjusting for various potential confounders, it was found that women with the highest dietary glycemic load had twice the CHD risk of those with the lowest glycemic load(44).

USDA food intake data shows that the carbohydrate consumption of Americans declined from the early 1900's to the mid-sixties, at which point it reversed direction and once again began to climb (see Figure 18b). The upward trajectory of carbohydrate intake turned sharply skyward in the early eighties, just as the low-fat, high-carbohydrate propaganda machine began hitting its full stride. Regrettably, most of this increased carbohydrate intake has come, not from fresh fruits and vegetables, but from refined sugars and white flours. The

Figure 18b. Average daily U.S. intake of carbohydrate, fat and protein between 1970-2000.

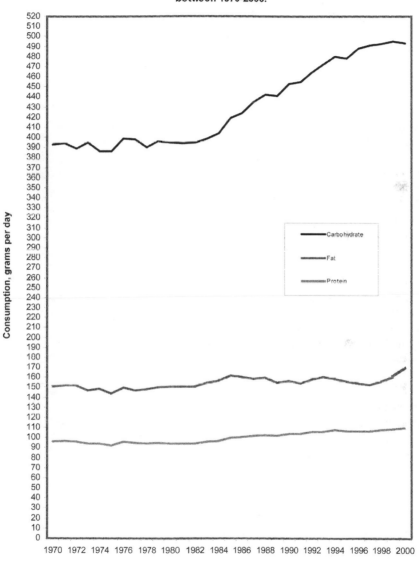

Source: USDA US Food Supply database: http://www.cnpp.usda.gov/nutrient_content.html

consumption of high fructose corn syrup, which is now the most commonly-used sweetener in the U.S. food industry, rose from nil in 1966 to twenty-nine kilograms per person in 2000!(45)

Even the most biased pro-carbohydrate commentator must admit that the campaign to fight heart disease by promoting low-fat, high-carbohydrate "nutrition" has failed miserably. The rise in refined carbohydrate consumption, coupled with a decrease in physical activity, corresponds almost perfectly with the concomitant increase in diabetes and obesity--both of which markedly increase the risk of heart disease. Little wonder that we have seen absolutely no decline in CHD incidence!

The cholesterol-phobic promoters of the pro-carbohydrate paradigm may soon be able to lay claim to another highly dubious achievement--America's first sustained drop in life expectancy in the modern era. In the March 17, 2005 issue of the *New England Journal of Medicine*, a research team headed by S. Jay Olshansky, PhD, from the University of Illinois reported that, if the current runaway rate of obesity and diabetes is not reversed, life expectancy for the average American could decline by as much as five years over the next few decades(46). Richard M. Suzman, Ph.D., Associate Director of the NIA for Behavioral and Social Research notes that an effect on life expectancy may already have begun. The sharp increase of obesity among people now in their sixties, he suggests, may be one reason why recent gains in U.S. life expectancy at older ages have been less than those of other developed countries(47).

Cut the Carbs

Reducing one's carbohydrate consumption, even when overall calorie intake is maintained, lowers blood glucose and improves numerous other indices of glycemic control, including daylong and post-meal glucose levels, excessive insulin secretion, and loss of insulin sensitivity.

High-carbohydrate diets can produce improvements in blood sugar control if overall caloric intake is reduced to levels that induce weight loss. In head to head comparisons, however, the research consistently shows that calorie-restricted low- and moderate-carbohydrate diets do a better job of restoring glycemic control than similarly-restricted high-carbohydrate diets. The greatest improvements of all are seen on low-carbohydrate diets(48-59).

Clinical studies have repeatedly shown that when people reduce their calorie intake, they experience improvements not only in blood sugar control, but also weight loss, blood pressure and blood markers of inflammatory activity. In animal studies, calorie-restriction repeatedly reduces cancer incidence and even extends overall life span.

There's just one wee problem with deliberate calorie-restriction--few of us are willing to do it for any length of time! After all, it involves eating less food, something that most of us deep down inside simply do not want to do.

While the short-term efficacy of calorie-restricted weight loss diets has been well documented in clinical research, their long-term track record is dismal. More often than not these diets draw us into a battle with some very formidable opponents, including ravenous hunger, temptation, and the evolutionary-programmed urge to eat up during times of abundance in order to compensate for periods of food scarcity.

This is where low-carbohydrate diets have been shown to possess another valuable advantage. In many clinical trials comparing high and low carbohydrate diets, individuals following the former were explicitly instructed to restrict their overall caloric intake in order to induce weight loss, while those on the low-carbohydrate diets were instructed only to restrict carbohydrate intake. Despite having no limitations placed on protein, fat or overall calorie intake, these low-carbohydrate dieters have typically reduced overall calorie intake to similar or lower levels as high-carbohydrate dieters intentionally restricting overall calories!(60-64) Among the reasons for this unintentional calorie-restriction effect are: 1) the clinically-demonstrated satiety value of increased protein intake; 2) a superior stabilizing effect on blood sugar levels, which helps to avert the hunger pangs of reactive hypoglycemia, and; 3) a shift by the body towards the increased utilization of fat, a more stable and longer-lasting fuel source than glucose.

So what kind of fasting blood glucose reductions can one expect after commencing a calorie-restricted low-carbohydrate diet? The following studies give us some indication:

- Atherosclerotic patients placed on an 1800-calorie high-fat, low-carbohydrate diet, consisting of meat, eggs, fresh fruit, and non-starchy vegetables, observed a reduction in average fasting glucose from 106.1 mg/dl (5.9 mmol/l) to 98.3 mg/dl (5.5 mmol/l) after only six weeks(65).
- A study of 102 obese males and females found that twelve weeks of a diet containing 80-100 grams of protein, but only 20-30 grams of carbohydrates, reduced average fasting glucose levels from 126 mg/dl (7.0 mmol/l) to 96 mg/dl (5.4 mmol/l). In other words, three months on a low-carbohydrate diet reduced fasting blood glucose levels from the diabetic category back into the normal range!(66)
- One of the most tightly controlled dietary intervention studies was conducted with obese volunteers who received dietary treatment whilst staying in a hospital ward. The average fasting blood glucose of these individuals was at the high end of the normal range, but was reduced further after six weeks of either a fifteen percent or forty-five percent carbohydrate

diet (both containing 1,000 calories per day), and two hours of exercise per day. Subjects on the low-carb diet reduced their fasting blood glucose from an initial 95 mg/dl (5.3 mmol/l) to 79 mg/dl after six weeks, while those on the forty-five percent carbohydrate diet reduced their blood sugar levels from 96 mg/dl (5.4 mmol/l) to 89 mg/dl (5.0 mmol/l). The low-carbohydrate group also experienced significantly greater reductions in fasting insulin, indicating superior overall glycemic control in the low-carbohydrate group(67).

- In hyperinsulinemic men, fasting blood glucose levels were reduced from 97.6 mg/dl (5.5 mmol/l) to 89.6 mg/dl (5.0 mmol/l) after four weeks of a twenty-five percent carbohydrate diet, but were virtually unchanged in a group who followed a fifty-eight percent carbohydrate diet for the same period(68).

- After six months on a thirty-seven percent carbohydrate, forty-one percent fat weight-loss diet, fasting blood glucose among diabetic subjects fell an average 26 mg/dl compared to only 5 mg/dl among those following a fifty-one percent carbohydrate, thirty-three percent fat diet(69).

It should be mentioned that, while high-carbohydrate diets can improve glycemic control at reduced calorie intakes, albeit on a lesser scale than low-carbohydrate diets, they consistently *worsen* blood glucose metabolism when consumed at maintenance-level calorie intakes in both diabetic and healthy individuals. Carbohydrate-restricted diets, in contrast, continue to exert favorable effects on glycemic control even when overall calorie intake is not reduced(70-75).

When diabetic subjects, most of whom were using oral blood-sugar lowering drugs, were placed on a maintenance-calorie diet containing only twenty-five percent carbohydrate for eight weeks, their fasting blood glucose dropped from a hefty average of 262 mg/dl down to 172 mg/dl. When they were subsequently placed on a fifty-five percent carbohydrate diet for twelve weeks, their fasting glucose shot back up to 231 mg/dl(76).

To reduce elevated blood sugar levels and improve overall glycemic control:

- Eat a moderate- to low-carbohydrate diet. Obtain the bulk of these carbohydrates from low and 'No' glycemic, nutrient-rich vegetables and fresh fruits (see Chapter 26 for details on how to construct a healthy reduced-carbohydrate diet);
- Exercise regularly;
- Maintain healthy sleeping habits;
- Do your utmost to minimize the amount and impact of stress in your life;
- Be especially vigilant to avoid stress during and after eating (see Chapter 14).

Chapter 19

"Tell me what you eat, and I will tell you what you are."
Anthelme Brillat Savarin

A Matter of Fats

Why the type of fat you eat is far more important than the amount.

It is extremely ironic that the two most vilified macronutrients in modern history--protein and fat--have been clearly identified by scientists as absolutely essential to human health. While scientists have yet to unearth an 'essential' dietary carbohydrate, they have indeed discovered *essential fatty acids* and *essential amino acids.* Without a steady dietary supply of the latter two, the maintenance of good health is virtually impossible.

The essential fatty acids (EFAs) are those that belong to the polyunsaturated family of fats, and are known as *omega-6* and *omega-3* fatty acids. The main omega-6 fatty acids are *linoleic acid* (LA) and *arachidonic acid* (AA). LA occurs naturally in a wide variety of plant and animal foods, including meat, poultry, eggs, nuts, seeds and grains, while AA can only be found in animal foods. The major sources of omega-6 fatty acids in today's Western diet are polyunsaturated vegetable oils, such as those derived from soy, corn, sunflower, safflower, cottonseed and peanut.

Omega-3 fats are also found in both animal and plant foods. The omega-3 *alpha-linolenic acid* (ALA) is found in foods such as walnuts, flaxseeds, pumpkin seeds and meats. Animal tissues can also contain several other types of omega-3 fatty acids, the two most important being *docosahexanoic acid* (DHA) and *eicosapentanoic acid* (EPA). While the most concentrated dietary source of DHA and EPA is brain tissue, the best-known source is fatty fish.

While ALA must be obtained from the diet, DHA and EPA can be produced inside the body using ALA as the raw material. Unfortunately, the conversion rate is pitifully low. Only six percent of ALA is converted to EPA and a meager four percent is converted to DHA--and that's with a favorable background diet high in saturated fat, which improves the conversion rate. On a diet rich in omega-6 fatty acids--the kind of diet most Westerners eat--the elongation of ALA into EPA and DHA is reduced by forty to fifty percent!(1,2)

While polyunsaturated fats are absolutely vital for human health, they are required only in very small amounts. Many lipid researchers believe they should comprise no more than 4.5 percent of our total daily calorie intake. Furthermore, omega-6 and omega-3 fatty acids are required by the body in roughly equal amounts.

In addition to a dramatic increase in refined carbohydrate intake, the last one hundred years has seen a steep rise in the consumption of polyunsaturated vegetable fats. This increase in polyunsaturates has come almost entirely from linoleic acid-rich vegetable oils and margarines. The consumption of omega-3-rich foods during this same period, however, has remained low. The end result is an excessive intake of omega-6 fats, a woefully inadequate intake of omega-3 fats, and a striking departure from the ideal ratio of omega-3 to omega-6 fats.

Analysis of primitive hunter-gatherer diets reveals that the average omega-6 to omega-3 ratio fell somewhere between 1:1 and 3:1. The typical standard Western diet features a ratio of 15:1 or more, a huge departure from that consumed by our ancestors! This imbalance is compounded by the fact that, inside our bodies, a high intake of omega-6 fatty acids actively inhibits the absorption of omega-3 fatty acids, causing our cells to become desperately starved of the latter(3,4). To understand what this all means for our cardiovascular health, we need to take a quick look at the all-important *eicosanoids*.

Eicosanoids: Tiny But Powerful

Eicosanoids are a class of lipids produced by our cells that possess potent hormone-like functions. Unlike other hormones (such as testosterone, estrogen or insulin) that are produced in one gland and then distributed throughout the body, eicosanoids act locally, influencing only the cells from which they originated and those nearby. Their localized influence--and the surprising lack of attention awarded to them by much of the research community--belies their universal importance. These metabolic mighty-mites exert a decisive influence on virtually all of the physiological processes that take place inside our bodies.

There are number of different types of eicosanoids, including *prostaglandins, thromboxanes* and *leukotrienes*. Some of these eicosanoids possess anti-inflammatory, artery-dilating and blood-thinning functions, while others have the exact opposite effect.

Because of their extreme importance and their widely differing functions, our well-being at any given moment is hugely dependent on the balance between these different types of eicosanoids. Thromboxanes are powerful instigators of blood clotting and arterial constriction, both lifesaving functions that prevent excessive blood loss when we cut or injure ourselves. If thromboxane production and activity becomes excessive, however, this group of eicosanoids quickly turns from friend to foe by increasing the risk of cardiovascular disease.

Thromboxanes are antagonistic to a prostaglandin known as *prostacyclin*, or PGI2, which inhibits blood clotting and is a powerful artery dilator. An imbalance between PGI2 and TXA2, the most potent of the thromboxanes, in favor of the latter will actively foster the initiation of inflammation, blood clot formation and arterial constriction.

Dietary Fats and Eicosanoids

For those wondering why I am discussing eicosanoids in a chapter about dietary fats, here's the critical link: the raw material for eicosanoid production comes from the fatty acids contained within our cell membranes, which in turn are derived from the polyunsaturated fatty acids (PUFA) we consume in our diets. Higher dietary intakes of a specific EFA--such as the omega-6 LA--leads to a higher concentration of that fatty acid in the cell membrane. The increased accumulation of this EFA occurs at the expense of other fatty acids--such as those belonging to the omega-3 family(5).

A proper ratio of omega-3 to omega-6 fatty acids, similar to that which we humans evolved on, results in a healthy balance of the various types of eicosanoids. An excess of omega-6 intake, however, suppresses the production of anti-inflammatory and vasodilatory eicosanoids like PGI2, while boosting the activity of pro-inflammatory, thrombotic and vasocontrictive eicosanoids like TXA2. The bottom line is that the typical Western diet--with its high intake of omega-6 fats and low intake of omega-3 fats--promotes excessive thromboxane formation, raising the risk of arterial spasm, blood clot formation and even cardiac arrhythmia(5,6).

The Real 'Artery-Clogging' Fat

While we have been warned beyond counting that saturated fat is an 'artery-clogger', scientists have shown that the fatty acids found within atheromas are predominantly of the 'heart-healthy' *unsaturated* variety. That's right--over fifty percent of the fatty acids in advanced atherosclerotic plaques are polyunsaturated, thirty percent are monounsaturated, and only twenty percent are saturated! When compared to normal arterial tissue, advanced plaque in the aorta contains a higher proportion of the omega-6 LA(7). These higher levels of LA in aortic plaque are reflected by similarly elevated levels in the patients' adipose tissue and blood, indicating a high dietary intake. No such correlation between the fatty acid content of plaque, blood and adipose tissue is observed for saturated fats(8).

What's more, researchers have found that the higher the LA content of atheromas, the greater the likelihood that their fibrous cap will rupture. As we discovered in Chapter 13, plaque rupture is the instigating factor that triggers a significant portion of heart attacks(9).

In a double blind, randomized trial reported in a 2003 issue of *The Lancet*, patients destined to undergo carotid endarterectomy (surgical removal of an advanced atherosclerotic plaque from the carotid artery) were randomized to consume either six grams of sunflower oil, fish oil or a placebo until surgery (the placebo was an 80:20 mix of palm and soybean oils; both sunflower and soy oils are rich in LA). The fish oil intervention supplied 1.4 grams of EPA plus DHA per day, and the median duration of treatment was 42 days. Even in this short time frame, the proportions of EPA and DHA became higher in the carotid plaques of the fish oil group than in either of the other two groups. In addition to being studied for their fatty acid content, carotid plaques were removed from fifty patients in each treatment group, and then graded according to the thickness of their fibrous caps. The researchers found that plaques from patients treated with fish oil were more likely to possess a thick fibrous cap, rather than a thin inflamed cap, when compared to those from the sunflower or placebo oil groups(10). This finding is of great importance because a thicker, more fibrous cap on an atheroma is less likely to rupture and instigate a life-threatening coronary event than a thinner, more fragile cap.

As Omega-3 Consumption Rises, CHD Decreases

It should comes as little surprise then, that in countries like Japan where dietary intake of omega-3 fats is higher than that seen in America, the CHD rate is much lower. Studies of the Greenland Eskimos have detected not only one of the highest average omega-3 intakes in the world, but an age-adjusted prevalence of CHD even lower than that of the Japanese(11).

It should also be of little surprise to learn that randomized clinical trials using omega-3-rich fish and/or fish oil supplements have shown substantial reductions in mortality amongst those with a prior history of CHD. The earliest of such trials was the Diet And Reinfarction Trial, which reported a twenty-nine percent reduction in all-cause mortality over a two-year period amongst male heart attack survivors who were advised to increase their intake of oily fish(12).

In a massive Italian trial, half of over 11,000 recent heart attack patients were randomly assigned to receive a dose of fish oil that supplied around 900 milligrams per day of EPA and DHA. They began experiencing reductions in both cardiovascular and total mortality only a few months into the trial. After 3.5 years, the modest dose of fish oil reduced the relative risk of cardiovascular mortality by twenty percent, and the risk of all-cause mortality by fifteen percent, a result comparable to that seen in similar-sized statin drug trials. The survival advantage in the fish oil group, by the way, had nothing to do with cholesterol lowering; after six months there was an increase in total cholesterol and LDL levels, which slowly returned towards initial values by the end of the follow-up period!(13)

Trans Fatty Acids--The Man-Made Mutant Fats

Thanks to cholesterol-phobia, there exists yet another class of industrially altered fats that have become extremely popular during the last century. These are the solidified vegetable fats found in margarines and shortenings that have been subjected to a process known as *hydrogenation*. During the production of margarines and shortenings, hydrogen gas is squeezed into liquid vegetable oils during an extensive manufacturing process, one that involves the use of extremely high temperatures, bleaches, dyes, and flavors. The result is a newly hardened, or hydrogenated, fat that supposedly constitutes a more wholesome alternative to butter.

Naturally occurring unsaturated fatty acids are characterized by a bent shape that gives oil its liquid consistency at room temperature. These natural unsaturated fatty acids are known as *cis fatty acids*, and these cis fats are incorporated into our cell membranes. During the hydrogenation process, the structure of unsaturated cis fatty acids is re-arranged, producing an unnaturally straight configuration. These artificially straightened fats are known as *trans fatty acids*. When we consume hydrogenated fats, cis fatty acids in our cell membranes are displaced by these unnatural *trans* fatty acids. Our cell membranes, in effect, become partially hydrogenated! The result is impaired function of the all-important cellular receptors on the membrane surface, the gatekeepers that regulate the entry of vital nutrients into the cells.

Research with both animals and humans suggests that the *trans* fatty acids found in processed vegetable fats contribute to some of our most common degenerative diseases, including heart disease. When a group of initially healthy Dutch men, aged sixty-four to eighty-four years, were followed for ten years it was observed that *trans* fatty acid intake was positively associated with the occurrence of CHD(14). Like most prospective examinations, this association was based upon a dietary survey given to the participants at baseline. However, studies examining blood and tissue concentrations of trans fatty acids, which accurately reflect dietary intake, have also detected an increased risk of CHD from the consumption of these 'bizzarro' fats.

Researchers in Seattle, Washington analyzed the trans fatty acid content of red blood cell membranes in first-time heart attack victims, and compared the results with samples obtained from healthy volunteers. Higher cell membrane levels of *trans linoleic acid* were associated with a three-fold increase in the risk of cardiac arrest(15). University of Oslo researchers similarly found adipose tissue levels of both *trans* and plant-derived polyunsaturated fatty acids to be higher in those suffering a first heart attack(16).

In experimental studies, subjects fed margarine made from hydrogenated soybean oil experienced increased production of *interleukin-6* and *tumor necrosis factor alpha*--both pro-inflammatory agents involved in the promotion of atherosclerosis. Subjects consuming the same number of calories from non-hydrogenated soybean oil or saturated fats did not experience these negative changes(17). In another study, female subjects were fed diets high in partially hydrogenated oils, polyunsaturated fats, or palm oil in a randomly alternating fashion. Levels of *tissue plasminogen activator* (tPA), a naturally occurring anti-clotting substance that is also used as a life-saving drug immediately after heart attack occurrence, decreased significantly on the partially-hydrogenated oil diet. Levels of tPA, by the way, remained highest on the palm oil diet--the diet highest in saturated fat(18).

Laboratory experiments conducted by lipid researcher Fred Kummerow show that *trans* fats increase the calcification of the endothelial cells that line our arteries--a hallmark development in atherosclerosis. He found that magnesium blocked this reaction, and concluded that trans fat consumption combined with dietary magnesium deficiencies--a common characteristic of modern diets--may accelerate the development of arterial plaque(19).

In another experiment, Kummerow and his team found that sows fed a diet of ten percent hydrogenated fat during pregnancy and lactation gave birth to piglets whose aortic cell membranes contained a significantly higher concentration of LA than piglets from sews fed butterfat or small amounts of corn oil(20). Hardly a positive development, given what we know about the harmful effects of excess LA on eicosanoid activity.

Trans fats have been repeatedly shown to raise blood levels of lipoprotein-(a), a potentially atherogenic substance receiving increasing attention from researchers. Researchers have also observed that trans fats tend to increase LDL and lower HDL cholesterol levels, a change allegedly associated with an increased risk of heart disease(21). Ironically, the saturated fats that health officials continually berate actually lower lipoprotein (a) and raise HDL, leading some researchers to suggest that margarine should be reformulated from highly-saturated tropical fats like palm and coconut oil!(22)

Trans Fats--Man Made Versus Natural

Trans fats occur in miniscule quantities in nature. They are formed in the rumen of cattle, and small amounts can be found in milk and meat. In contrast to man-made *trans* fats, the natural *trans* fatty acids found in milk and meat may actually be a boon to health. The *trans* fat *conjugated linoleic acid*, for example has been shown to exert anti-cancer effects in animals and appears to slightly enhance fat loss and muscle gain in humans.
Unfortunately, the overwhelming majority of *trans* fatty acids in the modern diet are derived from hydrogenated oils, and the wide array of foods to which these fats are added. Because of their ubiquitous presence in the food supply,

the average American now takes in around eight to fifteen grams of trans fats daily. Some of the commonly consumed foods containing hydrogenated fats include fried foods, baked goods, frozen dinners, chips, cookies, crackers, pastries, cake mixes, and peanut butter. Refined liquid polyunsaturated oils that have undergone high temperature processing--i.e. virtually all commercially available oils--also contain trans fats and are found in many, many more food items.

Destructive Legacy

The excess consumption of omega-6 polyunsaturated fats is yet another destructive legacy of the irrational anti-saturated fat bias of health authorities. For years, they enthusiastically urged us to consume omega-6-rich vegetable oils in place of animal and tropical oils. When increasing evidence began to mount that these oils did not prevent heart disease, but may in fact cause CHD and cancer, these same authorities quietly altered their dietary guidelines to recommend no more than ten percent of calories be consumed as polyunsaturated fats.

The ten percent limit on polyunsaturated fats nominated by the AHA may still be too high; rodent studies have shown these oils can induce tumor development at relatively low thresholds, and lipid researchers believe that no more than 4.5 percent of calories should come from polyunsaturates(23,24). Furthermore, the reasons for the guideline changes were never explained to the public. As a result, millions of people continue to consume polyunsaturated vegetable oils in complete ignorance of their potentially dangerous qualities. In order to maintain a favorable EFA ratio and avoid the harmful effects of trans fatty acids:

- Avoid polyunsaturated vegetable oils and the numerous foods in which they are found--all the omega-6 fats you need can be obtained from fresh whole foods like meats, eggs, nuts, and seeds.
- Be sure to consume long-chain omega-3 fats on a regular basis. Given that the richest sources of long-chain omega-3's--brains and fatty fish--are items that are not regularly consumed by most Americans, and the concern about contamination of seafood with environmental pollutants, the easiest and safest way to achieve regular omega-3 intake is via fish oil supplementation.
- Avoid packaged foods that contain the words 'vegetable oil', 'hydrogenated' or 'partially hydrogenated' on their labels.

Now it's time to learn about a substance that most people know little about, one that plays a pivotal role in the health of our arteries.

Chapter 20

"There is nothing so powerful as truth,--and often nothing so strange."
Daniel Webster

Just Say Yes to NO

Why your arteries can't live without nitric oxide.

At first glance, nitric oxide (NO) sounds like the last thing you would want inside your body. It is found in automobile exhaust fumes and plays a major role in the formation of smog. When encountered externally, it is a highly reactive gas that irritates the lungs and causes nasty chemical burns. NO formed within our bodies, however, is an entirely different animal.

Inside the body, NO facilitates healthy nerve, immune, kidney, and gastrointestinal function. It helps women give birth by relaxing the uterus. During sexual arousal, NO enables the blood vessels of the penis to dilate, allowing an influx of blood that results in an erection. Indeed, the popular impotence drug Viagra works by inhibiting the breakdown of NO. This unlikely gas also plays a monumentally important role in proper cardiovascular function.

NO: An Artery's Best Friend

NO is formed thanks to the actions of nitric oxide synthase (NOS), an enzyme found in endothelial cells--the cells that line the surface of our blood vessels(1). NOS converts L-arginine, an amino acid found in meats, nuts, fish, eggs and cheese, to NO. Once formed, this vital gas then goes on to perform a number of critical functions that help to keep our cardiovascular systems in peak working order. If NO levels in our arteries decline and remain at sub-optimal levels, then heart disease and stroke become increasingly likely outcomes.

One of NO's functions is to relax the muscle cells found in the walls of arteries. Endothelium-derived NO, in fact, is the most potent natural vasodilator known. With each pulsation of blood, the endothelial cells release a puff of NO. This NO diffuses into the underlying muscle cells, causing them to relax and thus allowing blood to easily pass through the vessel. Nitroglycerine, which is often prescribed for angina pain, delivers its benefits by generating nitric oxide, which relaxes the walls of the coronary arteries and arterioles.

NO also blocks the release of inflammatory substances from endothelial cells, making it a potent inhibitor of inflammation in blood vessels. In addition, NO produced by endothelial cells diffuses into the bloodstream, where it inhibits the aggregation of blood platelets and thus prevents inappropriate clotting.

Dysfunctional Arteries

One of the earliest occurrences during the development of CHD is what researchers refer to as 'endothelial dysfunction'. This arises when endothelial cells begin to abandon their beneficial activities, such as promoting arterial relaxation, impairing excessive blood clot formation, inhibiting the proliferation of smooth muscle cells within the artery, and limiting the permeability of the artery wall in order to prevent entry by unwanted visitors. Instead, endothelial cells turn into malfunctioning entities that promote arterial stiffness, blood clot formation, and smooth muscle cell accumulation. Dysfunctional endothelial cells also act like magnets for inflammation-promoting white blood cells, drawing them from the bloodstream into the artery wall. In light of the above, one might expect to see an increase in both atherosclerosis and acute coronary events when NO levels decline. That is exactly the case.

Low NO levels are a strong predictor of CHD risk. In a study of patients referred for cardiac catheterization, those who suffered an acute coronary event within two weeks of their examination had markedly lower NO production by blood platelets than patients with stable or no angina. After adjustment for other confounders, low NO levels imparted a four-fold risk of suffering an acute coronary episode. In the patients with angiographically-proven atherosclerosis, low platelet NO production was again associated with a four times greater risk of an acute coronary syndrome, whereas extent of atherosclerosis was not. Cholesterol levels, by the way, were not an independent predictor of risk(2).

In healthy people, infusion of the neurotransmitter *acetylcholine* into the bloodstream causes arteries to widen, but in patients with artery disease, the exact opposite occurs--arteries constrict and even go into spasm. Acetylcholine infusion is thus often used as a test of arterial function and to measure blood flow in clinical research. When researchers administered acetylcholine to CHD-free individuals, CHD patients with mild arterial narrowing, and CHD patients with severe artery blockage, the neurotransmitter produced the expected vasodilation in the healthy controls. In the CHD patients with mild arterial impairment, acetylcholine produced artery constriction in all but one patient. Among those with severe arterial obstruction, vasoconstriction was observed in every instance, and five of the eight patients suffered from arterial spasm that temporarily blocked blood flow. When given NO-boosting nitroglycerin, however, all the subjects' arteries underwent dilation(3).

Such findings strongly suggest that deficient NO production acts as a direct precursor of acute coronary events such as angina episodes and potentially fatal heart attacks.

Additionally, these findings may help explain why obstructive sleep apnea, which temporarily deprives the body of NO, increases the risk of cardiovascular disease(4). The cardiovascular damage arising from low NO levels also goes a long way towards explaining the link between erectile dysfunction and increased CHD risk. Penile tissue, after all, relies on a good dose of NO in order to achieve erection. In a study of 260 diabetic men, the prevalence of erectile dysfunction was significantly higher in patients with silent coronary artery disease than in those free of CHD (33.8 percent versus 4.7 percent)(5). In another study, CHD patients with one occluded artery had more frequent and firmer erections, and fewer difficulties achieving an erection, than men with two or three narrowed arteries(6).

Measuring NO

One way of gauging NO levels in the body is to measure blood levels of *asymmetric dimethylarginine* (ADMA)(7). ADMA inhibits the production of NO from L-arginine, and is elevated in patients with endothelial dysfunction and atherosclerosis(8).

In young, clinically asymptomatic adults, high ADMA levels were a significant independent predictor of impaired endothelial function, whereas triglycerides, blood pressure, and total, LDL and HDL cholesterol were not(9). In patients with angina and positive exercise stress tests, coronary angiography showed that higher blood levels of ADMA and lower levels of L-arginine were associated with more severe atherosclerosis(10).

Among 116 middle-aged subjects with no symptoms of coronary artery disease, increasing blood levels of ADMA were significantly correlated with greater carotid artery thickness, as measured by high-resolution ultrasonography. Plasma ADMA was not associated with triglycerides or total, LDL or HDL cholesterol(11).

In patients with kidney failure, cardiovascular disease is a common cause of death. When Italian researchers followed 225 dialysis patients for almost three years, sixty-four percent of subsequent deaths were from cardiovascular causes. Blood ADMA concentrations were a strong and independent predictor of overall mortality and cardiovascular outcome(12).

When Your Body Says No to NO

What causes NO levels to drop, you ask?

Free radicals.

Yes, those nasty little critters that directly attack our tissues also cause mayhem by depleting our bodies of NO. Free radicals directly inactivate NO, and they also convert NOS from an enzyme that converts L-arginine into NO into one that simply creates more free radicals!(13)

Our body is equipped with several key antioxidant enzymes that eliminate NO-depleting free radicals. Unfortunately, these can readily be exhausted by such factors as poor dietary habits, high blood sugar levels, and cigarette smoking. When concentrations of these vitally important antioxidant enzymes are deficient, then endothelial cell dysfunction and its resultant consequences are a virtual certainty. Luckily, there are several things we can do to bump up the levels of NO in our arteries.

Reason # 5,632 Why You Should Exercise Regularly

Exercise is well documented to reverse endothelial dysfunction, improve arterial blood flow, and even prevent excessive blood clot formation(14). Exercise also causes HDL cholesterol levels to rise while total and LDL cholesterol levels fall, leading many researchers to assume that it lowers CHD risk by lowering cholesterol. Again, they're wrong. By imposing moderate sheer stress on the vascular walls, exercise stimulates the release of NO. After as little as twelve weeks, the paradoxical vasoconstriction induced by acetylcholine in CHD patients is attenuated, blood flow improves, blood pressure is lowered, and antioxidant defenses are substantially bolstered(15,16). In hypertensive patients, exercise also lowers blood pressure(17).

In an experiment with atherosclerosis-prone mice given an NOS inhibitor, arterial lesion formation increased over 270 percent in those that remained sedentary. The mice that ran on a treadmill twice daily for an hour at a time, however, had a rate of lesion formation similar to those not given the NOS antagonist(18). In obese women with endothelial dysfunction, a one-year weight loss program of exercise, diet and behavioral counseling resulted in a minimum ten percent reduction in initial body weight. Accompanying this favorable body composition change was a substantial drop in inflammatory white blood cell levels and a dramatic improvement in endothelial function. In fact, after one year, a three-gram dose of L-arginine was able to elicit the same artery-widening response in the obese subjects as that seen in lean control subjects(19).

Obese men who undertake a similar program may receive an unexpected but very welcome side benefit. As part of a randomized clinical trial, fifty-five obese men with erectile difficulties lost weight by dieting and exercising and experienced improvements in penile function. No significant improvement was noted in the control group. After two years, seventeen men in the intervention group no longer met the criteria for erectile dysfunction compared to only three of the control subjects(20). Losing excess weight can benefit a whole lot more than just your arteries!

Eat Your Antioxidants

Increases in NO levels may largely explain the reduced CHD risk produced by diets high in antioxidant-rich non-cereal plant foods. When healthy subjects consumed high doses of purple grape juice for fourteen days, blood platelet-derived NO production increased by an impressive 170 percent. Blood antioxidant activity rose, superoxide radical formation decreased, and blood platelet aggregation was inhibited, indicating that the antioxidants found in purple grapes reduce the risk of blood clot formation(21).

Vitamin E is a potent antioxidant found in especially high amounts in nuts and seeds. The vitamin E found in these foods is made up of a variety of compounds known as *tocopherols* and *tocotrienols,* and is especially high in gamma-tocopherol. Commercially available vitamin E supplements, on the other hand, contain predominantly alpha-tocopherol. When researchers compared the effects of a mixed tocopherol supplement that was high in gamma-tocopherol with an alpha-tocopherol supplement and a placebo, they found that both of the vitamin E supplements increased NO levels in healthy adults. The mixed tocopherol supplement, however, produced greater increases in NO and was also more effective in preventing blood platelets from clumping together(22). These findings may explain why most clinical trials using alpha-tocopherol supplements have failed to reduce cardiovascular mortality. The highest concentrations of gamma-tocopherol can be found in sesame seeds, pecans, walnuts, pistachios and pumpkin seeds. Pine nuts, brazils and cashews also contain respectable amounts.

Human and animal experiments indicate that regular garlic intake may inhibit blood clotting and impair atherosclerotic plaque formation(23-25). In healthy adults aged 50 to 80 years, aortic stiffness increased by a significantly lower amount among those who took at least 300 milligrams of a standardized garlic powder daily for two years compared to matched control subjects who did not take garlic(26). Elevations in NO levels may help explain the pungent bulb's beneficial cardiovascular properties; incubation of human tissues with garlic extract has shown it to increase nitric oxide synthase activity(27).

Blood Sugar and NO

In laboratory experiments, glucose directly attacks NO when it is exposed to human endothelial cells at levels similar to those seen in the blood of diabetic patients(28). Lab studies also show that increased glycation (resulting from elevated blood sugar levels) causes red blood cells to bind more tightly with NO, preventing it from exerting its beneficial anti-clotting and artery-relaxing effects(29).

In studies with real live human subjects, high blood sugar levels quickly lower NO activity and produce rapid deterioration of endothelial function. When acute hyperglycemia was deliberately induced in healthy subjects via a glucose infusion, it took only thirty minutes for significant increases in blood pressure, heart rate, blood catecholamines, and platelet aggregation to occur, while blood viscosity significantly increased by sixty minutes. Blood flow in the legs was also measured, and found to be significantly impaired after ninety minutes(30).

To maintain healthy NO levels, keep your blood sugar level in the normal range. If it is high, use a carbohydrate-restricted diet (and the appropriate medication if necessary) to bring it back under control.

Cigarette Smoking: Just Say NO

If any of you reading this happen to smoke cigarettes--*stop!* Yes, I know, it's easier said than done, but do it--any way you can! Along with becoming diabetic, obese, alcoholic or highly stressed, cigarette smoking ranks as one of the worst possible things you can do for your health.

After smoking a single cigarette, blood concentrations of NO plummet, as do the concentrations of important antioxidants like ascorbic acid, cysteine, methionine, and uric acid. They do not return to normal until sixty minutes later, so it is little wonder that cigarette smokers exhibit lower NO release, increased susceptibility to artery constriction and blood clotting, excessive free radical activity, greater adhesion of white blood cells to the vascular wall, and a frightening 250 percent jump in cardiovascular disease risk(31-39).

These detrimental effects of smoking are also observed in passive smokers, albeit to a lesser extent. Despite a strikingly consistent epidemiological relationship between passive smoking and cardiovascular disease, apologists for the tobacco industry claim that the link is still controversial(40-43). Don't be fooled; young adults exposed to environmental tobacco smoke display significantly impaired endothelium-mediated blood flow when compared to non-passive smokers. The extent of impairment is directly related to the degree of exposure to secondhand smoke(44).

To ascertain the effects of passive smoking on antioxidant defenses and free radical activity, Finnish researchers analyzed blood samples collected from healthy, nonsmoking subjects before and after spending thirty minutes in a smoke-free area or in a room for smokers. This relatively brief exposure to environmental smoke caused an acute decrease in blood ascorbic acid and antioxidant activity, increased LDL oxidation, and evidence of increased lipid peroxidation(45). Researchers from the New York University Medical Center found that cockerels exposed to concentrations of environmental smoke equal to or even below that seen in bars experience accelerated arteriosclerotic plaque development(46).

The good news is that by throwing your cigarettes away and abandoning this destructive habit for good, you body quickly begins to reverse the damage caused by smoking. Japanese researchers have shown that smoking cessation leads to almost immediate improvements in NO levels and blood platelet function. They took twenty-seven healthy male medical students who smoked at least fifteen cigarettes per day for more than five years and randomly divided them into two groups. One group quit smoking for four weeks, while the second group quit for two weeks, but then resumed smoking at day fourteen. In both groups, blood platelet function and NO status significantly improved throughout the nonsmoking phase. In the group that resumed smoking at day fourteen, however, NO levels quickly returned to baseline levels, as did the tendency for platelets to clump together(47).

Chinese researchers found that blood samples from smokers showed initially significantly higher free radical concentrations at baseline, but after a year of complete smoking cessation these levels were no longer significantly different from those seen in non-smoking control subjects(48).

These improvements could quite literally save your life. In 2000, the *Archives of Internal Medicine* published a pooled analysis of prospective studies that examined the effect of smoking cessation after heart attack. A dozen studies, ranging in length from two to ten years and involving data from almost 6,000 patients in six countries, were included in the review. All twelve studies found that, on average, those who quit smoking after a heart attack nearly halved their risk of dying from a subsequent coronary episode when compared to those who kept smoking. The mortality benefit was consistent regardless of gender, duration of follow-up, location, and time period(49).

Keep Your NO Gas Tank Full

Compared to the gigantic amount of attention lavished upon cholesterol since the 1950's, serious research into the cardiovascular effects of NO is a relatively recent phenomenon. Most people, including many medical and health practitioners, are completely unaware of the pivotal role this colorless gas plays in ensuring healthy cardiovascular function. Anything that depletes your body of NO is likely to increase your risk of heart disease and stroke, so be sure to keep your NO gas tank full by eating antioxidant-rich foods, exercising regularly, keeping your blood sugar level in the normal range, and avoiding the hell out of cigarette smoke.

Chapter 21

"Science is not just an end result, but an ongoing process of change and the willingness to reevaluate old beliefs (theories) in the light of new information."
Tom Billings

The Infection Connection

Do infections cause heart disease?

In the days before sanitation, hygiene, and antibiotic use became commonplace, infection was the most prolific cause of death. Nowadays, when most people think of infections they tend to think of nasty short-term afflictions that can leave one feeling pretty rotten, but pose little long-term threat if attended to promptly. Thanks to some rather surprising new research findings, this mindset is currently undergoing a major shake-up.

A rapidly-expanding volume of research is implicating common infectious agents--including the respiratory bug *Chlamydia pnuemoniae,* the ulcer-causing *Helicobacter pylori* bacteria, herpes viruses such as cytomegalovirus and *Herpes simplex,* and even dental infections--as playing a direct role in the instigation and progression of CHD.

The most widely studied of these potential CHD-causing microbes is *Chlamydia pneumoniae (C. pneumoniae),* an extremely common source of respiratory infection. *C.pneumoniae* infection can vary in severity, sometimes producing little or no symptoms, other times causing life-threatening pneumonia or bronchitis. It is responsible for approximately ten percent of all pneumonia cases worldwide. In industrialized countries, approximately fifty percent of the population is in possession of *C.pneumoniae* antibodies by early adulthood. Men have a greater prevalence of antibodies than women, and re-infection throughout life appears to be common(1).

This ubiquitous bug first came under the CHD spotlight in 1988 when Finnish Professor Pekka Saikku and his colleagues observed a much higher prevalence of the newly-isolated *Chlamydia TWR* strain in CHD patients than among CHD-free controls(2). In 1992, the same group of researchers reported that participants of the Helsinki Heart Study who suffered a fatal or non-fatal coronary event were much more likely to show antibodies to *C.pneumoniae* than men who remained event-free(3). Since these seminal reports, dozens more published papers have reported that patients with cardiovascular disease have higher *C. pneumoniae* antibodies than healthy control patients(4). A review of thirteen published studies in which researchers went hunting for the organism in arterial tissues showed that the organism could be detected in over half of all atheromas, but in only five percent of adjacent, lesion-free, arterial tissue samples(5). Furthermore, researchers have found that *C. pneumoniae* can either initiate atherosclerotic lesions or cause exacerbation of existing lesions in both rabbits and mice(4).

Periodontal diseases, such as gingivitis and periodontitis, are chronic bacterial infections that affect the gums and bones supporting the teeth. In gingivitis, the gums redden, swell and bleed easily, but there is often little or no discomfort. Gingivitis is often caused by inadequate oral hygiene, and is reversible with professional treatment and good oral care at home. If gingivitis is left untreated, plaque can spread and grow below the gum line, resulting in periodontitis. In this condition, toxins produced by the bacteria in plaque irritate the gums, causing a chronic inflammatory response in which the tissues and bone that support the teeth are broken down and destroyed. Gaps form between the teeth and gums, which then become infected. As the disease progresses, these gaps deepen and even more gum tissue and bone are destroyed. Eventually, teeth can become loose and often have to be removed. Factors that promote periodontitis include cigarette smoking, stress, certain medications, diabetes, poor nutrition, pregnancy, and genetic susceptibility. Periodontitis is found in fifteen percent of all adults in the 21-50 age range, and in thirty percent of those over 50 years of age(6). In the U.S., forty percent of all adults have lost some or all of their teeth as a result of periodontitis(7).

For people wishing to avoid CHD, a trip to the dentist is likely the last thing on their mind, but maybe it shouldn't be; researchers have found a consistent link between poor oral health and increased cardiovascular disease risk. One of the earliest studies in this area was a comparison of oral health in 100 heart attack patients with a similar number of randomly selected controls; dental health was significantly worse in the heart attack patients than in the controls(8).

A twelve-year follow-up study of over 45,000 male health professionals initially free of cardiovascular disease found that subjects with a history of periodontal disease had a forty-one percent greater risk of CHD than those without. The loss of one or more teeth during the follow-up period imparted a similar CHD risk increase(9). When researchers from the School of Dental Medicine at the State University of New York in Buffalo examined fifty human atheroma specimens, they found that forty-four percent were positive for one or more strains of periodontal bacteria(10). A similar experiment by Canadian researchers detected periodontitis-causing bacteria in over half of the carotid atheroma samples they tested(11). These observations show that periodontal bacteria can indeed make their way from the oral cavity into the bloodstream, where they may proceed to wreak havoc on our arteries.

Some scientists believe that infectious agents may promote CHD by directly attacking the arterial wall, by promoting inflammation and blood clot formation, and by triggering plaque rupture(12,13).

It is a well-established fact that viral infections can attack the heart, leading to conditions such as cardiomyopathy, so it is not exactly a huge leap of faith to assume that infections could do the same to our arteries. Conclusive proof that infections cause CHD must come from controlled trials with human subjects. Obviously, deliberately infecting human subjects with harmful microbes so that their subsequent coronary event rates can be compared with an infection-free control group is out of the question. The best alternative devised so far is the administration of antibiotics to antibody-positive CHD patients in randomized, placebo-controlled trials. Numerous such trials have been conducted, with mixed results; some have shown a reduction in coronary events in patients randomized to receive antibiotic treatment while others have shown no difference(14,15).

The largest study to date, the WIZARD trial, randomized 7,747 heart attack patients who tested positive for *C.pnuemoniae* antibodies to receive either a three-month course of the antibiotic azithromycin or placebo. Overall, the result was disappointing; after an average follow-up of fourteen months, there was a non-significant seven percent reduction in cardiovascular outcomes (death, recurrent heart attack, re-vascularization operations, and hospitalization for angina) among the antibiotic recipients. However, among certain sub-groups, the results were indeed promising; among antibiotic-using diabetics, there was a nineteen percent reduction in risk of cardiovascular events, while in current smokers, risk was reduced by twenty-four percent. In patients who had diabetes *and* smoked, those taking azithromycin had an annual event rate of 14.6 percent, compared to 53 percent for those taking placebo, a noteworthy difference(16). Both diabetes and cigarette smoking substantially increase one's susceptibility to infection(17,18); in the Third National Health and Nutrition Examination Survey, *H.pylori* infection in diabetic men was significantly associated with CHD prevalence, but not in non-diabetic men(19).

There are a number of problems with the antibiotic trials conducted so far. In some of the trials, researchers did not even test to see if the antibiotic treatment actually eradicated the infection being treated. In others, testing showed that antibodies to the infection were not significantly reduced after antibiotic treatment. Obviously, if the infection is contributing to patient's coronary disease, little will be achieved from a therapy that fails to eradicate the responsible microbe.

The importance of ascertaining the effectiveness of antibiotic treatment was highlighted by Spanish researchers when they randomized *H.pylori*-positive patients to receive either a seven-day course of omeprazole, amoxicillin and metronidazole or placebos. After one year, there was no significant difference in coronary event rates between the antibiotic and placebo groups. However, one-third of the antibiotic-treated patients were still positive for *H. pylori*. The researchers then re-analyzed event rates according to *H.pylori* status and discovered that there was indeed a marked difference. Coronary events recurred in 55 percent of patients with persisting H. pylori infection compared 25 percent of patients in whom H. pylori was either absent or eradicated!(20)

Beasts of Burden

Another potentially confounding factor is the fact that is that it is one's total infectious burden that is the most important determinant of microbe-induced cardiovascular disease risk, not just the presence of any single bacteria or virus. In a representative study, 233 patients at a Washington DC cardiovascular research unit underwent coronary angiography to determine the presence of coronary artery disease, then were tested for a variety of bacterial and viral antibodies. The prevalence of CAD was 48, 69, and 85 percent in individuals with antibodies to two or less pathogens, to three or four pathogens, and to five pathogens, respectively. A similar association was also detected between increasing pathogen burden and C-reactive protein levels(21). As such, future trials seeking to reduce the incidence of CHD via antibiotics should take each patient's overall burden of infectious agents into account.

Research examining therapeutic treatment of infections in cardiovascular patients is still in its infancy. The best strategy at this point is to strengthen one's immune system through healthy living and eating in order to avoid infections in the first place, and to increase the body's resilience to any infections that do take hold. For those who have already succumbed to CHD and wish to discuss the role of antibiotic therapy with their doctor, clinical research indicates that certain antibiotics may be best left out of the discussion. Three clinical trials have observed increased cardiovascular and/or overall mortality in patients given the drug clarithromycin, while a large study of Medicaid patients revealed a doubling in the death rate from sudden cardiac mortality among those currently using erythromycin(22-25).

Flu Vaccine For CHD Prevention?

Deaths from cardiovascular disease tend to be much higher in winter, a phenomenon that appears to be largely due to influenza outbreaks(26). Researchers have also observed that cardiovascular mortality increases during influenza epidemics. This increase occurs abruptly with no lag period, a pattern that strongly supports the contention that infections may promote acute cardiac events by stimulating blood clot formation in coronary arteries(27-29). In case-control studies, influenza vaccination has been associated with a substantially reduced risk of heart attack, stroke and cardiac death(30-34).

In 2002, Argentinian researchers set out to test the possibility that influenza vaccines may improve the clinical outlook of heart attack patients. In a controlled pilot study, they randomized 301 patients to serve either as controls or to receive a single flu vaccination injection. After one year, recurrent heart attacks, re-hospitalization, and death rates were all lower in the vaccine group. Cardiovascular death had occurred in twenty-six (seventeen percent) of the controls, but only nine (six percent) of those who had received the flu shot (one patient in each group died from non-cardiovascular causes)(35).

Prevent Infection-Related Heart Disease--Raise Your Cholesterol!

If and when future trials confirm the infection hypothesis, it will be a moment of great irony in the history of cardiovascular research. There is now compelling evidence to show that low cholesterol levels *increase* the susceptibility to infectious disease, while high cholesterol levels appear to protect against infection! Before we discuss the research in this area, let's quickly look at some of the different types of microbes that may be affected by blood cholesterol levels.

Scientists often refer to different bacteria strains as 'Gram-negative' or 'Gram-positive'. Gram-negative organisms include *Salmonella, Shigella, Escherichia coli* and *Pseudomonas*, while Gram-positive organisms include *Staphylococcus, Streptococcus, Clostridium* and anthrax. These alternate categories arise from differences in the structure of these organisms' cell membranes. The cell membranes of gram-negative organisms contain what is known as *endotoxin*, or *lipopolysaccaride* (LPS), while Gram-positive microbes contain *lipoteichoic acid* (LTA). LPS and LTA are the virulent factors that trigger the inflammatory response and cause much of the unpleasant symptoms of infection.

In laboratory experiments, LPS and LTA rapidly bind to and are subsequently inactivated by HDL and/or LDL(36-39). In addition, *Staphylococcus aureus alpha*-toxin, a toxin produced by most strains of Gram-positive *Staphylococcus* bacteria that causes damage to a wide variety of cells, is bound and almost totally inactivated by LDL(40). When specially bred hypercholesterolemic mice are injected with Gram-negative bacteria, they experience a significantly lower and delayed mortality than normocholesterolemic control mice(41). When low cholesterol levels are induced in rats by administering 4-aminopyrolo-(3,4-D)pyrimide (which prevents the liver from secreting cholesterol) or estrogen, they are accompanied by markedly increased endotoxin-induced mortality. Administration of a cholesterol and triglyceride mixture prior to infection reduces the rats' mortality substantially(42).

In 1996, Dutch researchers reported on an experiment involving some rather brave subjects. Eight healthy male volunteers were studied on two occasions, separated by a 'wash-out' period of six weeks. On one occasion the subject was given an infusion of HDL then injected with *Escherichia coli* endotoxin, on the other a placebo infusion was given prior to administration of the endotoxin. Compared to placebo, the HDL infusion dramatically reduced the endotoxin-induced inflammatory response and lowered the prevalence of flu-like symptoms, including chills, nausea, vomiting, myalgia and backache(43).

When healthy adult men with a low cholesterol average of 151 mg/dl were compared with similar-aged men whose total cholesterol averaged 261 mg/dl, the former showed evidence of markedly lower immune function. Relative to the high cholesterol group, the hypocholesterolemic men had significantly fewer circulating lymphocytes, fewer total T cells, and fewer CD8+ cells, all important components of the body's infection-fighting arsenal(44). In men with high cholesterol, mononuclear cells (lymphocytes and monocytes) exerted a far more robust immune response than those in men with lower cholesterol levels(45). During acute infections, cholesterol synthesis increases, but the disappearance rate of cholesterol from the bloodstream is also increased, probably explaining why total cholesterol may either go up or down in an unpredictable manner during the course of various infectious diseases(46,47).

A vast sum of epidemiological evidence supports these laboratory findings. A pooled analysis of nineteen prospective studies, presented at the NHLBI's Conference on Low Blood Cholesterol and Mortality in 1990 and including 68,406 deaths, found that as total cholesterol went down, mortality from respiratory and gastrointestinal diseases--most of which are initiated by infectious organisms--went up. It is unlikely that the low cholesterol levels were due to these diseases because the inverse correlation remained even after excluding deaths that occurred during the first five years(48).

In a more recent study of over 120,000 men and women followed for fifteen years, a strong inverse association between baseline total cholesterol and the risk of being admitted to hospital due to an infectious disease was observed. Total cholesterol was inversely and significantly related to urinary tract, venereal, musculoskeletal, and overall infection incidence among men; and to urinary tract, all genito-urinary, miscellaneous viral infections, and overall infection incidence among women. Again, the significant inverse association with all infections persisted after excluding the first five years of follow-up(49).

Among 2,446 unmarried men with a self-reported history of sexually transmitted disease or liver disease, up to fourteen years of follow-up showed that those with total cholesterol levels below 160 had a sixty-six percent greater relative risk for HIV infection than men with cholesterol levels between 160 and 199. A similar excess risk of AIDS and AIDS-related death was observed. It's unlikely that the lowered cholesterol levels were due to HIV itself because those diagnosed with HIV during the first four years were excluded from the calculations(50). An inverse association between total cholesterol and AIDS mortality was also found in a follow-up of the MRFIT screenees(51).

Low cholesterol levels are also predictive of decreased survival among patients with postoperative abdominal infections, chemotherapy patients with very low white blood cell counts (who run a high risk of dying from bacterial infections), and edematous chronic heart failure who show raised plasma concentrations of bacterial lipopolysaccharide(52-54).

Remember that most cardiovascular events occur in the elderly. The overwhelming majority of prospective studies involving elderly people show that elevated cholesterol levels do not raise their risk of CHD or stroke(55-75). In fact, many of these studies show that raised cholesterol levels in senior citizens are predictive of *increased* survival and greater longevity. It's no secret that immune function declines with age, and that the elderly are more susceptible to infection-related mortality. Among a cohort of 724 Dutch seniors, mortality was significantly lower among those whose total cholesterol was 251 mg/dl (6.5 mmol/l) or greater than those with a cholesterol level of 193 mg/dl (5.0 mmol/l) or less. Each 39 mg/dl (1 mmol/l) increase in total cholesterol among this group corresponded to a fifteen percent decrease in overall mortality. This improved survival was due in large part to a significant reduction in death from infectious disease and cancer(74).

Considering the available evidence, doing everything you can to avoid succumbing to chronic infections seems a very wise strategy. There are numerous strategies that can be implemented towards this end:

- Avoid high blood sugar, refined carbohydrates, polyunsaturated vegetable oils, deficient dietary protein intakes, smoking, recreational drugs, excessive alcohol, insufficient sleep, and make every attempt to minimize exposure to both acute and chronic stress, as all these have been repeatedly shown to impair the immune system's response to invading pathogens(76-95).

Minimizing exposure to pathogens in the first place is also very important:

- Wash your hands thoroughly before preparing and consuming food and after visiting the restroom (it's amazing how many folks don't do this), adhere to a daily oral care routine that includes brushing and flossing, avoid promiscuity and practice safe sex, be uncompromising about eating only the freshest perishable food (if in doubt, throw it out), and stay as far away as possible from coughing, sneezing and wheezing work mates!

In the next chapter, we'll look at a nutrient that may hold the key to unraveling one of the great unsolved medical mysteries: why premenopausal women have far lower rates of CHD than similarly aged men!

Chapter 22

"In nature, there are neither rewards nor punishments--there are consequences."
Robert G. Ingersoll

The Irony of Iron

Can you get too much of a good thing?

For many years now, scientists around the world have been perplexed by the lower CHD risk experienced by premenopausal women. Because the risk of heart disease increases dramatically after menopause, it was long believed that the hormone estrogen conferred favorable cardiovascular benefits. In fact, some researchers were so convinced of estrogen's protective properties that they conducted clinical trials in the early sixties examining the effects of estrogen therapy in *men*. This line of investigation was short-lived; not only did estrogen fail to prevent CHD, many of the hapless gents in these trials experienced feminizing side effects that included impotence and breast growth.

Researchers quickly gave up on the idea of employing estrogen as a weapon against CHD in men, but remained convinced that it explained the lower risk of CHD in premenopausal women. On the basis of such conviction, millions of women around the world began taking hormone replacement therapy for the prevention of heart disease, despite fears that it could potentiate hormone-dependent malignancies such as breast cancer.

In 2002, the popularity of hormone replacement therapy (HRT) suffered a massive blow when the results of two large-scale clinical trials using estrogen and progestin were published. One of these showed no reduction in either primary or secondary CHD events in women taking the two hormones, while another was stopped early after researchers observed an *increase* in CHD, stroke and breast cancer in the HRT group(1,2). In 2004, the published results of a trial using estrogen only also failed to show any protection against CHD(3).

The failure of estrogen replacement to reduce cardiovascular incidence should come as little surprise. Any belief that estrogen, the dominant sex hormone in females, confers protection against heart disease in women, yet testosterone, the dominant sex hormone in males, fails to provide cardio protective effects in men defies logic. This is especially so in light of the abundant evidence showing high testosterone levels are a boon to male health and vitality. As with vanishing estrogen output in women, declining testosterone levels in men are closely linked to many of the deleterious effects of the aging process. If estrogen protects women from heart disease, then there is no reason to conclude testosterone would not do the same for men.

The Iron Connection

High estrogen levels are not the only way in which the biochemistry of premenopausal females differs markedly from that of males. Up until menopause, women regularly menstruate, a process that results in significant blood loss. As this blood is shed from the body, so too are substantial quantities of the mineral iron.

A highly accurate and widely used indicator of bodily iron status is *serum ferritin*, which measures the concentration of iron in the blood. In teenage males and females, serum ferritin levels average around 21-23 mcg/l. This rises to around 94 mcg/l in males aged 18-45, and 124 mcg/l in men over 45, but remains in the vicinity of 25 mcg/l among premenopausal women. After menopause, where the CHD risk in females rises to match that experienced by males, the average serum ferritin level is around 89 mcg/l(4,5).

With advancing age, iron stores steadily rise from the teenage level because the body has few outlets for disposing of excess iron. This characteristic may have been advantageous to Paleolithic humans, where several factors acted in concert to challenge their iron status, including 1) the highly-active Stone Age lifestyle; 2) a lack of readily available first aid kits to curtail prolific bleeding from traumatic injury, and; 3) infection with iron-depleting parasites, especially hookworm (hunter-gatherer populations, and individuals in developing countries, are often afflicted with hookworm, which can double and even triple daily iron losses (6,7)). Despite deriving a significant portion of their daily sustenance from iron-rich red meats, Stone Age humans would have had little opportunity to develop the elevated iron stores commonly seen among the modern-day inhabitants of industrialized nations.

Most people are aware of the consequences of insufficient iron intake, but few realize that excess iron can act as potent pro-oxidant--that is, a promoter of harmful free radical activity. High iron intake and/or high bodily iron stores have been implicated as possible culprits in the development of cancer, diabetes, and CHD.

In 1981, South Carolina scientist Jerome L. Sullivan, M.D., Ph.D., proposed that decreased iron stores could explain the low incidence of CHD in premenopausal women(6). Sullivan cited evidence from the Framingham study showing that women of child-bearing age who underwent hysterectomy--which brings menstruation to a permanent halt--suffered a marked increase in CHD, even when their ovaries (which produce most of a woman's estrogen) were left intact.

For over a decade, Sullivan's hypothesis was largely ignored by cholesterol-obsessed CHD researchers and health authorities. Things began to change in 1992 when Finnish Professor Jukka Salonen and his team published the results of the first epidemiological study which supported Sullivan's theory(9). Salonen and his colleagues had followed almost two thousand men aged 42-60 years, with no symptoms of CHD at initial examination, for an average of three years. After adjusting for a multitude of possible confounding factors, men with a serum ferritin reading greater than or equal to 200 mcg/l had a 2.2-fold relative risk of heart attack compared with men sporting lower blood ferritin levels.

However, since the publication of this hallmark study, scores of researchers have performed similar investigations with wildly conflicting results. Some have found evidence of a harmful link between iron and CHD, some have found no relationship, while others have even detected protective associations!(10)

By now, readers should hardly need reminding of the many limitations of epidemiological research. Most prospective studies have attempted to ascertain the relationship between iron and CHD risk by using a single measurement of iron status at baseline. Even levels of serum ferritin, regarded as the most reliable marker of iron status, can fluctuate markedly within individuals over time. Consequently, it is possible that the true relationship between iron and CHD risk--be it positive, negative or neutral--has been masked by the failure to monitor long-term iron status. Furthermore, most of these studies utilized cut-off points for serum ferritin levels that were likely far too high to detect any benefit. The oft-used cut-off point of 100 mcg/l, for example, is still well above the mean level of 89 mcg/l in post-menopausal women—a level accompanied by significantly greater CHD risk than that seen in premenopausal women, whose average serum ferritin is only 25 mcg/l.

Back to the Lab

Given that iron is well-known to possess potent pro-oxidant effects, it is hardly unreasonable to suspect that high bodily stores or a high intake of iron could increase one's risk of free radical-mediated diseases(11).

Hemochromatosis, or iron overload, is a well-recognized condition that most commonly results from an inherited disorder of iron metabolism. Like many nutrients, iron is absorbed from the diet through the small intestine, and the amount absorbed is determined by the body's requirements. Individuals with hereditary hemochromatosis absorb more iron than their body needs. Because the body does not have any way to increase excretion of this excess iron, a gradual build-up in tissues and organs occurs. Complications include arthritis, diabetes, liver cirrhosis, alterations in skin pigmentation, cardiac arrhythmias and heart failure.

Animal Studies

Studies with animals support the notion that excess iron has a destructive effect on cardiovascular health. When Taiwanese scientists fed either high-iron or low-iron diets to a special atherosclerosis-prone strain of mice for three months, they observed that cholesterol concentrations remained similar on both diets. However, lipoproteins isolated from the iron-restricted group were much less prone to oxidation, indicating that the low-iron diet reduced free radical activity. When the researchers inspected the animal's arteries, they found that the atherosclerotic lesions seen in mice fed a low-iron diet were significantly smaller than those found in their cousins on the high-iron diet(12).

More recently, the same group of researchers observed that atherosclerotic lesions in both young and old mice placed on low-iron diets showed substantially greater collagen content, making them less likely to rupture(13).

These cardiovascular effects appear to be largely free radical-mediated, and may therefore be prevented in rodents by ensuring they receive a high antioxidant intake. When rats were given identical diets that differed only in iron content, researchers observed that increased iron intakes produced greater levels of lipid peroxidation and depleted blood levels of antioxidants, as expected. However, adding antioxidants to the rats' drinking water attenuated these effects, raising the possibility that differences in antioxidant intake may also help explain the on-again, off-again epidemiological relationship observed between iron and cardiovascular disease(14).

Human Studies

What about controlled human studies? What do they tell us about iron's impact upon our hearts and arteries?

Well, in CHD patients and diabetics with endothelial dysfunction, marked improvements in blood flow are observed after administration of deferoxamine, an iron-binding agent that reduces blood iron levels. When a nitric oxide (NO) inhibitor is co-administered with deferoxamine, no improvement in blood flow is observed, indicating that iron possesses the ability to inhibit NO release(15,16).

Iron-binders are not the only way to reduce bodily iron levels; phlebotomy (blood withdrawal) can also be used to lower iron stores. Diabetic patients who had 1,500 milliliters of blood drawn over a two-week period showed greatly improved arterial dilation for as long as four months after the procedure. Insulin sensitivity also improved markedly, indicating a beneficial effect of the iron-depletion procedure on glycemic control(17,18).

Another group of researchers subjected type 2 diabetics and glucose-intolerant individuals to repeated phlebotomy, with an eye to bringing their blood iron levels as low as possible without inducing actual iron deficiency. When this goal was achieved, the researchers proceeded to measure the patients' blood glucose control and several other markers of cardiovascular disease risk. The iron depletion procedure significantly reduced blood glucose and insulin responses to oral glucose testing, as well as blood levels of fibrinogen and glycosylated hemoglobin (HbA1c). Also noteworthy is the fact that iron depletion increased HDL cholesterol levels while lowering LDL and total cholesterol levels(19). Here again we have another demonstration of how changes in blood cholesterol are likely to be a mere side effect of underlying processes that really do impact upon heart disease progression.

In addition to improving arterial function and blood glucose metabolism, reducing iron stores may also be highly beneficial for patients suffering from liver disorders. A study of patients with non-alcoholic fatty liver disease who underwent repeated phlebotomy experienced substantial reductions in the key liver enzyme *serum alanine aminotransferase* (ALT), suggestive of improved liver function. Significant improvements in blood glucose metabolism were also observed(20).

What about CHD? Well, a clinical trial examining the utility of iron depletion in the secondary prevention of CHD is now underway. As part of the feasibility investigations for this trial, researchers conducted a pilot study known as the Iron (Fe) and Atherosclerosis Study (FeAST). The results from this three-month trial were promising; among vascular disease patients who had sufficient blood removed to reduce their average serum ferritin level from 125 mcg/l to 52 mcg/l, only one (3.4 percent) experienced an adverse cardiovascular event (angioplasty). In the control group, eight patients (42 percent), experienced heart attack, heart failure, unstable angina, or dysrhythmia (a type of abnormal and potentially fatal heart rhythm)(21).

What to Do About Iron?

Before acting upon any of the iron-lowering suggestions that follow, you *must* ascertain your current iron status, which can be readily achieved by having your doctor order a simple serum ferritin blood test. The 'normal' range for serum ferritin is 12-300 mcg/l for males and 12-150 mcg/l for females.

Be forewarned: even if your test results show serum ferritin levels at the high end of the standard range, your doctor is likely to tell you that your iron status is 'perfectly normal'. Most doctors remain blissfully unaware that reducing serum ferritin levels to the low end of the normal range has, in clinical studies, brought about significant improvements in blood glucose control, liver function, kidney disease and even cardiovascular outcomes.

The standard procedure for lowering elevated blood iron levels is phlebotomy. Unfortunately, given the current poor state of knowledge among most physicians about the adverse affects of 'high-normal' levels of iron, few will be prepared to arrange a course of regular blood withdrawal unless your serum ferritin level clearly exceeds the upper limit.

One way in which you can have blood regularly drawn without too much fuss is to become a blood donor. However, standard blood donation procedures only allow the withdrawal of a maximum of 500 milliliters of blood every eight weeks. Depending on your initial serum ferritin level, this may be too infrequent to produce any meaningful reduction in iron stores. In one experiment, an average total of three 500 milliliter withdrawals, performed every two to four weeks, was required to reduce mean serum ferritin levels from 85 mcg/l to 27 mcg/l(22). In another, an average of seven to eight 500-milliliter withdrawals every two to four weeks was required to lower serum ferritin levels from 272 mcg/l to 14 mcg/l(19).

The above observations may explain why research examining the effect of donating blood on cardiovascular disease risk has yielded conflicting results. While some highly publicized studies have found a lower risk for blood donors, others have not(23-27). Depending on the donor's initial iron status and the frequency of withdrawal, standard blood donation may not consistently lower serum ferritin levels sufficiently to provide any meaningful protection against cardiovascular disease(28).

For those who cannot or will not give blood, or for whom standard blood donation occurs too infrequently to keep serum ferritin levels at a low level, there exists another option. This involves use of a substance known as IP-6, or *inositol hexaphosphate.* IP-6, which occurs in foods and is more commonly known as *phytic acid* or *phytate,* possesses the ability to bind to iron and promote its excretion from the body. While IP-6 supplements have been used empirically to lower iron stores, little published data exists on their use in humans. If laboratory studies are anything to go by, IP-6 may be a more potent iron-binder, and a more effective inhibitor of iron-induced free radical formation, than the more widely used drug deferoxamine(29).

In animal studies, phytic acid has also shown benefits against leukemia, breast, colon, liver, prostate and skin cancers(30). Phytic acid is commonly found in whole cereal grains and legumes, but please do not try and prevent cancer by eating more of these foods; in rodents, purified IP-6 dramatically reduces tumor incidence, whereas high cereal fiber diets providing a similar amount of IP-6 do not(31,32). In human trials, increased wheat fiber intake has failed miserably to protect against colon cancer or adenomatous polyp formation(33).

If you decide to try IP-6, don't start taking it every day for the rest of your life; use it only in short-term cycles, the length of which must be ascertained by monitoring one's serum ferritin status. Suggested dosages range between 1.6 to 2.4 grams per day. To minimize IP-6's interference with the absorption of other important minerals, take it away from food on an empty stomach--first thing in the morning is ideal. Regular serum ferritin tests will be necessary to determine just how effectively your IP-6 dose is lowering your iron levels. If you have any sign of renal impairment, the use of IP-6 should be approached with caution, as the iron it ejects from the body will need to pass through the kidneys.

How Low Should You Go?

How low should you aim to go when reducing elevated serum ferritin levels? At present, there is no consensus as to what constitutes and 'ideal' level of serum ferritin. We do know that premenopausal women, with an average serum ferritin reading of 25 mcg/l, suffer a very low rate of CHD. When this rises to 89 mcg/l after menopause, their CHD risk quickly rises to match that of similarly aged males. The promising results of the FeAST pilot trial were achieved by lowering mean serum ferritin levels from 125 mcg/l to 52 mcg/l, while another study produced significantly lower morbidity and mortality in diabetic kidney patients by reducing average serum ferritin levels average of 301 mcg/l to 36 mcg/l(34). Some health agencies have decreed a cut-off point for iron deficiency of 15 mcg/l, while others have set the upper limit of deficiency at 20 mcg/l. Given the currently available evidence, maintenance of serum ferritin levels between 25-50 mcg/l seems the most prudent course of action.

Iron and Exercise

Exercise greatly increases the utilization of iron, and may thus help prevent the build-up of high bodily iron stores. A Finnish study showed that men who exercised more than 2.6 hours each week, or more than three times per week, had a seventeen to twenty percent lower serum ferritin concentration than those who did not(35).

Generally speaking, the higher the frequency of training, the lower the serum ferritin levels; a study of highly active men found that mean serum ferritin levels were 86 mcg/l in those training four times per week, 49 mcg/l in those training seven to nine times per week, and 31 mcg/l in those training ten to fourteen times per week(36).

The effect of exercise on iron status may also contribute to the reduced cardiovascular mortality that is associated with higher levels of physical activity(37).

Before You Iron Out the Iron...

It must be noted that there are certain groups for which this low-iron approach may not be suitable, most notably pre-menopausal women. In this group, iron deficiency is common, as evidenced by a high frequency of serum ferritin readings under 20 mcg/l. A recent, randomized, double-blind Swiss study of women aged between 18-55 who had sought medical advice for fatigue, found that most of the women had low blood concentrations of iron. After four weeks, a significantly greater number of women receiving iron supplements reported a decrease in fatigue symptoms than those receiving placebo(38). Australian women complaining of fatigue showed similar improvements when treated with either iron supplements or a high-iron diet(39).

Because exercise increases the need for iron, and because iron deficiency is not uncommon among female athletes, physically active premenopausal women should be especially careful about getting enough of this mineral. Researchers have shown that iron-deficient women experience greater fitness gains in response to endurance exercise when receiving extra iron(40).

Women looking to boost their iron status should look to meat, especially red meat, as it is the richest dietary source of readily absorbed iron. When the iron status of previously sedentary women was challenged with twelve weeks of aerobic exercise, a high red meat diet protected iron stores more effectively than iron supplements(41). Trying to boost one's iron status with plant foods and dairy products won't work; individuals on lacto-ovo vegetarian diets consistently exhibit lower blood levels of iron, even when consuming similar total amounts of this mineral as omnivores(42-44). It is highly ironic that young women are the group most likely to shun red meat, but also the group benefit most likely to benefit from its consumption!(45)

To avert the possibility of fatigue, individuals engaged in strenuous exercise or competitive sport may need to have a smaller volume of blood withdrawn at each donation. Blood withdrawal shortly before an important competitive event or during intense phases of training should be strictly avoided.

Know Your Iron Status

When it comes to iron, the research shows that you can indeed get too much of a good thing. Every individual seeking to avoid heart disease should be aware of their iron status; along with measurement of one's blood sugar status, this may provide useful diagnostic information that no amount of cholesterol testing could ever dream of delivering.

SECTION THREE:
Preventing Heart Disease the Drug-Free Way.

Chapter 23

"A wonder drug is a drug you take and then wonder what it is going to do to you."
Author unknown.

Disrobing the Drug Myth

Do drugs really provide the most effective protection against CHD?

I'm sure you've heard it: The claim that by popping those miraculous golden drugs known as statins, your risk of succumbing to heart disease will be slashed by a massive one-third! According to drug company-sponsored spin doctors, taking statins is the most powerful thing one can do to reduce the occurrence of CHD.

Not true.

When Statins Work--And When They Don't

Take a good look at Table 23a, which lists the major controlled, randomized clinical statin trials conducted as of mid-2006(1-14). It shows that among people with CHD or considered to be at high risk of CHD, the effect of statins on the incidence of CHD mortality ranges from virtually nil (in the ALLHAT trial) to a noteworthy forty-six percent (the LIPS trial). The reduction in overall mortality produced by statins ranges from none (ALLHAT) to twenty-nine percent (the 4S trial). As Table 23a clearly shows, statins can in no way be guaranteed to produce a one-third reduction in CHD or all-cause mortality in high-risk patients. Nor can they be counted on to reduce overall mortality in stroke patients; while the SPARCL study showed a twenty percent reduction in cardiovascular mortality, there was no reduction in overall mortality.

Now, let's take a look at the studies that involved healthy people with the non-disease of 'hypercholesterolemia'. The first of these, the EXCEL trial, provides no figures for CHD mortality, but did report that overall mortality in the four groups taking various doses of lovastatin was 150-300 percent *higher* than that seen in the placebo group after one year. Despite the fact that the EXCEL trial continued for many more years, no further mortality data has ever been reported.

In the AFCAPS/TexCAPS trial, lovastatin reduced CHD mortality by a statistically insignificant twenty-seven percent, but overall mortality was similar (four percent higher in the lovastatin group). In the WOSCOPS trial, pravastatin decreased CHD and overall mortality by twenty-seven and twenty-one percent, respectively, but neither figure was statistically significant. In the Japanese MEGA study, cardiovascular and overall mortality rates were lower in the pravastatin group. However, the total number of deaths in both groups was very low compared to those seen in studies with Western subjects, and the differences between the two groups were not statistically significant. There exists little evidence to show that statins can extend the lives of people without clinical signs of CHD.

Statins Do Not Increase Survival in Women

When the mortality figures from all the trials which included women are tabulated separately by sex, they show no longevity benefit for the fairer sex whatsoever. Yes, you read right--despite the fact that around half of the millions of statin prescriptions written each year are handed to female patients, these drugs show no overall mortality benefit regardless of whether they are used for primary or secondary prevention. In women free of CHD, statins fail to lower both CHD and overall mortality, while in women with CHD, statins lower CHD mortality but increase the risk of death from other causes, leaving overall mortality unchanged(15).

Statins Do Not Increase Survival in the Elderly

The elderly are another group for whom it remains to be proven that statins offer any life-extending benefit. The only statin study dealing exclusively with seniors, the PROSPER trial, found that pravastatin did indeed reduce the incidence of coronary mortality. However, this decrease was almost entirely negated by a corresponding increase in cancer deaths. As a result, overall mortality between the pravastatin and placebo groups after 3.2 years was virtually identical.

The results from placebo-controlled trials indicate that statins can lower the risk of CHD death in males and the elderly. But when it comes to the more important benchmark of overall mortality, favorable outcomes have been established only in patients already at high risk of heart disease; namely, those with pre-existing CHD, hypertension, or diabetes.

In CHD-free non-diabetic men, in females with and without heart disease, and in the elderly, it is extremely doubtful whether statins can lower overall mortality at all, let alone by one-third. Two of the four statin trials involving healthy subjects indicate that statin use may *increase* overall mortality.

One thing is certain: the ingestion of statins by healthy people dramatically increases their risk of muscle weakness and pain, cognitive dysfunction and

Table 23a. CHD and Overall Mortality Risk in Randomized Clinical Statin Trials						
Trial	Trial participants	Number of participants (drug/control group)	CHD deaths (drug/ control group)	Total deaths (drug/ control group)	Relative risk for CHD mortality	Relative risk for total mortality
EXCEL Lovastatin 20-80mg Double-blind, 1 year*	Healthy males and females with high cholesterol.	6600/1650	?	?	?	+150-+300%
AFCAPS/ TexCAPS Lovastatin 20-40mg Double-blind, 5.2 years	Healthy males and females with normal cholesterol.	3304/3301	11/15	80/77	-27%‡	+3.9%
4S Simvastatin 10-40mg Double-blind, 5.4 years	Males and female CHD patients with high cholesterol.	2221/2223	111/189	182/256	-41%	-29%
WOSCOPS Pravastatin 40mg Double-blind, 4.9 years	Healthy males with high cholesterol.	3302/3293	38/52	106/135	-27%†	-21%
CARE Pravastatin 40mg Double-blind, 5 years	Male & postmenopausal female CHD patients with normal cholesterol.	2081/2078	96/119	180/196	-19%	-8%†
LIPID Pravastatin 40mg Double-blind, 6.1 years	Male & female CHD patients, all levels of cholesterol.	4512/4502	287/373	498/633	-23%	-21%
HPS Simvastatin 40mg Double-blind, 5 years	Males and females with CHD, other occlusive arterial disease or diabetes.	10269/10267	587/707	1328/1507	-17%	-12%
LIPS Fluvastatin 80mg Double-blind, 3.9 years	Male & female CHD patients with average cholesterol undergoing balloon angioplasty	844/833	13/24	36/49	-46%	-26%

Table 23a. CHD and Overall Mortality Risk in Randomized Clinical Statin Trials (cont.)						
Trial	Trial participants	Number of participants (drug/control group)	CHD deaths (drug/control group)	Total deaths (drug/control group)	Relative risk for CHD mortality	Relative risk for total mortality
ALLHAT Pravastatin 10-40mg 4.8 years.	Hypertensive males and females ≥55 years old, 15% with CHD, 35% with diabetes.	5170/5185	160/162	631/641	-1%†	-1%†
PROSPER Pravastatin 40mg Double-blind, 3.2 years	Elderly males & females aged 70-82 with pre-existing vascular disease (coronary, cerebral or peripheral) or heightened risk due to smoking, hypertension or diabetes.	2891/2913	94/122	298/306	-22%	-2%
ASCOT-LLA Atorvastatin 10mg Double-blind, 3.3 years.	Hypertensive males and females with normal cholesterol but at least three other CVD risk factors.	5168/5137	74/82**	185/212	-10%†	-13%†
CARDS Atorvastatin 10mg Double-blind, 5.5 years.	Male and female type 2 diabetics with no history of CVD and normal cholesterol levels.	1428/1410	21/25	61/82	-17%	-26%
SPARCL Atorvastatin 80mg Double-blind, 4.9 years.	Males & females, mean age 60, who suffered stroke or transient ischemic attack within 6 months prior to study.	2365/2366	78/98**	216/211	-20%	+2%
MEGA Pravastatin 10-20 mg, single-blind, 9 years	Healthy Japanese males & females with high cholesterol.	3866/3966	11/18**	55/79	-37%†	-28%†

*Figures for EXCEL derived from preliminary one year follow-up. No further mortality data has ever been published.
**Figures are for all cardiovascular deaths, not just CHD deaths.
† Difference not statistically significant.

memory loss, liver disorders, kidney failure and potentially-fatal rhabdomyolysis. Hardly what any rational individual would call an acceptable trade-off!

What About Aspirin?

It is fitting that statins are commonly dubbed *"the new aspirin"*, because the latter has also completely failed to demonstrate any overall mortality benefit in healthy people.

In clinical trials, aspirin has reduced cardiovascular mortality in patients with previous myocardial infarction, acute myocardial infarction, previous or acute stroke, and those with stable angina, peripheral arterial disease, and atrial fibrillation. In each of these high-risk categories, the absolute benefits of aspirin use have substantially outweighed its well-known downside: namely, the risk of serious bleeding injuries(16).

Overall, allocation to aspirin therapy among these high-risk patients reduces the risk of non-fatal heart attack by one third, and cardiovascular mortality by one sixth. Despite increasing the risk of hemorrhagic stroke, aspirin reduces non-fatal stroke by one quarter thanks to a favorable effect on ischemic stroke incidence. And despite a fifty percent increase in their risk of fatal bleeding episodes, aspirin lowers overall mortality in these high-risk patients by one-sixth.

Aspirin doses of 75-150 milligrams daily appear to be at least as effective as higher daily doses. In acute settings, such as immediately following a heart attack or stroke, an initial 'loading dose' of 160-325 milligrams may be required(16,17). A review of trials involving pravastatin also suggests that those simultaneously taking aspirin along with this statin drug may enjoy further reductions in cardiovascular risk than if either drug were taken alone(18).

The greatest benefit from aspirin use is seen in the first month after an acute coronary or cerebral event; researchers from the UK's Antithrombotic Trialists' Collaboration, who periodically conduct sweeping reviews of the clinical evidence pertaining to anti-platelet agents like aspirin, have estimated that:

- Among one thousand acute heart attack patients who are given one month of higher dose aspirin and then continue to take low dose aspirin on a longer-term basis, about forty would avoid a serious cardiovascular event during the first month and about a further forty would avoid a cardiovascular event in the next couple of years;

- Similar-sized long term benefits are likely to be seen if anti-platelet therapy is started soon after stroke or transient ischemic attack and continued long term;
- In patients at intermediate risk, such as those with no previous cardiovascular event but with stable angina, atrial fibrillation, or peripheral arterial disease, anti-platelet therapy for a couple of years would be expected to prevent about ten to fifteen vascular events for every one thousand patients treated.

The effect of aspirin in diabetics requires further research; in one trial, a hefty 650-milligram dose of aspirin per day reduced the occurrence of fatal and nonfatal myocardial infarction by seventeen percent, while overall mortality was lowered by a more modest nine percent(19). Another trial involving a much lower dose of aspirin (100 mg daily) showed a twenty-three percent increase in cardiovascular mortality among diabetics, although the relatively small number of participants rendered this difference statistically insignificant. No difference in death from other causes was observed, although the incidence of gastrointestinal bleeding was far higher in the aspirin group than in the control group (eight versus one cases, respectively)(20).

Patients with heart failure, as opposed to CHD, should *not* take aspirin; a recent controlled trial of almost 300 heart failure patients comparing aspirin (300 mg/day), warfarin, or no anti-clotting treatment found that significantly more patients randomized to aspirin were hospitalized for cardiovascular reasons, especially worsening heart failure(21).

What About Healthy Folks?

One of the first trials to have tested aspirin in people free of CHD was the six-year British Doctors Study, which found no significant reduction in heart attack incidence, cardiovascular mortality nor overall mortality among physicians randomized to 500 milligrams of aspirin daily. By the end of the study, forty-four percent of the aspirin group had to discontinue aspirin because of side effects, the most common being dyspepsia(22).

A year after the British study was published, researchers reported the results of the Physicians' Health Study, in which half of the participants had been randomized to take 325 milligrams every other day for five-years. Although the rate of heart attack was significantly lower in the aspirin group, there was no reduction in cardiovascular mortality. Overall mortality also remained unchanged. Side effects were more common in the aspirin group, including gastric ulcers, gastrointestinal bleeding, hemorrhagic stroke, and other bleeding disorders(23).

While neither of the aforementioned trials produced any significant reduction in overall mortality, the contrasting effects of aspirin on heart attack incidence are worthy of further comment. In the British study, the doctors were given plain old aspirin, whereas in the Physicians' Health Study aspirin was delivered in *buffered* form. Not insignificantly, the buffering agent was magnesium, a mineral deficient in the average Western diet but absolutely critical for cardiac health. This important factor was completely overlooked--as was the lack of effect on cardiovascular or total mortality--by those who foolishly began recommending aspirin for virtually everyone based on the Physicians' study results.

The Thrombosis Prevention Trial (TPT) randomized men to receive either seventy-five milligrams of aspirin per day or placebo for 6.8 years. Aspirin reduced the incidence of heart attack by twenty-four percent, but had no effect on total mortality(24).

In the Hypertension Optimal Treatment (HOT) trial, all the participants had high blood pressure and nearly half were female. The daily seventy-five milligram dose of aspirin reduced heart attack incidence by thirty-five percent, but again there was no significant effect on overall mortality after 3.8 years(25). Minor bleeding injuries were significantly higher among aspirin users in both the TPT and HOT trials.

In the Women's Health Study, over 39,000 initially healthy females 45 years or older were randomly assigned to receive 100 milligrams of aspirin every second day or placebo. They were then monitored for ten years, with researchers recording the incidence of major cardiovascular events, cardiovascular deaths, and all-cause mortality.

Compared with placebo, aspirin had no effect on the risk of fatal or nonfatal heart attack or death from cardiovascular causes. Researchers did observe a seventeen percent reduction in the risk of stroke in the aspirin group, owing to a twenty-four percent reduction in ischemic stroke incidence (aspirin conferred a statistically insignificant twenty-four percent increase in hemorrhagic stroke risk). Gastrointestinal bleeding requiring transfusion was forty percent more frequent in the aspirin group than in the placebo group. As for aspirin's effect on overall mortality, there was none--all-cause death rates were similar between the placebo and treatment groups(26).

Stopping Aspirin

If you have been taking aspirin and wish to stop, it is important that you seek the assistance of a competent medical practitioner. In 2004, a group of researchers compared over 8,000 first-time heart attack patients with healthy controls to see if sudden discontinuation of nonsteroidal anti-inflammatory drugs (NSAIDs) like aspirin conferred any increased risk. They found a fifty-two percent increased risk of heart attack in those who stopped taking NSAIDs within four weeks of their cardiac event. The risk was highest in subjects with rheumatoid arthritis, systemic lupus erythematosus and for subjects who discontinued therapy with NSAIDs after previous long-term use(27).

There are natural therapies, which we shall discuss in the coming chapters, that also exert anti-clotting actions. Again, it is advised for anyone who stops taking NSAIDs like aspirin to be monitored by a knowledgeable professional as they transition from this drug to less toxic natural strategies.

The Bottom Line

In trials lasting up to six years, statins have demonstrated the ability to reduce cardiovascular and overall mortality in individuals with pre-existing CHD, and may also impart similar benefits to high-risk hypertensives and diabetics. Their use is not without considerable risk--statins frequently produce muscle weakness, lethargy, liver dysfunction and cognitive disturbances ranging from confusion to transient amnesia. They have shown themselves capable of producing severe rhabdomyolysis that can lead to life-threatening kidney failure. Even in high-risk patients, their use should be instituted with the utmost caution and close monitoring should be maintained at all times.

Excepting those with hemorrhagic stroke and heart failure, aspirin has been shown in clinical trials to reduce cardiovascular and overall mortality in patients with pre-existing cardiovascular disease. In these patients, their benefit outweighs a significantly increased risk of fatal bleeding. Aspirin may also be of benefit to diabetic patients at higher dosages, although the evidence is too scanty at present to draw any firm conclusions.

For the rest of us, the ability of these drugs to reduce cardiovascular mortality is highly doubtful, and they appear to be next to useless for decreasing overall mortality. Listening to the numerous 'experts' that urge healthy people to take these drugs appears to do little more than relieve of us our hard-earned money and expose us unnecessarily to their potentially-life-threatening side effects.

What then, can we do to truly lower our risk of heart disease and stroke?

Find out in the next chapter.

Chapter 24

"Leave your drugs in the chemist's pot if you can heal the patient with food."
Hippocrates

If Not Drugs, Then What?

Clinically-proven drug-free methods for preventing CHD

The first thing we need to do when devising a safe and effective drug-free CHD-fighting strategy is to list the interventions that have actually been shown in randomized clinical trials to lower both CHD and overall mortality. Table 24a presents just such a list. It reports the results of trials that successfully utilized various non-drug strategies--including dietary modification, nutrient supplementation, and exercise--in individuals with or considered to be at high risk of CHD(1-8).

Letting The Cat Out of the Bag

Looking through Table 24a, we can quickly see why drug companies don't want you to know about these non-drug interventions--the reductions in coronary and overall mortality they impart are of a similar magnitude as those conferred by statins, and in some cases they are superior. What's more, the substantial mortality benefits derived from these natural agents are not accompanied by an increased risk of cancer, heart failure, muscle damage, cognitive dysfunction, liver abnormalities, kidney failure or premature death. In fact, many of the strategies in Table 24a--such as eating a vegetable, fruit and nut-rich diet, exercising, and regularly consuming omega-3-rich foodstuffs like fatty fish/fish oil--are things that we should all be doing anyway. All of these will not only reduce our risk of heart disease, but will also protect us from a plethora of other nasty ailments, including cancer, diabetes and cognitive decline.

Let's take a closer look at the benefits afforded by these strategies.

Increased Intake of Long-Chain Omega-3 Fatty Acids

Clinical trials utilizing the sole intervention of increased fatty fish or fish oil intake have produced reductions in CHD deaths of one-third and have lowered overall mortality by twenty-one to thirty percent.

The benefits of EPA and DHA-rich items like fish and fish oil are not confined to the cardiovascular system. In epidemiological studies and animal experiments, increased intakes of long-chain omega-3 fatty acids have been

Table 24a. CHD & Overall Mortality Risk in Non-Drug CHD intervention trials						
Intervention (Study)	Trial participants	Number of participants (intervention/ control)	CHD deaths (intervention/ control)	Total deaths (intervention/ control)	Relative risk for CHD mortality	Relative risk for total mortality
Reduced total fat & processed food intake, increased omega-6 & omega-3 fat/fruit/vegetable/ complex carbohydrate intake (Semi-blind, 3.4 yrs)	Males with CHD	26/24	1/2	1/3	-50%‡	-66%‡
Increased omega-3 & monounsaturated fat/fruit/vegetable, legume/bread intake, decreased saturated fat intake (Semi-blind, 2.4 yrs)	Recent heart attack patients, 9% female	302/303	3/16*	8/20	-81%	-60%
200-400g fatty fish per week or 500mg fish oil daily (Semi-blind, 2 yrs)	Males recovering from heart attack	1015/1018	78/116	94/130	-33%	-30%
Fish oil (supplying 900mg EPA + DHA daily) (Partial blind, 3.5 yrs)	Recent heart attack victims, 14% females	5666/5658	209/258	477/554	-32%	-21%
100mg coenzyme Q10, 100mcg selenium (Placebo-controlled, 1 yr)	Acute myocardial infarction patients, 18% females	32/29	0/6	1/6	(Cannot be calculated)	-83.3%
100mcg selenium daily	Acute myocardial infarction patients, 22% females	40/41	0/4**	0/4	(Cannot be calculated)	(Cannot be calculated)
4g L-carnitine daily (Non-blind, 1yr)	Recent heart attack victims, 29% females	81/79	0/3	1/10	(Cannot be calculated)	-90%
Exercise (Meta-analysis of 14 trials, 6 months to 5 years in length)	Total of 2,576 CHD patients, <6% females	N/A	N/A	N/A	-35%	-27%

*Figure includes all cardiovascular deaths; separate figures for CHD deaths not provided in published paper.
** Figure includes all cardiac deaths; separate figures for CHD deaths not provided in published paper.
‡ Not statistically significant due to low number of deaths in both groups.
† Difference not statistically significant.

associated with lower rates of cancer, depression and mental illness, adverse pregnancy outcomes, infectious disease, osteoporosis, lung disease, menstrual pain, cognitive decline in the elderly, eye damage, childhood asthma and attention-deficit hyperactivity disorder(9-35). In clinical trials with human subjects, researchers have observed benefits from long-chain omega-3 supplementation in the treatment of asthma, Alzheimer's, rheumatoid arthritis, depression, schizophrenia, infant health, pregnancy outcomes, kidney disease, menstrual problems, ulcerative colitis, Crohn's disease and cystic fibrosis(36-56).

Clearly, regular long-chain omega-3 intake is a boon to both cardiovascular *and* overall health. There are, however, legitimate concerns regarding the consequences of ingesting fish contaminated with environmental pollutants such as mercury, lead, and organochlorines like PCB and dioxin. The worst offenders are larger fish varieties, which, because of their position higher up the aquatic food chain, accumulate greater levels of these toxins. An analysis of various fish species revealed that tilefish, swordfish, king mackerel and shark contained the highest levels of methylmercury, while salmon, tuna, halibut, and catfish were amongst those showing the lowest levels of contamination(57).

In addition to avoiding large fish, it would also be wise to steer clear of farmed fish. A comparison of farmed versus wild salmon samples from around the world showed that the concentration of organochlorines was significantly higher in the former--an important finding, considering that around half of all the salmon sold globally is farmed(58).

The safest, most convenient, and least expensive solution to the problem of ensuring regular long-chain omega-3 intake is to take fish oil supplements. Modern processing of these oils tends to eliminate their mercury content; lab testing of numerous popular brands of fish oil has shown them to be free of detectable mercury(59-61). As for organochlorines, an analysis of various fish and cod liver oils by European researchers found that salmon oils originating from the US and Norway had non-detectable amounts of PCBs and negligible amounts of other organochlorines. Cod liver oil supplements from the UK, on the other hand, had the highest amounts.

The average salmon oil capsule supplies 300 milligrams of EPA and DHA, meaning that three capsules a day are necessary to emulate the dosage successfully used in the GISSI trial. Some users of encapsulated fish oil experience an unpleasant fishy aftertaste. Believe it or not, the best way to counter this problem is to thoroughly chew the capsules before swallowing. While this may not sound especially appetizing, high quality fish oil preparations will not impart any fishy taste when ingested in this manner.

Because long-chain omega-3 supplements effectively reduce blood clotting, fears have arisen about a possible harmful interaction in patients already taking blood-thinning medications. Published reports have not shown any increase in bleeding episodes among patients taking fish oil along with anti-coagulant agents like aspirin and warfarin(62-64). Nonetheless, anyone taking these drugs who wishes to begin taking fish oil should work closely with their doctor. One case report appearing in the medical literature describes a female patient taking warfarin who doubled her fish oil dose without telling her pharmacist. Subsequent testing revealed an increase in bleeding time that necessitated a reduction in her warfarin dosage(65).

Because they suffer a dramatically higher incidence of CHD, diabetics are a group that may especially benefit from fish oil supplements. However, some studies have found that fish oil may cause fasting blood glucose levels to rise in type 2 diabetics. However, the ingested amounts of EPA and DHA in most of these studies were higher than those used in successful CHD intervention trials(66). Diabetics should gradually build up their dosage of EPA and DHA, all the while keeping a close eye on their fasting blood glucose levels. In contrast to the situation with type 2 diabetics, a review of the literature suggests that similar dosages of fish oil help to lower fasting blood glucose in type 1 diabetics(67).

One final word of caution regarding fish oil supplements. There is one clinical trial that did not emulate the positive results of the GISSI and DART trials. In the DART-2 study, the group assigned to fish/fish oil consumption not only failed to lower their cardiovascular and all-cause mortality, they actually experienced increased cardiac mortality(68).

Numerous factors have been posited to explain the puzzling discrepancy between the results of DART-2 and the original DART study. One of these is that DART-2 was conducted under less-than-ideal conditions, a fact acknowledged by the DART researchers themselves. Due to funding issues, they were forced to perform DART-2 in two phases. Only 1,111 patients were enrolled during the first phase of the trial (1990-1992), which was then halted for twelve months due to lack of funding. The remaining 2,003 patients were then recruited during the second phase spanning from 1993-1996. To determine compliance, the researchers measured and compared blood levels of EPA--but not DHA--during the first phase only, and in a mere sixty-eight subjects from the fish oil and control groups. These blood EPA measurements were taken at baseline and then again at six months, even though patient follow-up ranged from three to nine years. Therefore, we have no idea whether most of the subjects actually consumed the fish/fish oil as instructed, and we have no knowledge of the subjects' long-term compliance. Although *mean* EPA levels were higher after six months in the tested fish/fish oil patients, *individual* blood EPA concentrations varied widely, indicating that many of the subjects had *not* complied with the fish/fish oil recommendations. Furthermore, no mention is made by the authors of DHA status, despite the fact that DHA is the predominant long-chain omega-3 fat found in cell membranes, and that that EPA and DHA may have differing effects upon the cardiovascular system(69).

Other questions also remain: What was the background omega-6 intake of the subjects assigned to fish oil? The authors do not report giving the fish oil subjects any advice to simultaneously lower their background omega-6 intake. If the subjects in DART-2 were consuming higher background levels of omega-6 fatty acids than the original DART participants, then any potential beneficial effect of the omega-3 fatty acids found in fish may have been negated. Indeed, FAO food disappearance data indicate that the consumption of omega-6 rich vegetable fats in the UK (the DART trial was conducted in Wales) rose through the 1980s and 1990s, while animal fat consumption declined(70). Given that increased linoleic acid intakes reduce cell membrane concentrations of omega-3 fats, while saturated fats enhance omega-3 status, this is not a trivial consideration. Improving one's omega-3:omega-6 ratio doesn't just involve taking extra omega-3s; it also requires minimal consumption or avoidance of omega-6-rich vegetable fats and the abundance of processed foods that contain them.

Also, the trial was not blinded. The authors themselves postulated that regular fish consumption or use of fish oil capsules could possibly have influenced the patients' or their physicians' behavior towards intake of medication or other issues related to diet and lifestyle.

All the aforementioned confounders notwithstanding, is there any actual property of fish/fish oil that could potentially have contributed to the negative results of the DART-2 study? One possibility proposed by the DART researchers is that, while fish oil is well-known among researchers to possess anti-arrhythmic effects, in susceptible patients they may exert pro-arrhythmic actions(71). In the original DART study, most of the men consumed fish, whereas in DART-2, a far greater proportion of men consumed encapsulated fish oil. Interestingly, in DART-2, most of the excess mortality risk was born by men consuming fish oil capsules instead of fish. When fish is eaten in solid form, its constituent nutrients are broken down and absorbed at a controlled rate. The authors speculate that if the men assigned to fish/fish oil in DART-2 were taking their entire daily dose of fish oil all in one 'hit', on an empty stomach, that this may have triggered a prompt and unnaturally large increase in blood omega-3 levels, one sufficient enough to disturb heart rhythm(72).

Such an explanation must be considered speculative, especially in light of DART-2's numerous other flaws. Nonetheless, as a precautionary measure, fish oil should always be consumed with food (preferably fat-containing meals) and, if possible, the dosage should be divided between meals. Multi-gram dosages of EPA and DHA should be avoided, unless one has an inflammatory condition that necessitates such high dosages and is being supervised by a knowledgeable medical practitioner.

Exercise

Overall, clinical studies utilizing exercise as the only intervention in CHD patients have elicited thirty-five percent and twenty-seven percent reductions in CHD and overall mortality, respectively. Again, these mortality benefits are similar in magnitude to those observed with statins.

In addition to dramatic cardiovascular improvements, exercise is highly effective for weight loss, improving glycemic control, attenuating and reversing the age-related decrease in muscle mass and strength, alleviating depressive symptoms, and increasing bone mineral density(73-76). Epidemiological studies have consistently linked regular physical activity with a lower risk for various types of cancer(77).

Don't waste time debating whether you should do resistance training (such as weight-lifting) or aerobic exercise--research shows that the greatest benefits are derived from a program that incorporates both(78).

Diets Rich in Vegetables, Fruits, and Omega-3 Fatty Acids

Diets that emphasize not only regular omega-3 intake but also vegetables and fruits have produced reductions in coronary and overall mortality of up to eighty-one percent and sixty percent, respectively. Mortality reductions of this degree are far greater than those seen in any of the statin trials.

In addition to protecting against CHD, a dietary pattern characterized by high fruit and vegetable intake is associated with lower incidence of stroke, cancer, Alzheimer's and osteoporosis(79-91). As with fish oil, boosting your intake of non-cereal plant foods is a win-win proposition; numerous prospective studies have shown that those who eat the most fruits and vegetables tend to live the longest(92-94).

Supplementation With Coenzyme Q10, Selenium, and L-carnitine

The studies in Table 24a involving supplemental coenzyme Q10 (CoQ10), selenium, and L-carnitine suggest that striking reductions in cardiovascular and overall mortality can be achieved by administering these nutrients to CHD patients.

Enthusiasm for the large death rate reductions observed must be tempered by the fact that the aforementioned nutrients were all tested in small trials. Whether such marked reductions in mortality can be replicated in trials with larger numbers of participants remains to be seen. What we do know at present is that:

- All of these nutrients play crucial roles in maintaining healthy cardiovascular function;
- They are often deficient in cardiovascular patients;
- The proposed mechanisms by which fortification of these nutrients may provide cardiovascular benefits are indeed scientifically plausible.

CoQ10, for instance, is found in every cell in the body with the highest concentrations occurring in the heart, liver and kidneys. Unfortunately, our C0Q10 status becomes progressively poorer with advancing age. At 40 years of age, levels of CoQ10 in the average person's heart are twenty-five percent lower than what they were at age 21; by age 80, CoQ10 levels have typically declined by fifty-seven percent!(95)

In patients with CHD, CoQ10 at daily doses of 100-200 milligrams has been shown to significantly lower blood pressure, free radical activity, blood sugar and insulin levels, and lipoprotein(a)(96). In order to ingest such high levels of CoQ10, supplementation is essential. The average diet supplies around three to five milligrams of CoQ10, a figure that can be bolstered somewhat by consuming organ meats such as liver, kidney and heart(97). Research suggests that CoQ10 in soft gels and powdered capsules is absorbed with greater efficiency than that found in hard tablets(98,99). For optimal absorption it may also be wise to consume CoQ10 supplements with a fat-containing meal.

No serious side effects have been noted with high dose CoQ10 therapy, although increases in nausea have been observed in trial participants taking 100 milligrams per day. There has been some concern that CoQ10 could interfere with the actions of blood-thinning medications, but a four-week double-blind trial found that 100 milligrams daily did not in any way impair the efficacy of the widely prescribed anti-coagulant warfarin(100). As with fish oil, anyone taking anti-coagulant drugs should have their doctor keep an eye on their bleeding time and clotting markers as a precautionary measure.

CoQ10 does not adversely impact upon glycemic control in diabetic patients; some studies have actually detected an improvement in glycemic control and/or endothelial function in diabetics taking 100-200 milligrams of CoQ10(101-105).

Because cholesterol-lowering drugs can severely deplete the body of CoQ10, supplementation may literally prove to be a lifesaver for those taking statins. Italian researchers found that while C0Q10 levels dropped in patients taking twenty milligrams of simvastatin per day, they actually increased in patients who took 100 milligrams of CoQ10 along with their simvastatin(106).

In 2005, Texas cardiologist and researcher Peter Langsjoen published a report on fifty patients who had discontinued statins and commenced taking CoQ10. The patients were identified after Langsjoen screened all 328 new patients presenting at his cardiology clinic between January 2002 and December 2003, and identified 50 patients who were taking statin drugs at the time of their initial visit. As all 50 patients presented with one or more statin-related adverse effects as their chief complaint, statin drug therapy was discontinued. Langsjoen instructed all the patients to begin taking CoQ10 daily, at an average dose of 240 milligrams per day.

After an average follow-up of twenty-two months, the prevalence of fatigue dropped from 84% to 16%, myalgia from 64% to 6%, dyspnea from 58% to 12%, memory loss from 8% to 4% and peripheral neuropathy from 10% to 2%. There were two deaths from lung cancer and one death from aortic stenosis but no strokes or myocardial infarctions. Measurements of heart function either improved or remained stable in the majority of patients. Langsjoen and his co-authors concluded: *"... statin-related side effects, including statin cardiomyopathy, are far more common than previously published and are reversible with the combination of statin discontinuation and supplemental CoQ10. We saw no adverse consequences from statin discontinuation."*(107)

In addition to its coronary benefits, CoQ10 supplementation also improves immune function and has shown promise in the treatment of cancer, heart failure, periodontitis, early stage Parkinson disease, and mitochondrial disorders that leave sufferers feeling chronically weak and fatigued(108-116).

Super Selenium

Selenium may be one of the lesser-known trace elements, but is nonetheless critical for good health. It forms an essential part of the antioxidant enzyme *glutathione peroxidase,* and works synergistically with vitamin E to scavenge free radicals from our bodies. Glutathione peroxidase and other selenium-containing compounds are involved in regulating nitric oxide levels in arteries, the adhesion of cells to artery walls, of apoptosis (cell death), and of eicosanoid production. Therefore, they are an important determinant of cardiovascular health(117).

That selenium may offer protection against CHD may come as a surprise to many, for this trace element has been most widely researched for its potential in cancer prevention. Selenium's cancer-fighting prowess was demonstrated among 1,300 skin cancer patients randomized to receive, in double-blind fashion, a daily 200-microgram selenium supplement or an identical placebo. After an average treatment period of four and a half years, selenium supplementation produced a thirty-seven percent reduction in total cancer incidence and a fifty percent decrease in overall cancer mortality! Prostate cancer incidence was reduced by sixty-three percent, colorectal cancers by fifty-eight percent, and lung cancer was cut by forty-six percent among those receiving selenium. It is interesting to note that all of the participants of this trial were recruited from the eastern coastal plain of the U.S., an area characterized by low soil selenium levels and high rates of cancer mortality. Also noteworthy was the fact that at the commencement of the study, the subjects' average blood selenium levels were 114ng/ml. While in the lower range of the normal levels reported for U.S. citizens, this figure was nonetheless nowhere near the 30ng/ml limit considered indicative of overt selenium deficiency(118).

An intervention trial undertaken among over 130,000 residents of Qidong County in China, an area afflicted by high rates of hepatitis B infection and liver cancer, found that liver cancer incidence was reduced by thirty-five percent in selenium-supplemented residents during eight years of follow-up. After selenium was withdrawn from the treated populations, their liver cancer rates began to climb back to former levels. The same group of researchers also performed a clinical study among 226 Qidong County Hepatitis B patients who took either 200 micrograms of supplemental selenium or an identical placebo tablet daily for four years. During the treatment period, none of the subjects in the selenium group developed liver cancer, whereas seven of 113 placebo subjects were diagnosed with this malignancy(119).

Linxian County, also in China, suffers one of the world's highest rates of esophageal and stomach cancer rates in the world. In the mid-eighties, researchers wondered if vitamin and mineral supplementation would prove to be of any benefit in reducing Linxian's disproportionately high cancer rates. In 1986, they began giving over 29,000 Linxian residents one of four different vitamin/mineral combinations, or a placebo. When the trial finished in 1991, those receiving a selenium, beta carotene, and vitamin E formulation experienced a twenty-one percent lower rate of stomach cancer, a thirteen percent reduction in total cancer incidence, and a nine percent reduction in all-cause mortality. None of the other supplement combinations produced any significant reductions in cancer or all-cause mortality(120).

In 2004, French researchers published the results of the SU.VI.MAX study, a randomized, double-blind, placebo-controlled trial involving over 13,000 healthy adults aged 35-60. The participants took a single daily capsule containing 120 milligrams of ascorbic acid, 30 milligrams of vitamin E, 6 milligrams of beta carotene, 100 µg of selenium, and 20 milligrams of zinc, or a placebo. After 7.5 years of supplementation, cancer and overall mortality rates in men were significantly reduced, by thirty-one and thirty-seven percent, respectively!(121)

Low selenium intakes have been linked to diabetes, poor immune function, AIDS, asthma, thyroid disorders, male infertility, spontaneous abortions, cognitive impairment, depression, anxiety, and hostility(122-130). In addition to lowering cancer rates, double-blind trials have shown that selenium supplementation produces significant clinical improvements in asthmatic patients, distinct improvements in mood and anxiety levels, improved immune function and, when combined with zinc supplementation, marked reductions in infectious illnesses among institutionalized elderly subjects(131-136).

The amount of selenium found in plant and animal foods is largely dependent upon the selenium levels of the soil in which they are grown or raised. Unfortunately, soil levels of selenium throughout most of the world--including Australia, England, New Zealand, and much of China and the U.S.--are quite poor. Recent estimates suggest that selenium deficiency affects up to one billion people worldwide. To make matters worse, researchers have found that the selenium content of the average diet is in decline. The estimated average selenium intake in cancer-prone countries ranges from 12-43 micrograms in England, 75 micrograms in Australia, and upwards of 60 micrograms in the US. The Japanese, whose cancer rates are relatively low compared to most Western countries, have estimated average selenium intakes range between 104-127 micrograms. In Venezuela, where total cancer rates are even lower than those of Japan, average selenium intakes range between 200-350 micrograms(129,137,138).

Brazil nuts are by far the richest food source of selenium, averaging 543 micrograms per ounce. If you don't eat Brazil nuts on a regular basis, and unless you live in a region with high selenium levels in the soil and water, then supplemental selenium is a wise idea. While selenium intakes over 1,000 micrograms per day are not recommended because of toxicity concerns, supplementation with the 100-200 microgram amounts used in clinical trials has not been associated with any adverse effects. For those wondering which of the myriad types of available selenium supplements they should buy, the successful CHD and cancer intervention trials have used selenium-rich yeast, sodium selenite and l-seleno-methionine.

L-Carnitine

L-carnitine is an amino acid whose presence is absolutely essential for the fat-burning process to proceed. It assists the transport of fatty acids across the cell membrane and into the mitochondria, the 'engine rooms' of our cells, where they are used to produce the ultimate cellular energy source, adenosine triphosphate (ATP). Mitochondrial fat burning is the primary fuel source in heart and skeletal muscle, which should provide a pretty strong clue as to just how important optimal intakes of this nutrient are.

A review of the scientific literature shows that this remarkable amino acid has generated clinical benefits in heart failure, impotence, chronic fatigue syndrome, male infertility, and pregnancy outcomes. L-carnitine also enhances exercise tolerance in patients with angina and respiratory disorders(139, 140).

The primary source of L-carnitine is meat, with lamb being an especially potent source. However, unless you eat several kilograms of meat on a daily basis, achieving a daily intake of four grams--the amount used in the successful study shown in Table 24a--necessitates the use of carnitine supplements. In addition to regularly eating meat, avoiding low-fat intakes and keeping a lid on carbohydrate consumption can also help improve your carnitine status. In healthy men receiving the same amount of dietary carnitine, blood levels of this crucial amino acid rose significantly in those following a high-fat, low-carbohydrate diet, while no change in carnitine levels were observed in individuals on a high-carbohydrate, low-fat diet(141).

Better than Statins

The strategies discussed in this chapter have each been shown to lower CHD and overall mortality to a degree similar or superior to that seen with statin drugs, the establishment's current darlings when it comes to fighting CHD. There also exists the very real possibility that the combination of all these interventions together could lead to even more pronounced reductions in cardiovascular and all-cause mortality--reductions of a magnitude that would simply blow those seen with statin and aspirin therapy right out of the water.

Unlike statins or aspirin, these non-drug interventions do not increase the risk of adverse effects but actually lower the risk of other ailments including diabetes, cancer, arthritis, asthma, depression, and pregnancy complications. As such, they deserve top billing in any regimen designed to prevent CHD.

That most health authorities, medical professionals, and laypersons know so little of these low-risk but highly-effective approaches is a shameful indictment on the current state of our Big Pharma-dominated health care system.

An important part of piecing together an effective anti-CHD strategy is not only establishing what does work, but also what doesn't. By doing so, we can make sure our time, effort and financial resources are directed only towards productive interventions. To this end, we will take a look in the next chapter at some highly touted 'heart-healthy' interventions that have not been demonstrated to lower CHD nor overall mortality.

Chapter 25

"There are in fact two things, science and opinion; the former begets knowledge, the latter ignorance."
Hippocrates

Heart Frauds

Identifying the unproven and the useless

"Eating Fiber Reduces Heart Disease", exclaims the press release for a large epidemiological study by Harvard researchers; *"foods containing soy protein...may reduce the risk of CHD",* states the Food and Drug Administration (FDA); *"...some experts now 'prescribe' olive oil as an excellent way to cut the risk of first time as well as subsequent heart attacks and strokes",* writes a best-selling author.

Dietary fiber, olive oil, and soy foods are just a few of the substances that have been vigorously promoted as effective CHD-fighters. Despite such enthusiastic claims, there is a complete lack of clinical evidence to show that these and many other highly-hyped interventions can actually reduce coronary or all-cause mortality. Let's take a closer look at some of these unproven strategies.

The Fiber Fallacy

Attempting to convince the average dietitian that whole-grain cereal products are not a health-enhancing food is a task only slightly less difficult than trying to convert the Pope to atheism. Whole-grain cereals are repeatedly promoted as the holy grail of healthy eating, a concept completely unsupported by clinical evidence. In fact, as any Paleontologist worth his salt could tell you, humans were never even meant to eat cereal grains. We only started doing so in earnest around 10,000 years ago, when a mix of population pressure, climate change, and declining availability of large wild game precipitated the onset of the Agricultural Revolution.

When it comes to the alleged ability of cereal fiber to prevent heart disease, there is plenty of epidemiological evidence to suggest this is true. Epidemiological studies, however, are invariably subject to a whole host of confounding factors that can never be fully accounted for, no matter how hard their authors try. In the case of cereal fiber consumption, it is well known that those who eat whole-grain and whole-meal foods tend to be more health-conscious than those who eat refined cereal products.

In the Iowa Women's Health Study, for example, which examined cereal grain intake among over 34,000 women, researchers found that *"higher whole-grain intake was associated with having more education, a lower body mass index and waist-to-hip ratio [and] being a non-smoker, doing more regular physical activity, and using vitamin supplements and hormone replacement therapy."*(1) In addition, those who ate more whole-grains also ate less refined-grains and less sugar. Simply abstaining from smoking and engaging in regular exercise, two of the qualities more common among whole grain consumers, will dramatically improve one's odds of avoiding CHD. It goes without saying that clinical trials in which these other confounding variables are controlled would be a far better way to tease out any heart-healthy effect of cereal fiber.

Only one controlled clinical trial has ever tested the claim that cereal fiber reduces heart disease. The Diet And Reinfarction Trial (see Chapters 8 and 23) examined the effect of either increasing fish or fish oil intake, replacing saturated fat with polyunsaturated fat, or increasing fiber consumption among over 2,000 male heart attack survivors. The men in the fiber group increased their consumption of wholemeal bread, high-fiber breakfast cereals, and wheat bran. They also suffered the highest death rate in the study.

After two years of follow-up, 123 men in the fiber group had died, compared to only 101 given no fiber advice. In comparison, only 94 in the fish group died, compared to 130 given no fish advice, while no change in mortality was observed among the fat advice group(2). This is the only controlled trial that has examined the effect of unrefined grain consumption on CHD. The fact that it completely fails to support the theory that increased cereal fiber intake protects against heart disease has proved to be of little deterrence to dietitians and health authorities who regularly make just such a claim.

Another group of British researchers tested the hypothesis that dietary fiber might protect against the development of CHD via reductions in platelet aggregation and blood clotting. They fed volunteers white bread for three weeks and brown and wholemeal breads for a further three weeks each. No change was seen in platelet function. A further experiment in which the subjects were fed an additional thirty-six grams per day of pectin (a soluble fiber found in oat bran and vegetables) showed that, while serum cholesterol concentrations were significantly lowered, platelet aggregation, platelet fatty acid composition, blood clotting times, and bleeding times remained unchanged(3).

Diabetics are another group who are urged by their dietitians to increase cereal fiber intake, but the findings of Canadian researchers would suggest that whole-grain products are best left off the diabetic menu. Twenty-three type 2 diabetic men and women completed two three-month phases of a randomized crossover study. In the test phase, high-fiber bread and breakfast cereals were provided, giving an extra nineteen grams per day of cereal fiber. During the control phase, only four grams per day of additional cereal fiber was given. No differences were seen in body weight, fasting blood glucose or glycated hemoglobin (a measure of long-term glycemic control). No favorable effect was found for any of the following CHD risk markers: serum lipids, apolipoproteins, blood pressure, serum uric acid, clotting factors, homocysteine and C-reactive protein. Oxidation of LDL cholesterol, implicated in the development of CHD, was actually higher in the fiber-rich phase than during the low-fiber phase(4).

So much for the hypothesis that fiber reduces heart disease...

Protection from cancer is another claim frequently made for high-fiber cereal foods; colon cancer in particular, we are repeatedly told, would be dramatically reduced if only we would all start eating more whole-grains. While epidemiological studies backing this notion are easy to find, none of the numerous controlled intervention trials conducted in this area support the possibility that high wheat fiber intakes prevent the progression of colon cancer(5).

When you set about ridding all the refined and processed garbage from your diet, be sure to replace it with fresh meats, eggs, fruits, nuts and vegetables. Cereal grains, whole or otherwise, should *not* form the foundation of a healthy diet--in fact, many researchers question whether we should be eating them at all. If you must eat cereal grains, keep your intake low and emphasize gluten-free and low-lectin varieties like rice and millet (lectins are anti-nutrients found in most cereal grain and legume varieties that may negatively influence immune function).

Soy: Savior or Serpent?

In October, 1999, the FDA authorized the following health claim for foods containing soy protein: *"...foods containing soy protein included in a diet low in saturated fat and cholesterol may reduce the risk of CHD..."* The FDA approved this health claim for soy protein in response to a petition by Protein Technologies International, one of the world's largest soy producers(6). It should be clearly noted that there is no evidence whatsoever that soy protein has ever prevented even a single heart attack. The heart-healthy claim for soy was predicated almost entirely upon studies showing that soy protein consumption lowers blood cholesterol levels(7). Evidently, forty-years worth of non-supportive results from dietary cholesterol-lowering trials mattered little to the FDA. The regulatory behemoth recommended that consumers incorporate at least twenty-five grams of soy protein into their diets each day--the minimum amount determined to be necessary for cholesterol reduction.

To date, there has not been a single controlled dietary intervention trial examining the impact of soy upon CHD incidence or mortality. A number of studies have been conducted examining the impact of soy upon various parameters of CHD risk, such as arterial function and LDL oxidation, but the results of these are a mixed bag. Some of these studies have shown soy intake reduces LDL oxidation (8-10). Some researchers have presented evidence suggesting soy intake may improve arterial function(11). Others however, have found no difference(12,13), and some researchers have found evidence of worsening arterial function among subjects consuming soy protein(14,15).

Researchers who tested soy's ability to counteract blood platelet aggregation, a measure of blood-clotting potential, could not detect any benefit in healthy men consuming soy protein isolate(16). Overweight and obese women who consumed either red meat or soybeans as their major protein source for sixteen weeks experienced similar reductions in weight, blood pressure, and improvement in measurements of arterial function(13). Other researchers have found that soy protein raises levels of lipoprotein(a), a compound implicated in the development of CHD(14,17).

Apart from the obvious financial benefits to those who profit from the sale of soy foods and isoflavone supplements, there is little reason at present to promote soy as a heart-healthy food. Whether soy can in fact reduce CHD mortality is completely unknown, and research on soy's influence upon various measures of cardiovascular health is conflicting. Indeed, some evidence suggests that soy consumption may actually have adverse effects on the cardiovascular system.

In a strain of mice especially prone to hypertrophic cardiomyopathy, feeding males a soy-based diet resulted in dilation and heart failure. However, males fed a milk protein (casein) diet did not deteriorate to severe, dilated cardiomyopathy. Remarkably, their left ventricle size and contractile function were preserved, and several other indicators of pathological decline in cardiac function were prevented(18).

The multinational giants who control the soy industry have been extremely successful in favorably manipulating public perception of soy. By sponsoring research, then relentlessly promoting the results of what appear to be supportive studies, they have convinced millions of people around the world that soy is a wonderfully healthy 'super-food'. The soy-marketing machine has aggressively publicized studies suggesting a possible protective effect of soy on cancer, but numerous studies suggesting that it may *increase* cancer have not enjoyed such enthusiastic promotion(19-28).

Experimental, clinical and epidemiological evidence has also linked soy with immune impairment, thyroid dysfunction, Type 1 diabetes, lowered testosterone levels in males, and even hypospadias (birth defects of the penis)(29-54). Soy consumption has also been shown to interfere with iron absorption, even when its considerable phytate content is removed. As such, it is a highly questionable food choice for premenopausal women, a group that is often troubled by sub-optimal iron status(55). Soy foods are also unusually high in aluminum, a metal that has been implicated in promoting Alzheimer's disease(56). Individuals who are susceptible to kidney stones have been warned against consuming soy foods due to their high concentrations of oxalate, a compound that can bind with calcium in the kidney to form kidney stones(57).

No one can predict with any certainty just what the long term effects of consuming soy in the amounts recommended by the FDA will be. While the Chinese and Japanese are eagerly proffered as shining examples of the long-term safety of soy, their daily consumption of this staple is much lower than what we have been led to believe. Recent studies indicate that the median intake of soy protein among Chinese women is ten grams, a lot less than the twenty-five gram amounts currently being promoted for 'disease-fighting' purposes(58). The Japanese eat even less; a survey of over 4,800 Japanese adults showed that the average intake of soy protein was eight grams among men, and 6.9 grams among women(59).

Until scientists can conclusively establish the long-term safety of consuming soy, the use of soy foods, soy protein, and soy isoflavone supplements should be avoided. The exception is small amounts of traditional soy condiments such as miso and soy sauce, which when used in small amounts are unlikely to be problematic due to their miniscule soy protein and isoflavone content.

Oily Claims For Olive Oil

After realizing that they made a big mistake by prematurely endorsing polyunsaturated vegetable oils, health authorities quietly stopped recommending their copious consumption. Instead, they began promoting a new variant of saturated fat restriction: the low-fat, high-carbohydrate diet. Again, their foolishness has been highlighted by the startling increase in diabetes and obesity that has closely followed the population's ready acceptance of the low-fat paradigm. Not yet ready to discard this whole idiotic anti-saturated fat charade, many authorities and researchers are now slowly discarding the high-carbohydrate theory and turning towards monounsaturated fat-rich foods. The best known and most widely promoted of these has been olive oil.

Olive oil, we are told, is a major reason why the Italians, Spaniards, and Greeks enjoy such low rates of heart disease. Before you fall for such hype and begin smothering your food with this 'liquid gold' in the hope of avoiding heart disease, be aware that only one randomized, blinded, clinical trial has ever examined the effect of olive oil on CHD mortality. This study, conducted by British researchers and published in 1965, compared three diets over a two-year period: An olive oil-enriched diet, a corn oil-enriched diet, and a control diet containing a typical amount of animal fat. The results were hardly supportive of the widely accepted notion that olive oil is the most heart-friendly of fats.

After two years, nine coronary incidents had occurred in the olive oil group, twelve in the corn oil group, and six among the control group. Three subjects from the olive oil group and five from the corn oil group had died, whilst only one fatality occurred among those eating the animal fat-rich control diet. All deaths were due to heart disease(60). This may have been a relatively small study of short duration, but the step-wise increase in mortality that occurred with increasing dietary fat unsaturation fully concurs with what we know about the role of free radical damage in CHD and the increased susceptibility of unsaturated fats to oxidation. It also concurs with the results of controlled clinical trials showing saturated fat-rich diets to reduce markers of blood clotting and free radical activity when compared to diets dominated by monounsaturated or polyunsaturated vegetable oils(61-63).

The purported benefits of the Mediterranean diet are likely due not to monounsaturated fat consumption, but a high intake of antioxidant-rich vegetables and fruits, and consumption of foods that encourage a more favorable omega-6:omega-3 ratio. Next time someone tries to tell you a low intake of saturated fat is responsible for the low rates of CHD seen in Mediterranean countries, keep in mind that the French, copious consumers of saturated fat-rich butters, cheeses and pates, experience the lowest CHD death rates in all of Europe. As we learnt in Chapter 6, the widely proffered excuse that liberal red wine consumption explains this phenomenon doesn't wash--the Italians enjoy a per capita red wine consumption similar to that of their French neighbors, but have CHD mortality rates on a par with those seen in Greece and Spain, where far less wine is consumed.

The above is not meant to imply that olive oil should join omega-6-rich polyunsaturated vegetable oils and be completely abolished from our diets; the former is not as oxidation-prone as the latter, nor will it exert the same highly detrimental effects on the body's omega-6:omega-3 ratio. Plus, a modest amount of olive oil, along with a sprinkling of herbs and a little lemon juice, can go a long way towards spicing up an otherwise bland salad. Just don't overdo it, and don't fall for unfounded claims that fat from olives is somehow healthier than that from meats, eggs and dairy.

Cholestin Conjecture

Cholestin, or red yeast rice extract, is another cholesterol-lowering supplement that has been heavily promoted as an alternative to statins. Chinese researchers have reported that cholestin can lower levels of C-reactive protein, lipoprotein(a), and post-meal blood triglycerides(64,65). Whether these reductions in 'risk factors' translates to an actual decrease in mortality is anyone's guess--no controlled trial has ever been carried out to test this possibility.

Be warned--just because something is 'natural' does not mean it is safe. One of the active ingredients in red yeast rice extract is lovastatin, the same compound used in the statin drug Mevacor. Like statins, this supplement possesses the unwelcome ability to dramatically lower CoQ10 levels. When mice were given one of two red yeast rice extract doses--the lowest being equivalent to the average recommended human dose--liver and heart CoQ10 levels declined dramatically in both groups within thirty minutes! After twenty-four hours, levels of liver and cardiac CoQ10 were still reduced. Not surprisingly, the higher dose of red yeast rice exerted a greater suppressive effect than the lower dose(66). CoQ10 is extremely important for energy production and defense against free radicals. Anything that depletes our bodily levels of this important substance--especially in critical organs like the heart and liver--should be avoided like a bad smell.

Side effects from red yeast rice extract have already been reported in human patients. The December 2003 issue of the *Southern Medical Journal* reported on a middle-aged man with joint pain and muscle weakness that had begun a month after starting red rice extract. Laboratory testing revealed a moderately elevated creatine phosphokinase level, indicating that the extract was causing muscle damage. His symptoms and lab test abnormalities resolved upon discontinuing the supplement. Eight months later, the man resumed taking the product and his creatine phosphokinase level again headed north(67). In 2002, researchers from St. Michael's Hospital in Toronto reported a case of rhabdomyolysis in a renal-transplant recipient, which appeared after the patient began taking a herbal preparation containing red yeast rice. The condition resolved when consumption of the product was ceased(68).

Fire Your Shrink and Buy a Bike Instead?

Given that exposure to stress and depression greatly increase the incidence of CHD, it is not unreasonable to assume that stress management and psychological interventions could help prevent CHD mortality. However, a pooled analysis of trials involving psychological-based interventions in patients with CHD showed no reduction in cardiac or overall mortality(69). Only small improvements were noted in anxiety and depression, raising the possibility that these trials failed to produce favorable mortality outcomes simply because the psychosocial changes achieved were too small to be of any benefit.

Clinical trials suggest that some stress management techniques are better than others, and may indeed be of benefit when properly applied. In a randomized three-month trial that compared Transcendental Meditation (TM) with progressive muscle relaxation, the former reduced systolic pressure by 10.7 and diastolic pressure by 6.4, while the latter produced smaller reductions of 4.7 and 3.3, respectively(70). Another trial by the same researchers, involving hypertensive African American adults, found that those assigned to practice TM experienced a decrease in carotid intima-media thickness (a surrogate for coronary atherosclerosis) over a 6.8 month follow-up period, while those who took part in a *"CVD risk factor prevention education program"* experienced a slight increase(71).

The possibility that these changes could produce real reductions in mortality was raised when the researchers published long-term follow-up data for 202 elderly participants of two three-month TM trials. After an average of 7.6 years' follow-up, the TM group experienced a twenty-three percent reduction in all-cause mortality and a thirty percent drop in cardiovascular mortality(72). Excitement over these positive results must be tempered by the fact there was no direct contact with individual subjects after the initial three-month trials, so compliance rates with the prescribed treatments during the follow-up period remain unknown. High short-term compliance rates were reported in the original papers, and, according to head researcher Robert H. Schneider, M.D., *"experience suggests that long-term compliance with the TM program is relatively high, especially compared to compliance with modern medical treatments, which is notoriously low."*(73) Further research into the potential mortality benefits of Transcendental Meditation is certainly warranted.

When it comes to treatment for stress and depression, the most effective treatment may not be group therapy or lying on a psychiatrist's couch, but putting on your workout gear and raising up a good sweat! As we shall learn in Chapter 28, exercise produces substantial mood-enhancing effects that appear to surpass those of meditation and anti-depressant medication(74-78).

Fact Versus Faith

Every intervention discussed in this chapter has a devoted army of followers deeply committed to the belief that it can reduce the death toll from CHD. At present, their enthusiasm is not accompanied by supportive scientific data. Because misplaced faith, hope, and fantasy are of little use to those seeking to avoid the very real killer that is CHD, readers are advised to base their efforts on strategies that possess demonstrated efficacy.

In the next chapter, we will seek to answer one of the most commonly asked questions by those wishing to avoid CHD.

Chapter 26

"Opinions are like noses--everybody's got one."
Author unknown.

So What Should I Eat?

Constructing a heart-healthy diet you can live with.

When it comes to outlining the 'ideal' diet, there is no shortage of opinions, most of which wildly conflict with each other. Mainstream 'experts' insist that carbohydrates are the Holy Grail of nutrition, while others maintain they are to blame for the skyrocketing incidence of obesity and diabetes. Milk is enthusiastically lauded in some quarters as 'the perfect food' and denounced in others as a harmful toxin that was never meant to be consumed by humans. Dietitians and health authorities prescribe copious cereal grain consumption with an almost religious devotion, while an increasing number of researchers caution that these are a historically recent food to which we have not yet fully adapted. Proponents of vegetarianism rabidly assert that animal flesh ingestion explains much of our health woes, while scores of ex-vegetarians report how much better they felt after reintroducing meat into their diet...

Yes, if there is one thing you can count on each time you visit your local bookstore or log on to the internet in search of dietary guidance, it is the prospect of being confronted with a staggering array of starkly contrasting and confusing theories. While these will range from the scientifically plausible to the downright ridiculous, there is one common denominator among their promoters: Each is adamant that their theory is the ultimate path to nutritional utopia.

The aim of this chapter is not to present you with yet another one-size-fits-all 'ultimate' diet plan. Instead, it has been written with the knowledge that human beings vary widely in their individual metabolic requirements, digestive abilities, tastes and food preferences. Rather than campaign for a single dietary ideology, this chapter will discuss two extremely important characteristics of heart-healthy nutrition that can and should be adopted by virtually anyone, regardless of their individual dietary preferences.

These two crucial requirements of a truly heart-healthy diet are:

1) It must keep blood glucose levels well within the normal range.
2) It must deliver as many protective vitamins, minerals, trace elements, amino acids, and plant phenols per ingested calorie as possible.

As readers have already learnt throughout this book, the importance of these characteristics in preventing heart disease is underscored by a huge volume of supportive scientific research. Let's see how we can all best incorporate them into our daily diets.

Requirement #1: Keeping a Lid on Blood Sugar

After reading Chapter 18, you should hold no doubts about the importance of keeping blood sugar levels safely inside the normal range. Without question, the single most effective dietary strategy for lowering elevated blood glucose is to cut your carbohydrate intake. At maintenance calorie levels, a reduced carbohydrate intake will lower elevated blood sugar levels, while a high carbohydrate diet similar to that advised by the AHA and the American Diabetes Association (ADA) will typically raise blood sugar levels.(1-5)

The latter organization even admits as much; in one of the most bizarre and self-contradictory pieces of nutritional advice this author has ever read, the ADA states that: *"Yes, foods with carbohydrate--starches, vegetables, fruits, and dairy products--will raise your blood glucose more quickly than meats and fats, but they are the healthiest foods for you."* They allude to the deleterious consequences of following such advice when they admit: *"Your doctor may need to adjust your medications when you eat more carbohydrates. You may need to increase your activity level or try spacing carbohydrates throughout the day."*(6)

If you are diabetic and proceed to eat more carbohydrates, your doctor may indeed need to adjust your medication dosage--upwards! And don't expect exercise to negate the effects of a high carbohydrate intake; a study with type 1 diabetics who exercised three or more times a week found that a modest increase in carbohydrate ingestion from fifty to fifty-nine percent of calories bumped up blood glucose levels by an average ten percent, increased insulin requirements by fifteen percent, and lowered athletic performance by six percent(7).

Living La Vida Low-Carb

If one chooses to go the reduced-carbohydrate route, just how much carbohydrate should be eaten each day?

For our purposes, a true low-carbohydrate diet can be categorized as one that supplies less than 100 grams of carbohydrate per day. It is below this level that noticeable increases in blood ketones--metabolic byproducts of the fat-burning process--become apparent. Very low-carbohydrate diets are those that supply fifty grams of carbohydrate or less per day (these figures, by the way, are for total carbohydrate intake, not 'net carbs', the latter being a controversial method of calculating carbohydrate intake promoted by certain popular low-carb authors). Very low carbohydrate diets, or "ketogenic" diets, result in far greater levels of blood ketones than diets supplying over fifty grams of carbohydrate per day.

Very low-carbohydrate ketogenic diets have been clinically demonstrated to be effective for weight loss and improving glycemic control. The problem with these diets is that many people will temporarily experience a number of untoward effects. Lethargy, mental fogginess, irritability, halitosis, cramping, carbohydrate cravings and declining athletic performance are some of the undesirable, albeit transient, effects that can soon occur after reducing carbohydrate intake to very low levels. This occurs because the body is making the transformation from burning primarily glucose for fuel to burning fat. This metabolic shift requires the up-regulation of hormones, neurotransmitters and enzymes that are responsible for efficient fat burning. This process seems to take longer in some people than others, temporarily leaving them in an energy-deficient state. After successfully completing this metabolic transition, many people find they have greater--and much more stable--energy levels than ever before.

A number of popular low-carbohydrate diet plans--whose authors are under the erroneous impression that ketosis is a critical component of successful weight loss--feature a two-week 'induction' phase, where carbohydrate intake is suddenly cut to twenty grams or less per day. This is done to plunge the body into ketosis and *"kickstart"* the weight loss process. This is not a particularly intelligent strategy. If you have been on a high-carbohydrate diet for most or all of your life, you cannot expect to make this metabolic shift smoothly overnight. The initial lethargy that frequently accompanies the early stages of adopting a very low-carbohydrate ketogenic diet is often exacerbated by the fact that many beginning low-carb dieters are also simultaneously cutting their caloric intake. This scenario simultaneously presents the body with two major metabolic challenges at once. If you are intent on adopting a very low-carbohydrate ketogenic diet, it is strongly recommended that you lower your carbohydrate intake gradually, rather than rudely shocking your body with a massive overnight cut in carbohydrate intake.

After thoroughly examining the literature, and contemplating the personal experiences of hundreds of individuals that I have personally trained, consulted and corresponded with, I firmly believe most people are best served forgetting about ketogenic diets. My advice is to throw away the Ketostix, and settle on a daily carbohydrate intake of sixty to eighty grams. At this level you will still derive the considerable benefits of low-carbohydrate nutrition without the uncomfortable side effects that can initially accompany very low-carbohydrate diets(8,9). A similar level of carbohydrate intake is advised by Wolfgang Lutz, M.D, an Austrian physician who has prescribed low-carbohydrate diets for over four decades to thousands of patients with much success(10).

A common criticism of low-carbohydrate diets is that they are deficient in phytochemical-rich plant foods. Like most criticisms of low-carb nutrition, this is pure hogwash. The next time someone tries to tell you that low-carbing means eating nothing but meat and eggs, keep in mind that a seventy-five gram daily carbohydrate limit allows the consumption of:

100g fennel
100g Romaine lettuce
100g red tomato
(the above items used in a salad and seasoned with lemon juice, olive oil and herbs)
100g broccoli
100g cauliflower
100g pumpkin
70g walnuts
200g blueberries

or

100g avocado
100g strawberries
100g red cabbage
70g (1 small bulb) onion
3g (1 clove) garlic
308g (2 fruits) pomegranate.

The above examples, which are only two of hundreds of possible combinations, allow for the daily consumption of 681-870 grams of fruits, nuts and vegetables--easily exceeding the 400-500 gram amounts that have successfully improved antioxidant status in controlled clinical trials. In fact, anyone who structures their low-carbohydrate diet correctly should find themselves eating more antioxidant-rich non-cereal plant foods than ever before. Even very low-carbohydrate diets still allow for the consumption of significant amounts of nutrient-rich vegetables, especially ultra-healthy greens.

If you are diabetic or have elevated blood sugar levels, just how low your carbohydrate intake must go is something that should be ascertained by keeping a close watch on your blood sugar levels. All things being equal, the lower the carbohydrate intake, the greater the reduction in blood glucose(11).

The exact amount of carbohydrates ingested will depend, of course, on body size, activity levels, and individual metabolic requirements. Highly active individuals should be aware that reduced carbohydrate intake will typically need to be offset by increased fat intake in order to avoid impaired recovery and reduced athletic performance. Many people will find that a little fine-tuning is necessary to determine their ideal carbohydrate level.

How do you figure out how many grams of carbohydrate you are consuming? You'll need to weigh your servings of carbohydrate-containing foods on a scale then use a nutrient database to determine how many grams of carbohydrate in that portion. Good nutrient guides are available at most bookstores. An even better option is the huge, and free, USDA National Nutrient Database at http://www.nal.usda.gov/fnic/foodcomp/search/ which enables you to retrieve the protein, fat, carbohydrate, vitamin and mineral content of thousands of different foods.

After you have become familiar with the carbohydrate content of the foods you eat, you can rely less on the scale and more on the 'eyeball' method to determine portion sizes.

The Higher-Carb Option

What about those who do not wish to follow a low-carbohydrate diet, who adamantly insist they cannot live without their bread and pasta? Luckily for these folks, there are still a number of available strategies that can help keep blood sugar levels in the normal range. Foremost among these is the abandonment of highly refined carbohydrates.

Whereas our hunter-gatherer ancestors subsisted entirely on freshly killed meats and gathered plant foods, today's diet is predominated by foods that have undergone extensive processing and that are comprised of ingredients that were essentially alien to the human digestive tract prior to the Agricultural Revolution some ten thousand years ago.

If you choose to keep eating a high-carbohydrate diet, be sure to cut all the highly refined junk from your diet (this tends to happen on low-carbohydrate diets as a matter of course). That means ditching sugar, donuts, cakes, confectionery, sodas, fruit juices, flavored milks, biscuits, crackers, crisps, French fries, and all packaged products containing corn syrup, sucrose, fructose, dextrose (glucose), maltose, maltodextrin (glucose polymers), fruit juice concentrate, brown rice syrup, maple syrup, date sugar, cane sugar, corn sugar, beet sugar, succanat and lactose.

All of these foods provide an abundance of calories and quickly absorbed carbohydrates that send blood sugar levels soaring, but provide little in the way of protective micronutrients. Because they contain little to no fiber, and because they are all quickly consumed items that provide little satiety value, these foods are an open invitation to excess carbohydrate and calorie intake. Their unusually high concentration of sugars is delivered to us minus Mother Nature's usual safeguards against over-consumption.

A fresh cut of meat, in contrast, must be chewed thoroughly before being swallowed, placing a natural limit on the rate of ingestion. Likewise, the carbohydrate content of fresh fruits and vegetables not only tends to be lower than that of cereal products and sugar-rich foods, but it is also accompanied by substantial water content, and considerable roughage in the form of soluble fiber, both of which have the effect of slowing the rate of ingestion.

The ingestion of excess calories via a diet comprised entirely of fresh meats and whole plant foods is an exceedingly difficult undertaking; on a diet of calorie-rich, fiber-poor, processed garbage, it is effortless. Throw in a lack of physical activity with the latter, and you have all the makings for an epidemic of diabetes and obesity--which is exactly what has occurred over the last three decades.

If you cannot live without cereal grains, here's what I suggest you do: prepare only half the usual amount of pasta, rice, beans, etc, that you would normally eat, and fill the rest of your plate with fibrous and nutrient-dense vegetables, such as broccoli, Brussels sprouts, cabbage, carrot, cauliflower, squash, sweet potato, tomato, zucchini, or salad greens. When increasing your vegetable intake, don't look to white potatoes--the high carbohydrate content of this historically recent tuber is absorbed very quickly, causing abrupt spikes in blood glucose levels. Sweet potatoes, pumpkin or squash are all far better alternatives. As for snacks, use low-glycemic fruits and nuts as a superior alternative to sugar- and cereal-based products. Such changes will help guard against excessive carbohydrate intake, helping you to maintain a normal blood sugar level.

Requirement #2: Get the Most Nutritional Bang For Your Buck

In Chapters 15 and 16, we learnt how increasing meat and non-cereal plant consumption at the expense of cereals and legumes will dramatically increase one's intake of protective nutrients. We shall now discuss why shunning the low-fat fad will also help boost your intake of vital nutrients.

Fat increases nutrient absorption. Researchers have shown time and time again that consuming low-fat meals drastically reduces the absorption of vitally important fat-soluble vitamins and carotenoids in food(12-15). When subjects ingested equal amounts of lutein--a carotenoid that may protect against age-related macular degeneration and cataract--from eggs, spinach or supplements, it was observed that lutein absorption was significantly higher during the period of egg consumption(16).

In another study, researchers compared the absorption of carotenoids from salads that contained either zero, six or twenty-eight grams of canola oil. There was essentially no increase in blood carotenoid concentrations after the fat-free salad, while the reduced fat salad produced markedly lower blood carotenoid elevations than the high fat version(17).

Dramatic increases in fat-soluble antioxidant uptake were also observed when research participants were fed avocado. The addition of 150 grams avocado to salsa enhanced lycopene and beta-carotene absorption by 4.4 and 2.6-fold, respectively, compared to avocado-free salsa. In the same subjects, adding either twenty-four grams of avocado oil or 150 grams avocado to salad greatly enhanced alpha-carotene, beta-carotene and lutein absorption by 7.2, 15.3 and 5.1 times, respectively, compared with avocado-free salad!(18)

Animal fats contain important fat-soluble vitamins. It is in the fatty portions of meat, dairy and eggs where one finds the highest concentrations of fat-soluble vitamins such as A, D, E and beta-carotene(19). Stripping the skin from your chicken breast not only makes it less tasty, but also reduces its vitamin A content by seventy-eight percent! Skim milk yogurt, meanwhile, contains ninety-three percent less vitamin A than the whole milk variety!

Throwing away your egg yolks is likewise antithetical to the goal of optimal nutrition; while one large egg yolk contains 245 IU of vitamin A, 18 IU of vitamin D, and 186 mcg of lutein plus zeaxanthin, along with small amounts of other carotenoids and vitamin E, a large egg white contains none of these nutrients. Egg yolks, along with beef liver, are also an especially concentrated dietary source of *phosphatidylcholine* (lecithin) and *choline*, which the body requires for healthy liver function and for the formation of the key neurotransmitter *acetylcholine*. Lower levels of acetylcholine are associated with memory loss and cognitive decline(20). In experiments with rabbits and baboons, intravenous administration of lecithin has induced regression of arterial plaque(21,22).

Anthropologists have repeatedly documented how our hunter-gatherer ancestors consistently and deliberately emphasized fat-rich animal foods. These 'primitive' peoples knew that fat-rich meats were not only tastier but much more nutritious than their lean equivalents. Today, people think they are acting in an enlightened fashion when they trim the fat from meat and pour egg yolks down the sink. Voluntarily reducing the nutrient-density of the foods one eats is not in any way enlightened—it is downright stupid.

Saturated fats improve mineral absorption. Numerous animal studies have shown that saturated fat improves mineral absorption, and emerging evidence indicates this holds true for humans as well(23-25). A pilot study by researchers at the USDA Grand Forks Human Nutrition Research Center examined the effect of different fats and carbohydrate on performance and mineral metabolism in three male endurance cyclists. During alternating four-week periods, each subject consumed diets in which either carbohydrate, polyunsaturated, or saturated fat contributed about fifty percent of daily energy intake. Endurance capacity decreased with the polyunsaturated fat diet. The polyunsaturated diet also resulted in increased excretion of zinc and iron, while copper retention tended to be positive only on the saturated fat diet(26).

In men consuming diets containing forty-two percent of calories as fat, increasing linoleic acid intake from four to sixteen percent of energy, at the expense of saturated fat, resulted in a significant decrease in iron balance, hemoglobin levels, and red blood cell counts(27).

Saturated fats help improve omega-3 status. Saturated fat improves the body's conversion of plant-source omega-3 fats into the longer-chain varieties like EPA and DHA, while omega-6-rich fats impede the conversion process. In young males, elongation of alpha-linolenic acid (ALA) and linoleic acid (LA) to DHA, EPA and AA was reduced by forty to fifty percent when dietary LA intake increased from fifteen to thirty grams per day(28). When rats were supplemented with linseed oil, their serum and tissue content of the all-important omega-3 fatty acids increased, and omega-6 levels decreased, to a far greater extent on a saturated fat-rich (beef fat) diet than on a linoleic acid-rich (safflower oil) diet. By creating a more favorable omega6:omega-3 ratio, saturated fat may help guard against a plethora of deadly diseases, including CHD(29).

Saturated fats may protect against infection. Saturated fats are well known for their ability to raise both LDL and HDL cholesterol. As we learnt in Chapter 21, both HDL and LDL help to neutralize harmful bacteria. Animal studies show that high cholesterol improves survival in animals infected with deadly microbes, while humans given intravenous HDL prior to infection with *E.coli* endotoxin experienced less flu-like symptoms and a significant reduction in inflammatory immune system activity.

Certain saturated fatty acids may also exert direct anti-microbial effects. Dairy and tropical fats contain special types of saturated fats known as *medium-chain* and *short-chain* fatty acids, which, in laboratory research, have been shown to attack a wide array of gram-negative germs.

Whole milk consumption in children is associated with fewer gastrointestinal infections than is consumption of low-fat milk (30). Rats consuming diets high in milk fat show a significantly greater resistance to Listeria infection and higher survival rates than those whose diets were low in milk fat(31). Similar results have been observed in mice fed diets high in saturate-rich coconut oil(32).

Saturated and monounsaturated fats positively influence hormonal function.
Low fat diets have been shown to lower levels of testosterone, essential for
well-being in both men and women. Free testosterone elevates sex drive,
produces muscle growth, increases bone density, boosts immune function, and
may even protect against cardiovascular disease. Unfortunately, testosterone
levels tend to decline with age. A study with weight-training men showed
higher saturated fat and monounsaturated fat consumption to be positively
associated with testosterone levels. In contrast, higher dietary levels of
polyunsaturated fats relative to saturated fats were associated with lower
testosterone levels (33).

A number of other studies show that reducing fat intake from around forty
percent to 20-25 percent of calories decreases testosterone output in men. Low
fat diets also increase levels of sex hormone-binding globulin (SHBG), a
protein which binds to testosterone, thus reducing the amount of bioavailable,
or 'free', testosterone in the body. It is free testosterone that is responsible for
this hormone's favorable effects on growth, repair, sexual capacity and immune
function(34-36).

Saturated fats may protect the liver from foreign substances. Ingestion of
foreign substances can take a heavy toll on the liver, whose primary role is to
neutralize these toxins and aid in their removal from the body. In animal
experiments, diets enriched with saturated fatty acids (from beef tallow,
coconut and palm oils) protect against alcohol-induced liver injury, whereas
diets containing polyunsaturated fatty acids promote liver injury(37-40).
Epidemiological evidence also suggests that both saturated fat and cholesterol
protect against alcoholic cirrhosis while polyunsaturated fats promote
cirrhosis(41). The protective mechanism is believed to be saturated fat's ability
to reduce alcohol-induced free radical damage in the liver.

Saturated fats may assist bone growth. In animal studies, diets containing
saturated fat produce superior bone development than those containing
polyunsaturated fats(42,43) Among women followed through the transition
from pre- to post-menopause, increased intakes of unsaturated fats were
associated with greater bone loss in the hip and lumbar spine(44).

Animal fats contain CLA. Animal fat is the only significant dietary source of
conjugated linoleic acid (fish and vegetable foods contain only trace amounts
of CLA(45)), a unique fatty acid that has been shown repeatedly in animal
studies to protect against cancer(46). Research with humans indicates that CLA
may enhance immune function and, in diabetics, improve blood glucose
control(47,48). A double-blind study at Purdue University which compared the
effects of CLA supplementation with a safflower oil placebo in Type 2
diabetics found that after eight weeks, decreases in fasting blood glucose were

seen in nine out of eleven subjects taking CLA, but only two out of the ten subjects receiving safflower oil.

CLA has also shown the ability to simultaneously enhance muscle gain and accelerate fat loss in humans, although not all trials have been able to confirm this, and the effect observed in successful studies has been relatively small(49-58).

Saturated fat may protect against heart disease. Harvard researchers took 235 postmenopausal women with established coronary heart disease, and divided them into four categories according to their level of saturated fat intake. They then performed coronary angiographies at baseline and after a mean follow-up of 3.1 years, analyzing over 2,200 coronary artery segments in the process.

After adjusting for multiple confounders, increasing saturated fat intakes were associated with progressively less narrowing of the arteries and less progression of coronary atherosclerosis. Compared with a 0.22 mm narrowing in the lowest quartile of intake, there was no narrowing in the highest quartile of saturated fat intake!

Carbohydrate intake was positively associated with atherosclerotic progression, particularly when the glycemic index was high. Polyunsaturated fat intake was also positively associated with progression of atherosclerosis, but monounsaturated and total fat intakes were not associated with progression.

After examining the baseline data for the study subjects, it is apparent that the results can not be explained away by otherwise healthier lifestyles among those eating the most saturated fat; the high saturated fat group, in fact, had the greatest number of current smokers!(59)

Studies like this do not prove causation, but we do know that saturated fatty acids, because of their lack of vulnerable double bonds, are the least susceptible to free radical damage; polyunsaturates are the most vulnerable. We also know that increased carbohydrate consumption, especially of the refined variety, does an outstanding job of raising blood sugar and insulin levels, which accelerates glycation, free radical activity, blood clot formation, and arterial smooth muscle cell proliferation.

Furthermore, the contention that increased polyunsaturated fat and carbohydrate consumption can worsen cardiovascular disease is supported by evidence from clinical trials and by the observation that increasing heart disease incidence throughout the twentieth century has been accompanied by increasing polyunsaturate and refined carbohydrate consumption. Animal fat consumption, in contrast, has remained stable over the last 100 years.

Embrace the Fat—Gradually!

If you have succumbed to the low-fat fad and would like to reintroduce some healthy fats back into your diet, remember that a little commonsense goes a long way. A dinner consisting of the fattiest meat you can find, fried in spoonfuls of lard and accompanied by vegetables slathered with butter, all topped off with a whipped cream-laced desert is probably going a *wee* bit too far! Try gradually increasing your intake of fat, starting with an egg yolk a day at breakfast, a handful of nuts to accompany your chicken salad at lunch, and an untrimmed (or partially-trimmed) cut of your favorite meat dish for dinner. If you have been following a very low-fat diet for any length of time, a gradual approach is especially important in order to allow your digestive system to reacclimatize to the increase in dietary fat.

People often read my writings in defense of saturated fat and then ask me: *"So does this mean we can eat all the eggs, butter and fatty meats we want?"* No, it doesn't. Many people evidently wish to hear that it's OK to shovel as much food as they wish into their mouths and suffer no adverse consequences. Gluttony is never a good thing, no matter how wholesome the food. Eat until you are satiated, and no more. There is no benefit, and much potential harm, in eating beyond your physiological needs.

Grass-Fed is Best

A diet enriched in 'hunter-gatherer' foods can be utilized by just about anyone. Seek out the freshest meats, eggs, vegetables, fruits, and nuts that you can find and make them the mainstay of your diet. If possible, consume meat, eggs and dairy from animals that have been range-fed on grass instead of hastily fattened on grain. Grass, not grain, is the natural diet for herbivorous animals. Meat and dairy from grass-fed animals contain more CLA, vitamin E and slightly more omega-3 fats than that from grain fed animals(64-67). Eggs from freely foraging chickens contain up to eight times more omega-3 fats than regular supermarket eggs(68).

Return to Your Dietary Roots

Mainstream dietary guidelines have proven themselves to be a complete and utter failure in bolstering public health. In fact, they have directly exacerbated the very problems they were purported to solve. Despite a substantial drop in smoking rates, CHD incidence has not fallen since the launch of the anti-cholesterol/animal fat campaign, while obesity and type 2 diabetes have spiraled to unprecedented levels. A return to our dietary roots, to the natural foods that kept humankind going for almost 2.5 million years, is long overdue.

Chapter 27

"For every complicated problem there is a solution that is simple, direct, understandable, and wrong."
H.L. Mencken

Micronutrient Magic

A supplement routine that could truly save your life

On June 28, 2003, the *British Medical Journal* sent the media and medical professions into a frenzy when it proudly announced a *"remarkable"* breakthrough in the war against cardiovascular disease. The journal's editor, Richard Smith, gushed that *"It's perhaps more than 50 years since we published something as important"* and advised readers to safely file away the June 28 issue because *"It may well become a collector's item."*(1)

Why was the editor of one of the world's oldest and most widely read medical journals so excited? His unbridled exuberance stemmed from a paper appearing in the same issue titled *"A strategy to reduce cardiovascular disease by more than 80%"*. The paper was authored by two London researchers who had formulated what they termed the 'Polypill'(2). This latest of 'miracle' pills was a proposed combination of six ingredients: a statin, three blood pressure lowering drugs, folic acid, and aspirin.

According to the researchers, *"The Polypill strategy could largely prevent heart attacks and stroke if taken by everyone aged 55 and older and everyone with existing cardiovascular disease. It would be acceptably safe and with widespread use would have a greater impact on the prevention of disease in the Western world than any other single intervention."*

The hyperbole reached fever pitch when they claimed the Polypill would reduce coronary events by a staggering eighty-eight percent and stroke by a similarly impressive eighty percent. As for side effects, *"the Polypill would cause symptoms in 8-15% of people"*, meaning that the alleged benefits would far outweigh the expected risks.

What was truly *"remarkable"* about this paper was that these stunning claims were presented and hailed in a leading journal even though the Polypill had not been tested in even a single randomized controlled trial. The authors arrived at their startling figures simply by firing up their computers and calculating risk estimates using the average CHD and stroke reductions seen in randomized trials for each of the proposed Polypill ingredients (in the case of folic acid, which has failed to show any benefit in clinical trials, data from epidemiological studies was used instead). The predicted incidence of adverse symptoms was similarly calculated by adding together the side effect rates observed in randomized trials for each component.

The creators of the Polypill recommended that everyone over the age of fifty-five and every individual with existing cardiovascular disease begin taking their patented formulation when it eventually becomes available. *"One third of people taking this pill from age 55 would benefit, gaining on average about 11 years of life free from an IHD event or stroke"*, they claimed, adding *"There is no need to measure the four risk factors* [LDL cholesterol, blood pressure, platelet function and homocysteine] *before starting treatment, because intervention is effective whatever the initial levels of the risk factors, nor to monitor the effect of the treatment..."*

Perhaps Nicholas M. Regush, the late outspoken editor of *Redflagsdaily.com*, best summed up the audacious nature of the Polypill claims when he wrote: *"This has got to be one the most egregious presentations that I have ever come across in all my years as a health reporter, both in the print world and at ABC News in New York. That the authors actually appear to have the support of the editor of the British Medical Journal is truly amazing--and dangerous. All these so-called health professionals actually have convinced themselves that if you put six different drugs together, they will all add up to one big cure of sorts. This is not only junk science at its worst, but reveals the sloppy intellectual processes going on these days in medical science..."*(3)

The Polypill creators appear to be completely blind to the fact that neither statins nor aspirin have ever been shown to lower mortality in the elderly, women and non-diabetic individuals free of cardiovascular disease. They are evidently unaware that the reported incidence of side effects in carefully screened clinical trial participants with these drugs is far lower than that noted among the general population.

All of the Polypill ingredients, with the sole exception of folic acid, have been clearly documented to produce severe side effects in susceptible individuals. The authors did not consider the possibility that taking all these ingredients simultaneously could magnify the incidence of adverse events. The use of statins alone can cause liver toxicity and kidney failure--what would happen to the frequency rate of such outcomes when statins are taken in conjunction with four other potentially toxic drugs?

The 'New-Improved Polypill'--Cheap, Safe, and Effective

For those who don't want to become the unwitting guinea pigs in yet another overly optimistic mass social experiment, there exists a cheaper, safer and far healthier alternative to the Polypill. It involves the daily ingestion of a small handful of nutritional supplements, some of which, as we learnt in Chapter 24, have already established their mortality-lowering benefits in controlled clinical trials. I won't be so crass as to offer any wildly spectacular percentage mortality reductions for the supplement regimen outlined below, at least not until supportive clinical data are available. What I will say without any reservation is that all available evidence indicates the magnitude of reduction would be substantial. Make no mistake: the supplement regimen below *will* save lives. To make life easier for readers, I have not only presented the specific nutrients one should take daily, but the names of supplements containing these nutrients. The listed formulations contain the required amount of nutrients, are competitively priced, and come from reputable manufacturers. Without any further ado, here they are:

1) Multi-vitamin/mineral formula without iron or copper. A good multivitamin/mineral formula should form the foundation of any heart-protective nutrient supplementation regimen. Look for a product that is free of iron and copper (see Appendix F for more information about copper), but at least 100 micrograms of selenium.

Suggested product: Life Extension Two-Per-Day
Dosage: Two tablets daily
Cost: Twenty-six cents a day (120 tablets, $15.75)
Ingredients:
Vitamin A: 5000 IU
Vitamin C: 500 mg
Vitamin D: 400 IU
Vitamin E: 200 IU
Thiamine (vitamin B1): 75 mg
Riboflavin (vitamin B2): 50 mg
Niacin (vitamin B3): 50 mg
Vitamin B6: 75 mg
Folate: 800 mcg
Vitamin B12: 300 mcg
Biotin: 300 mcg
Pantothenic acid: 100 mg
Calcium: 20 mg
Iodine: 150 mcg
Magnesium: 100 mg
Zinc: 30 mg
Selenium: 100 mcg
Manganese: 2 mg
Chromium polynicotinate: 200 mcg
Molybdenum: 100 mcg
Potassium: 25 mg
Alpha-carotene: 50 mcg

Boron: 3 mg
Choline: 22.9 mg
Inositol: 50 mg
Xantopina® plus lutein extract: 12.5 mg
Lycopene: 2 mg
PABA (para-aminobenzoic acid): 30 mg

If you eat B-vitamin-rich meats such as liver on a regular basis, you may wish to opt for a formula rich in antioxidants, but void of B-vitamins. Optimum Nutrition Super Antioxidants is a suitable formula (as is Enajon Antioxidants for Australian readers). Both of these formulas are void of vitamin D, so if you opt for them then supplemental vitamin D during winter is advisable (NOW vitamin D 1000 IU is ideal). Enajon also contains no selenium, thus necessitating supplemental selenium. For Australian readers who desire a multi rich in B-vitamins, a good substitute for Life Extension Two-Per-Day is Golden Glow Super One a Day (www.goldenglow.com.au). Again, it is not as rich in selenium and contains no vitamin D, so extra supplementation of these nutrients is warranted.

2) Fish oil
Suggested product: NOW Molecularly Distilled Omega-3 (supplying 300mg EPA+DHA)
Dosage: One to three capsules daily
Cost: Six to eighteen cents a day (180 Softgels, $10.98)

3) Coenzyme Q10
Suggested product: Natrol CoQ10
Dosage: 100mg (one capsule) daily
Cost: Forty cents a day (30 x 100mg caps, $11.89)

4) Magnesium
Suggested product: NOW Magnesium Malate
Dosage: Three tablets daily (supplies 450mg elemental magnesium)
Cost: Ten cents a day (180 Tablets $6.19)

Optional Supplements

5) L-Carnitine (highly recommended for patients with existing cardiovascular disease)
Suggested product: NOW L-Carnitine
Dosage: Four grams (four capsules) daily
Cost: $1.72 a day (100 x 1000mg capsules, $42.98)

6) Garlic
Suggested product: Enzymatic Therapy Garlinase 4000

Dosage: Patients with atherosclerosis--one capsule daily; healthy individuals--one capsule on three alternate days per week.
Cost: Twenty-two cents a day (100 Tablets $21.78)

The regimen outlined above is free of iron but contains fish oil, coenzyme Q10, selenium, magnesium, vitamins C and D, and high potencies of vitamins B6, B12 and folic acid--the benefits of which we have already discussed throughout this book. What follows is a quick discussion of magnesium and garlic (for more information on L-carnitine, see Chapter 24).

Garlic

There's nothing smelly about garlic's beneficial effects on the cardiovascular system; in placebo-controlled clinical studies, ingestion of garlic has repeatedly produced anti-clotting, antioxidant and blood-thinning effects(4). In animal experiments, aged garlic extract significantly reduces both the build-up of lipid deposits in arteries and the thickening of arterial walls(5). Garlic may also help prevent atherosclerosis in humans; in a randomized, double-blind, placebo-controlled trial with patients showing advanced atherosclerotic arterial plaques, men randomized to receive 900 milligrams of garlic powder each day for four years experienced a smaller increase in plaque volume than those receiving a placebo. While women assigned to placebo also experienced increases in plaque volume, those assigned to garlic actually experienced a slight decrease(6). A small double-blind, randomized trial by Californian researchers found that patients taking a statin drug plus aged garlic extract experienced an average 7.5 percent increase in arterial calcification over one year, far better than the twenty-two percent increase seen among those taking a statin alone(7).

In patients with peripheral arterial occlusive disease, a significantly greater increase in walking distance was observed in those taking 800 milligrams of garlic powder for twelve weeks than taking a placebo. Diastolic blood pressure, blood platelet aggregation, and blood viscosity also decreased significantly(8).

Side effects from garlic and garlic supplement use are rare, but include gastrointestinal discomfort and nausea, bloating, headache, dizziness, and profuse sweating. Individuals taking anti-clotting or blood-thinning drugs should check with their doctor before using garlic, as garlic may amplify the effects of these drugs. The consequences of such interaction are potentially serious--at least one case of life-threatening hemorrhage has been reported in the literature(9-13).

In addition to its cardiovascular effects, regular garlic ingestion may deliver numerous other health benefits, including protection against cancer, age-related cognitive decline, liver damage, and even the common cold(14-28).

Chopping or crushing garlic releases an enzyme called alliinase, which rapidly converts alliin in garlic to allicin. Allicin is not only responsible for the characteristic odor of fresh garlic, but is also considered one of garlic's most important biologically active compounds. Alliinase, and thus allicin, can be activated only when garlic cloves are crushed or cut. Garlic must also be eaten raw to exert its full effect, as alliinase is quickly inactivated by heating, thus preventing the conversion of alliin to allicin. Researchers have found that microwave heating for as little as sixty seconds totally destroys alliinase activity. Unlucky rats fed cooked garlic and given a carcinogenic compound did not experience any of the considerable anti-tumor protection seen in similarly exposed rats consuming unheated garlic(41). Boiling or heating garlic at temperatures between 60–100°C can completely block its beneficial anti-microbial, antioxidant, and blood thinning effects(29-33).

All is not lost for those who cannot tolerate raw garlic. Crushing and/or cutting garlic at its top and allowing it to stand for ten minutes before cooking preserves up to seventy percent of its anti-carcinogenic properties(34).

When it comes to the 'stinking rose's' famous anti-social effects on breath odor, tooth brushing unfortunately has little effect--garlic's lingering impact on breath emanates from the gut, not the oral cavity. Ingestion of fresh parsley has been reported to alleviate garlic breath, otherwise there are always garlic supplements.

Magnesium

Deficiencies of magnesium have been implicated in diabetes, atherosclerosis, cardiac arrhythmia and acute myocardial infarction(35).

Coronary artery disease patients receiving 365 milligrams of magnesium citrate daily for six months showed significant improvements in exercise tolerance, exercise-induced chest pain, and quality of life compared to patients taking a placebo(36). A double-blind study involving patients with stable coronary artery disease, all of whom were taking aspirin, indicated that three months of magnesium supplementation could reduce thrombus formation by thirty-five percent compared to placebo treatment(37). In this patient group, magnesium supplements have also been shown to improve arterial dilation(38).

Magnesium is important for healthy blood sugar metabolism, and supplementation with this mineral has produced significant improvements in blood glucose control in both type 2 diabetics and non-diabetic insulin resistant subjects(39,40).

Magnesium deficiency is all-too-common in populations relying heavily on processed foods. A recent survey of U.S. adults found that the average daily intake of magnesium among Caucasian men is only 352 milligrams, and a mere 278 milligrams among African American men. Caucasian women consume an average of 256 milligrams per day, while African American women take in only 202 milligrams daily(41). The lower amounts of magnesium ingested by African Americans have been posited as a possible contributor to their increased susceptibility of hypertension, diabetes, and cardiovascular disease(42).

Coffee and tea drinkers may also be at increased risk of magnesium insufficiency. Acute ingestion of caffeine in amounts similar to those found in two to three cups of coffee (around 300 milligrams of caffeine) increases the urinary excretion of calcium, magnesium and sodium for at least three hours after consumption(43). Urinary excretion of zinc may also increase with caffeine intake(44). These increased urinary losses may potentially affect bone mass by increasing the release of minerals from bone into the bloodstream in order to maintain balance.

For those who can't or won't eat magnesium or calcium-rich foods on a regular basis (Brazil nuts, pumpkin seeds, halibut, tomato paste, spinach, artichokes, cashews, almonds are some of the foods particularly high in magnesium), or for diabetics and CHD patients who wish to ensure high levels of this mineral in their diets, magnesium supplementation is worthy of serious consideration. Few side effects have been noted with magnesium supplements, although excessive intake can cause diarrhea.

Effective CHD Prevention that Doesn't Cost the Earth

The daily cost of the above regimen, minus optional items, is eighty-two to ninety-four cents per day (depending on the dose of fish oil), or $299-$343 per year. In comparison, the *lowest* dose (ten milligrams) of the world's most popular statin drug, Lipitor, costs $2.49 per day, or $909 per year(45). If L-carnitine and garlic are included in the supplement mix, the daily cost is $2.63-$2.88, or $962-$1,051 per year(45).

These figures do not capture the full economic advantage of this supplement regimen; unlike statins, the above supplements do not cause muscle or tendon damage, immune suppression, cognitive dysfunction, neurological impairment, transient memory loss or life-threatening kidney failure. The above supplement routine offers protection against heart failure and cancer--unlike statins, which may actually increase the risk of these ailments. This regimen, therefore, may bring about further substantial savings in terms of alleviated future medical expenses.

Unlike statins, aspirin or anti-hypertensive drugs, the above regimen helps to ensure adequate intake of many important nutrients that are commonly deficient in the average Western diet. Even health-conscious individuals who eat a relatively nutritious diet will find it exceedingly difficult to obtain many of the above nutrients solely from food sources. Selenium, for example, is woefully deficient in much of the world's soil, in the plants that grow on this soil, and in the animals that graze upon these plants. Adequate intake of long-chain omega-3 fats from dietary sources would require the regular consumption of fatty fish, a staple that has become increasingly subject to contamination with environmental pollutants. The only other viable source of long-chain omega-3 fats is brain, which, while considered a delicacy in many cultures, is unlikely to win widespread appeal any time soon in most Western countries. The handful of foods that contain any meaningful amount of vitamin D--egg yolks, liver, full fat dairy products and cod liver oil--are shunned by much of the population. Not surprisingly, vitamin D deficiency is common during winter and in individuals who receive little sun exposure on their skin.

To make matters worse, the average vitamin and mineral content of America's vegetables has declined markedly over the last forty years. USDA figures show that, since 1963, the amount of vitamin A in apples has dropped from ninety milligrams to fifty-three milligrams, while nearly half the calcium and vitamin A in broccoli have disappeared. Cauliflower has lost almost half its vitamin C, along with its B1 and B2. Pineapple, meanwhile, has lost fifty-nine percent of its calcium. Collards aren't what they used to be, either. Their vitamin C content has plummeted by sixty-two percent, vitamin A by fifty-one percent, calcium by twenty-nine percent, potassium by fifty-two percent, and magnesium by a hefty eighty-four percent. The examples are endless, but the message is the same--modern farming methods, which involve the use of mineral-deficient fertilizers, not only produce a gradual depletion of nutrients from soil but also from the produce grown in that soil(46).

While sub-optimal intakes of these and other nutrients are an all-too-common reality in Western nations, there is no such thing as a statin, aspirin or anti-hypertensive drug 'deficiency'. Cardiovascular disease and most other degenerative illnesses arise because the body does not receive the appropriate amounts of macro and micronutrients, sleep, physical exertion and respite from mental stress that it needs to keep functioning at optimal capacity. Deluded hyperbole to the contrary notwithstanding, these diseases do not arise because of a lack of statins in the drinking water!

In the next chapter, we will learn how to go about implementing another important strategy that not only protects against CHD but also dramatically improves overall health.

Chapter 28

"Those who think they have not time for bodily exercise will sooner or later have to find time for illness."
Edward Stanley, Earl of Derby

An Exercise in Longevity

A little physical activity can go a long way.

We all know that we should exercise. We know that regular physical activity brings with it numerous benefits, including marked improvements in appearance, physical health and even mental outlook.

So why do so few of us do it?

Without question, the most commonly cited reason for not exercising is lack of time. While busy schedules certainly make it harder to find time for exercise, they by no means render the task impossible. The sad fact is that, even when we do have the time, the majority of us still don't exercise. For all our bleating about being short on time, most of us, given a spare hour or two, will watch TV, read the daily barrage of bad news in the papers, chat on web forums, go shopping for things we don't really need, or participate in a long list of other non-essential activities long before we will even think about getting up off our butts and raising a sweat.

It doesn't take a rocket scientist to work out the real reason why so much of the population gets so little exercise. The indisputable fact is that most people don't exercise simply because *they don't have to!*

The Sedentary Revolution

During almost our entire evolutionary history, humans had to physically exert themselves in order to obtain food and water. For our Paleolithic ancestors, regular physical activity was essential for survival. Since that time, industrialization has all but rendered the need for exertion obsolete. Except for the small proportion of us who still work in physically demanding jobs, vigorous activity is no longer an intricate part of life. It is now an optional activity, something that we refer to as 'exercise' and do only when sufficiently motivated.

Exercise requires effort, and humans are inherently lazy creatures. During the Paleolithic and Agricultural eras, where strenuous activity was an inescapable aspect of daily life, this trait actually served a protective function; it helped prevent us from 'overdoing it', from reaching beyond the body's capacity for self repair. Laziness ensured that an unavoidably high level of physical activity was balanced with sufficient recuperative downtime. Nowadays, overdoing it is typically the least of our worries; in our fully automated society, it is a lack of activity that is killing us.

Time is on Your Side

For those with truly busy schedules, the good news is that even relatively low levels of activity have been shown to improve health and lower both cardiovascular and overall mortality. What's more, you don't need to purchase fancy equipment or expensive gym memberships in order to achieve these benefits. Improved health can be attained with one of the simplest and safest physical activities known to mankind: brisk walking!

According to the Centers for Disease Control and the American College of Sports Medicine, each of us should engage in at least thirty minutes of moderate-intensity physical activity (e.g. brisk walking at 3-4 mph) on most, and preferably all, days of the week(1). Currently, only forty-five percent of Americans meet even these minimal guidelines(2).

Can the minimal amount of activity stipulated by these guidelines have any meaningful impact upon mortality? A review of the literature by researchers from the Harvard School of Public Health suggests they can. After analyzing numerous epidemiological studies, they found that activity levels similar to those recommended by the CDC and ACSM were associated with a significant twenty to thirty percent reduction in all-cause mortality. Further reductions were seen with increasing levels of physical activity, an effect seen in men and women, and in younger and older subjects. Of course, this association may be influenced by the fact that regular exercisers may also practice other health-enhancing behaviors, such as smoking abstinence and moderation in eating and drinking habits; however, when the researchers adjusted for such factors, the association remained. As the authors stated, *"The preponderance of evidence suggests that the risk of dying during a given period continues to decline with increasing levels of physical activity..."*(3).

Further weakening the *"I don't have time"* argument is a recent study showing reduced mortality in healthy male 'weekend warriors' who burnt at least 1,000 calories per week from sports or recreational activity one to two times per week. Compared to sedentary males, weekend warriors without any major CHD risk factors had a fifty-nine percent lower risk of dying when compared with sedentary men(4). If time restrictions dictate that you must schedule your major workouts on the weekend, please be especially vigilant in using proper exercise technique and thorough warm-ups in order to avoid injury (see below).

Despite the many benefits of regular exercise, its true importance appears to be widely under-recognized by those who disseminate medical information. When researchers conducted a review of medical journals commonly read by Australian physicians, spanning the period 1987-1997, they found that far fewer articles were written about physical activity (six percent) than high cholesterol (thirty-two percent), hypertension (forty-two percent), or smoking cessation (twenty percent). Similar findings were gleaned from a review of medical magazine articles, while a study of advertisements from these publications found that none pertained to exercise; most were for pharmaceutical approaches to lowering cholesterol, blood pressure and smoking cessation(5). These findings are of relevance not only to Aussie doctors; several of the reviewed publications were among those widely read by North American physicians.

Making Exercise a Part of Your Life

Given the minimal amounts of moderate activity required to induce health and mortality benefits, one can no longer cite lack of time or money, dislike of gyms, or fear of injury as excuses for not exercising. Anyone who owns a pair of walking shoes and who is prepared set aside a mere thirty minutes on most days for brisk walking, can significantly lower their risk of cardiac and overall mortality.

Keep in mind that the CDC and ACSM guidelines have been designed with the goal of ascertaining the least amount of exercise necessary to instigate health improvements. They are not intended for obese individuals looking to lose significant amounts of body fat, individuals wishing to attain high levels of fitness, or those wanting to build athletic-looking physiques. The CDC and ACSM guidelines may serve as a useful starting point for sedentary and unfit people seeking these outcomes, but a progression to exercise regimens of higher intensity and/or duration will be necessary if such goals are to be realized. A discussion of higher-level physical conditioning is beyond the scope of this chapter. The information presented here is intended simply to impress upon people that one need not become a gym junkie in order to lower their risk of heart disease.

Resistance Training Versus 'Aerobics'

I am often asked by potential exercisers whether they should do weight training or aerobic-type activities such as running, cycling, skipping, etc. My answer is always the same; for best results, do both! Numerous studies have shown additive benefits when both forms of exercise are employed. In patients with CHD, for example, those who undertook a relatively simple weight training routine after aerobic exercise experienced greater improvements in fitness, strength, fat loss and muscle gain than those who performed aerobics only(6).

Exercise When You're Not Exercising

Increasing the amount of activity in one's daily routine can go a long way towards improving one's fitness levels. Walking or cycling to work instead of driving, walking to the shops and carrying groceries home instead of throwing them in the back of the family wagon, and taking the stairs at work instead of the elevator are all practical methods for getting some meaningful physical movement back into your life.

For individuals who live in cold climates, or in neighborhoods where walking alone may pose a danger to one's imminent wellbeing, there are other options. Stationery bicycles can be purchased at relatively low cost, allowing you to exercise while watching your favorite shows on TV or listening to your favorite music. Anyone who lives in an apartment building has access to a great piece of training equipment: the stairwell! Skipping ropes, punching bags and wind trainers (an apparatus that allows you to turn your regular bike into a stationary cycle) are other low-cost indoor alternatives. Whatever form of exercise you choose, just do it, and do it consistently. The very minute you start exercising you activate the mechanisms that cause your body to become fitter, leaner and healthier.

Also remember that the benefits of exercise quickly disappear upon cessation. Studies of college alumni show that athletic activity during youth does not afford any protection against heart attack later in life; ex-varsity athletes enjoyed lower risk only if they maintained a high level of physical activity as adults(7). A nineteen-year follow-up of participants who participated in a randomized exercise trial during the seventies found that the initial reduction in mortality risk enjoyed by those in the exercise group gradually disappeared after the trial ended(8). All you aging ex-jocks who like to boast about what outstanding physical specimens you were in your youth, stop it, because nature isn't listening! If you want to fight off disease and early death with exercise, you need to get active *now!*

Exercise: Cardiac Fountain of Youth?

The outstanding ability of exercise to preserve healthy cardiac function was clearly demonstrated in a study that compared a group of twelve male and female masters athletes (average age 67.8 years), with twelve healthy sedentary senior men and women (average age 69.8 years) and fourteen young sedentary control subjects (average age 28.9 years). Six of the masters athletes, who participated in events from swimming to track, were nationally ranked competitors and six were regional champions. The sedentary participants had not engaged in regular endurance exercise throughout their life.

Researchers examined the function of the left ventricle--the heart's main pumping chamber--among the three groups. They found that not only were the older, sedentary individuals' hearts fifty percent stiffer than the masters athletes, but also that the hearts of the senior athletes were indistinguishable from those of the healthy younger participants(9).

As the researchers explained: *"It appears that lifelong exercise training completely prevented the stiffening of the heart muscle that has been thought to be an inevitable consequence of aging."*(10)

The Fast Route to Fitness

OK, so you are now convinced that exercise is necessary--but still adamant that your hectic schedule doesn't allow for even the minimal amounts prescribed in the CDC and ACSM guidelines. Well, what if I told you excellent improvements in fitness--superior to those obtained by traditional sixty minute training sessions--could be obtained in workouts lasting *sixteen minutes*? You might suspect I was some huckster using too-good-to-be-true fitness claims to extract some of your hard-earned dollars. No way; superior improvements in fitness can indeed be had from workouts lasting sixteen minutes—and these workouts do not require some highly-hyped contraption being peddled on late night infomercials.

High-Intensity Interval Training (HIIT) involves the repeated performance of short but intense bouts of exercise. These intense bouts are separated by intervals comprised of much lower intensity, which some researchers refer to as 'active recovery'. Perhaps the most famous HIIT regimen is the Tabata protocol, created by Dr. Izumi Tabata at the National Institute of Fitness and Sports in Tokyo, Japan. The Tabata protocol involves three phases, all performed in continuous sequence. The first phases involves riding on a stationary bicycle at only fifty percent of maximum effort for four minutes. This is then followed by a series of eight sprints in which you pedal as fast as possible for twenty seconds. These twenty-second sprints are each interspersed with active recovery intervals lasting ten seconds. During these ten-second 'rest' periods, you continue cycling but at only fifty percent of maximum effort. After the eighth and final sprint, you continue to cycle at fifty percent of maximum effort for another four minutes.

The superiority of HIIT was demonstrated when Tabata assigned active male subjects to one of two groups, each training five days per week for six weeks. One group performed sixty minutes of moderate intensity exercise (70% VO2max), while the other group performed Tabata's HIIT protocol. The group performing moderate intensity exercise improved their aerobic fitness, but made no improvements in anaerobic fitness (anaerobic refers to the generation of energy without utilization of oxygen by the muscles involved). The HIIT group, not only made greater improvements in aerobic fitness but also improved their anaerobic capacity by twenty-eight percent(11).

The Tabata protocol is hardly the only HIIT regimen to have shown its superiority in controlled trials. There is a wealth of research showing a variety of HIIT formats* to produce sizable fitness gains in a shorter time frame and with the use of briefer workouts(12).

Intense HIIT routines like the Tabata protocol are *not* for individuals whose cardiovascular systems have been compromised by heart disease. However, less intense HIIT-style protocols may benefit stable CHD patients. In a study by Canadian researchers, fourteen men with CAD who had undergone bypass surgery or angioplasty at least six months previously performed a sixteen-week exercise program. All the men were stable, 'highly functional' patients (i.e., all had a negative exercise stress test result and VO2peak greater than 9 METs). Twice a week, one group performed a ten-minute warm-up, thirty minutes of continuous aerobic exercise at sixty-five percent of heart rate/VO2 reserve, weight training, and a ten-minute cool-down period. The HIIT group used identical warm-up, weight training and cool-down procedures, but performed the aerobic portion using two-minute work phases (85-95% of heart rate/VO2 reserve) followed by two-minute recovery bouts (35-45% of heart rate/VO2 reserve). In addition to these twice-weekly workouts, both groups also engaged in three additional training days per week consisting of continuous exercise at sixty to seventy percent of heart rate/VO2 reserve.

After sixteen weeks, both groups had increased their fitness, but improvement in time to exhaustion was significantly greater in the HIIT group. Anaerobic threshold also increased to a greater extent in the HIIT group(13). No adverse effects occurred as the result of participating in either training program, but it must be remembered that the patients were all screened for participation and then monitored during the study by professional researchers. If you are a CHD patient, please do *not* 'self-experiment' with HIIT; consult with a qualified practitioner before commencing any exercise program.

Starting Out

During the first few weeks of your new exercise routine, slowly build the intensity and duration of your workout sessions. Your focus during this time should be on giving your body a chance to acclimate to the new movement

---

Some of these studies used shorter/longer work periods, and longer rest periods, than the Tabata format. The optimal ratio of work/rest will vary depending on such factors as fitness level and type of activity (for many people, sprint running will necessitate longer rest intervals than sprint cycling). For those looking to begin HIIT training, the Tabata protocol is a good—and clinically proven—starting point.

patterns and physical demands being placed upon it. As your fitness, strength and flexibility improve, you can gradually begin to increase the difficulty level of your workouts. It is highly recommended that, when commencing an unfamiliar physical activity, you seek out the assistance of a competent and knowledgeable instructor who can educate you on proper exercise selection and technique. Another recommended resource for the beginning exerciser is *Building Strength and Stamina* by Wayne Wescott (Human Kinetics, 2003). This easy-to-read book provides simple, time-efficient and effective strategies for improving both strength and endurance.

When performing strenuous activities, be it weight training or wood chopping, *always* warm up beforehand. Don't tell you yourself you don't have time to warm up; cut back on the strenuous component of your workout if necessary, but *never* commence a workout without first preparing your body for the increased physical demands about to be imposed upon it. If you have heart disease or even appear to be at high risk of heart disease, avoid strenuous activity wherever possible first thing in the morning. If you exercise early in the morning before work, try and allocate this time to moderate aerobic-type activities, and see if you can slot in your more intense cardiovascular and weight training workouts later in the day or on weekends.

When starting out, use the 'Talk Test' to ascertain how far you should push yourself during aerobic activities. To implement this test, exercise at a level where carrying a conversation requires effort but does not become difficult. When researchers instructed subjects using treadmills and stationary cycles to use the Talk Test guidelines, they observed that the resultant exercise intensities of the subjects were almost exactly correlated with their cardiovascular thresholds(14). As for weight training, the first month or two should be devoted to focusing on correct exercise technique and gradual increases in the weight lifted. Exercising to the point of momentary muscular failure (the point at which the exercise can no longer be continued in good form no matter how hard one tries) is something that should not be attempted by beginning exercisers until they have attained the requisite conditioning and mastery of exercise technique.

It is highly recommended that apparently healthy but relatively inactive individuals over forty undergo a physical examination by their doctor prior to starting a vigorous exercise program. Individuals of any age who smoke or have elevated blood pressure, diabetes, a family history of heart disease, or any chronic health condition would also be well advised to seek clearance from their doctor. It is especially important that anyone with a known history of heart disease or other heart problems have a medical evaluation that includes a graded exercise test before engaging in strenuous physical activity.

Chapter 29

"Accept that some days you're the pigeon, and some days you're the statue."
Author unknown.

No Worries

Taking the sting out of stress.

It is not just the number or severity of emotional challenges we face in life that determines whether we avert the harmful effects of stress, but also our ability to deal with them. Different individuals vary greatly in their response to stressful situations; an ordeal that would hardly cause one person to raise an eyebrow can send another into a blind fit of rage. The latter type of individual likely has some deep-seated emotional and psychological issues that need thorough redress, a process that can sometimes take years. Such firmly entrenched psychosocial issues cannot be resolved simply by popping a pill or eating 'heart healthy' foods, a major reason why stress has received so little attention from mainstream health authorities. It is much easier and far more profitable to instead rally the population into embracing cholesterol-lowering drugs and glorified low-fat pseudo-foods.

In this chapter, we will discover research-proven, drug-free methods for fighting stress. First, we'll explore some important psychosocial strategies, then we will examine dietary and lifestyle tactics for countering stress.

Psychosocial Interventions For Combating Stress

Place less emphasis on material goals, and more emphasis on family and friends. This author is not against the accumulation of worldly goods, and has no wish to join the legions of hypocrites who rally against the 'evils' of materialism from the comfort of their air-conditioned, fully appointed homes. There's little wrong with wanting material comforts. There is, however, plenty wrong with placing inordinate emphasis on the attainment of such material possessions, to the point where one overextends themselves financially. From a young age, our consumer-driven culture subjects us to a relentless deluge of marketing designed to make us feel grossly inadequate if we fail to purchase the latest widgets and gadgets. Not infrequently, our reward for succumbing to such clever manipulation is a high level of debt and constant worrying over financial matters.

Money problems are a major cause of psychological stress, one that could readily be reduced if people considered the wisdom of their purchasing decisions a little more carefully. Is it really worth plunging yourself into debt to own the latest SUV or a larger home--especially if your current car and place of abode are more than adequately fulfilling their respective roles?

It's not just major purchases that get people into financial strife--the cumulative cost of small, frequent and unnecessary expenditures can be horrendous. If you routinely smoke cigarettes, drink more than a glass or two of alcohol a day, or repeatedly make non-essential calls on your cellular phone, then you are quite literally throwing money into the wind. In *Getting Rich in America,* Dwight R. Lee and Richard B. McKenzie illustrate the potential financial benefits that await an eighteen year old who decides to remain smoke-free. If this individual diverts the $2.25 spent on cigarettes each day into a fund with an eight percent annual return, they will accumulate over $435,000 by the time they reach sixty-seven! This figure doesn't take into account any future increase in the cost of cigarettes, nor the increased medical bills that often arise after decades of smoking(1).

In addition to draining our finances, overemphasis on material acquisitions often draws us away from the things that matter the most--our family and friends. When you look back over your life during your last days, will you curse yourself for not having worked long enough to have afforded a wider screen TV--or for not having spent more time participating in your precious children's lives? Unlike cars, fancy clothes or appliances, your family and close friends are priceless and irreplaceable--don't neglect them, nor the development of your own character, just for the sake of having bigger and more expensive toys.

Learn to say no. There are only twenty-four hours in a day; continually committing yourself to a schedule that cannot possibly be completed in this time frame at a sane pace is a sure-fire route to becoming burnt out. Take inventory of your current commitments; see if there is anyway you can simplify, rather than further overload, your current schedule.

Spend quality time with quality people. Long-term prospective studies show that people with higher levels of social relationships and activities are significantly less likely to die during the follow-up period than socially isolated individuals, even after accounting for socioeconomic status and health practices(2,3).

Before you rush off to establish a giant, record-breaking social network, remember that it's not just the size of one's social circle that is important, but also the quality of the relationships. Social relationships characterized by negative, critical and/or demanding interactions are quite literally toxic; such social interactions are associated with elevated catecholamine levels, increased heart rate and blood pressure, and depressed immune function, whereas more positive, supportive social interactions are associated with the exact opposite profile(4).

Hang around with negative people long enough, and chances are you will become negative yourself; misery loves company. The world can be a scary place to navigate alone, but that doesn't mean you have to settle for second-rate relationships. If you have acquaintances who specialize in repeatedly pointing out your faults in order to make themselves feel better about their own shortcomings, or getting you riled up about past hurts or injustices that should have been forgotten long ago, it's time to seek out more positive company.

Be Happy--It's Healthy! Sheldon Cohen, PhD, and his team from the Department of Psychology at Carnegie Mellon University gave hundreds of healthy volunteers nasal drops containing rhinoviruses, then monitored them in quarantine for the development of a common cold. The researchers discovered that those with the most positive emotional style experienced a three-fold lower risk of catching a cold than those with negative emotional tendencies(5).

When faced with a chronic illness, some people understandably become disparaged. Others, however, maintain an optimistic outlook, seek to establish a sense of control over the illness, and work on restoring or enhancing their self-esteem. Among a sample of patients treated successfully with balloon angioplasty (a procedure used to widen narrowed arteries), those who displayed these positive characteristics were significantly less likely to experience progression of arterial disease or to require further surgery than those with a more negative outlook(6).

Be Pro-Active. Those who approach life in a pro-active manner, by conducting due diligence before making important decisions, greatly reduce their chances of getting into costly, aggravating and even fatal situations. For illustration purposes, let's apply this principle to a situation that many of us face at some point in our life--the decision to buy a new home. When in the market for a new abode, do you see a beautiful house in a seemingly nice area at what appears to be a very reasonable asking price, quickly warm to the idea of owning it, then rush in and make an offer? Or do you have an independent expert examine the property and give you an extensive, detailed report on its structural soundness? Do you speak to surrounding residents and other people who know the area? Such preliminary investigative work may save you from discovering after it's too late that your new neighbors stubbornly delight in subjecting you to the soothing tunes of Metallica at two o'clock in the morning and that your new street serves as the local drag-racing strip. Pre-inspection by a qualified expert may save you from tens of thousands of dollars in structural repairs, years of regret, and messy, drawn-out legal battles.

Employing this principal of pro-activity when making major financial purchases or investments, embarking on business ventures or entering into new relationships can save you from a ton of future stress. When making life-altering decisions, do your homework and don't rush in blind.

Learn, and practice, self-responsibility. Self-reliance was once considered a virtue in America, but modern-day 'intellectuals' and social commentators have since convinced many of us that self-responsibility is an outmoded concept promulgated only by heartless, uncaring ultra-conservatives. We are encouraged to view ourselves as victims, to find someone or something else to blame for our misfortunes. The end-result of this philosophical bankruptcy is the current welfare-burdened, litigation-mad society we see around us.

One can never entirely remove the possibility of bad luck in life, but accepting responsibility for your own actions instead of always seeking to blame others or outside circumstances will immediately bestow you with a life-enhancing sense of empowerment. Instead of merely accepting unfavorable circumstances, you begin to seek knowledge that will enable you to change, or at least better cope, with those circumstances. You begin to examine your own behavior and beliefs in order to learn what role they may have played in influencing the outcome of life events, and what you can do to favorably influence future outcomes. As a result, your character, resilience, confidence and efficacy as a person begin to grow in leaps and bounds.

Conversely, the belief that all your problems are at the behest of some external force becomes a self-fulfilling prophecy; like a rudderless boat in a choppy sea, your direction, progress and outcomes will indeed be largely determined by forces over which you exert little control. It is little coincidence that individuals who believe they are mere victims of circumstance often appear to have more 'bad luck' than those who take a pro-active approach to life. Such individuals are more prone to feeling powerless over the course of their lives. At best, these individuals will be more prone to experiencing frequent bouts of depression, moodiness, anger and frustration; in worst-case scenarios, suicide often becomes a very real option for alleviating their helplessness.

Instead of crying *"why me?"* when misfortune strikes, train yourself to ask more productive questions, such as, *"what can I do to stop this from happening again?",* and *"how can I best deal with this now that it has happened?"* Stop reading those useless star signs and start taking an active role in determining your own destiny!

If you get depressed, get busy! In their book *Managing Your Mind*, Gillian Butler and Tony Hope suggest that self-distraction should form the first line of defense against depression. They say, *"Fill your mind with something else, and give yourself a rest from dwelling on unhappy thoughts."*(7)

Many years back, one of my close cousins, who had been a model employee at his workplace of six years, lost his job after having a heated dispute with his newly-appointed supervisor, a confrontational individual who himself was later fired by senior management. My cousin's angst was compounded when he subsequently split up with his long-time girlfriend. He proceeded to slip into an extended state of melancholy, one marked by alternating bouts of despair, anger and self-pity. For several months, this previously upbeat young man became a walking gray cloud, bringing an aura of doom and gloom wherever he ventured.

One early summer's day, while I was preparing for a bike ride in the hills, my cousin came over to my house. His somber mood was in full force, but after much coaxing I somehow convinced him to jump on my brother's bike and join me on my ride. Thirty minutes later we were halfway up a particularly steep hill when my exhausted cousin suggested that maybe he should turn around and go back home. I won't repeat the exact words I used in response, but I did infer that his failure to accompany me to the top of the hill would cast serious doubts on his masculinity.

My cousin might have been depressed, but he wasn't about to be labeled a wuss--he leapt out of his saddle and started stomping down on the pedals with new-found vigor, almost as if he was literally channeling months of stress out through his legs and into the road. As I pedaled alongside him, egging him on, I heard something that I had not heard from my cousin in months; in between a string of profanities and labored breathing, I heard my cousin *laugh!*

When we returned home, my cousin confessed that he had forgotten just how much he loved escaping into the hills on his bike. He went home, pulled his bike out of his garage and immediately set about restoring it to full working order. As he became immersed in rebuilding his bike, shopping for parts and accessories and getting up to speed on the latest happenings in the world of cycling, the gray cloud that had stubbornly hung over his life for months gradually began to disappear. As my cousin became ensconced in his rekindled passion for cycling, he stopped dwelling on the disappointment of losing his job and girlfriend. Within weeks, he was back to his normal affable and buoyant self.

The next time you find yourself wallowing in the depths of despair and self-pity, throw yourself into a constructive activity that will help draw your mind away from whatever it is that is bothering you. This may be the last thing you initially feel like doing, but if you can just muster up enough energy to get started, then a return to a more positive frame of mind may only be a stone's throw away.

Lighten Up! As we learnt in Chapter 14, angry people tend to live shorter lives.

If you're one of those hot-headed folks that finds themselves fuming and wishing unspeakable evil on the driver in front because he has the temerity to obey the speed limit--or heaven forbid, drive at five miles per hour under-- when you happen to be running late for work, it's time for a major attitude overhaul. Ditto if you frequently find yourself agitated by the fact that spouses, children, friends, co-workers, employees, shop assistants, telephone operators, customers, etc, etc, don't always see things your way and/or don't always rush to accommodate your every demand.

Believe it or not, others have their own lives to worry about! We are all the product of a unique blend of accumulated life experiences, genetics, and parental, educational and other environmental influences. Each and every one of us has our own unique goals, desires, concerns, talents, likes and dislikes. Life in such a giant potpourri of individual differences is inevitable to have its bumpy moments. The total absence of conflict would be possible only in a world full of mindless automatons, a world in which most of us would hardly wish to reside.

Rather than launching into a tirade of abuse the next time someone accidentally cuts into your lane, you may instead like to recall how many times you have done the exact same thing (and you know you have)!

The above should not be interpreted as suggesting that we should put up with all manner of unreasonable behavior from others, and it certainly does not mean to imply that we should ignore malevolent actions that threaten our physical, mental or financial well-being. People should be allowed to do as they please, so long as their actions do not interfere with the rights of others to do the same. Your neighbor has every right to listen to music you abhor in the privacy of his own home, but when he keeps you awake at night by blasting his favorite tunes at full volume, its time to assert your right to peace and quiet. And on that note;

Be assertive, and pick your battles wisely. Avoiding unnecessary conflicts will go a long way to reducing the amount of stress you are subjected to, but that doesn't mean you should timidly tiptoe through life in a painstaking attempt to not pee anyone off. Turning yourself into a walking doormat might help avoid conflict in the short-term, but frustration and resentment will begin to bubble under your placid exterior. All too often, this volcano of suppressed emotion eventually explodes in a spectacular manner, manifesting itself in chronic disease, violence, and potentially fatal risk-taking behavior.

Learn the art of rational assertiveness. Don't let others walk all over you, and by the same token, don't treat every adverse event as if it were an imminent threat to your survival. I once worked at a gym where overdue payment reminders were routinely sent to customers with outstanding membership dues. Because most of these members were typically busy people who had simply forgotten about the outstanding debt, these reminders were deliberately worded in a manner that was as non-threatening as possible. As a result, the majority of recipients responded quite positively to these friendly payment reminders.

A notable exception was an extremely irate gentleman who came stampeding into the gym one day, loudly issuing threats and a string of obscenities at the startled receptionists, whilst madly waving an overdue payment notice that had recently been sent to his wife. After calming him down, the receptionists called one of the administrative assistants, who checked and found that the notice had been issued in error. The assistant politely reassured the gentleman that the gym records did indeed show receipt of full payment and sincerely apologized for the mix-up.

The problem was a simple error that was rectified within minutes, an outcome that would have been achieved just as easily had this individual remained calm. Had he engaged his rational faculties a little more carefully, he would have seen what most other people in the same situation saw: A relatively innocuous reminder notice. Instead he allowed his irrational tendencies to take over, triggering a primal fear response that caused him to feel unjustifiably threatened. As a result, he overreacted, employing the use of a cannon where a peashooter would have been more than ample. Continued on a long-term basis, such behavior not only makes you a laughing stock, it is a great way to court hypertension and ill health.

Next time you receive a final payment notice or an invoice billing you for items you don't recall purchasing, don't start acting like a cornered animal. Take a deep breath, then think about how you can calmly and rationally tackle the problem. Save the heavy artillery for when you really need it.

Diet and Lifestyle Interventions

Obviously, the best way to alleviate the effects of chronic stress is to avoid it in the first place. Of course, that's easier said than done when life often has the annoying habit of biting you in the butt just when things seem to be moving smoothly. The following are easily implemented interventions that not only help prevent stress but can minimize its effects after the proverbial horse has already bolted.

Get Physical! One well-known effect of vigorous exercise is that it stimulates the release of natural painkillers called endorphins, which produce feelings of euphoria and relaxation. Researchers have found that the mood-enhancing effects of exercise are similar--and possibly superior--to those of anti-depressant drugs and relaxation techniques like meditation(8-10).

In a recent study of patients with major depression, exercise was compared with the widely prescribed anti-depressant drug Zoloft over a period of sixteen weeks. The exercise group attended three supervised exercise sessions per week (each consisting of a ten minute warm-up, thirty minutes of continuous walking or jogging, then a five minute cool-down). While Zoloft produced a more rapid initial response, after sixteen weeks there were a similar number of patients in each group that no longer met the criteria for major depression(11). Six months after the study ended, those who had achieved remission in the exercise group enjoyed significantly lower relapse rates than subjects in the Zoloft group. In addition, those who kept exercising during the follow-up period were only half as likely to be diagnosed with depression at the end of that period(12).

If you're wondering whether you should do aerobic or anaerobic-type activities, a two-month study by Norwegian researchers found that both produced similar and significant improvements in depressed patients(13).

Avoid low-fat diets. In Chapter 3, we learnt how experiments with monkeys and humans have demonstrated a significant worsening of mood state and increased hostility during the consumption of low-fat diets(14,15). These undesirable effects were observed in healthy, psychologically robust volunteers; individuals with a history of depression or aggressive behavior should be especially wary of low-fat diet plans.

Avoid blood cholesterol-lowering treatments. The epidemiological link between low cholesterol levels and depression, suicide and other forms of violent death is well documented. Cholesterol-lowering drugs also possess the ability to worsen mood states in susceptible individuals (see Chapter 3).

Avoid low blood sugar. If you have ever been around a diabetic who was suffering from a severe bout of hypoglycemia, you will know that low blood sugar levels can rapidly induce an extremely sour demeanor in even the most agreeable of folks. While few non-diabetics will ever experience the terrifying sensation of severe hypoglycemia, the majority will indeed experience a more subtle and insidious form of low blood sugar--the kind that results from crash dieting or consuming too many carbohydrates. The latter initially causes excessively high blood glucose concentrations, to which the pancreas often 'hyper-responds' by secreting excessively large amounts of insulin, bringing blood sugar crashing down to below normal levels. This situation, known as *reactive hypoglycemia,* can quite literally result in an emotional roller coaster ride, where an individual feels fine one moment, but thirty minutes after a meal becomes listless, moody and touchy.

Take your fish oil. Scientists believe that changes in nerve and brain cell membrane fatty acid composition, caused by a distorted dietary omega-6:omega-3 ratio, can adversely affect the transmission of serotonin, an important neurotransmitter involved in regulating mood and sleep.

Epidemiological studies have found higher omega-3 intakes to be associated with lower prevalence of depression, hostility, seasonal affective disorder (SAD), and even homicide(16-21). Supporting this link are double-blind studies with omega-3 fatty acids that have observed significant improvements in sufferers of depression, bipolar disorder and even schizophrenics(22-25).

A study by Japanese researchers examined the effect of fish oil on psychological stress in Japanese medical students. The study began during the students' summer vacation and ended three months later during their end-of-year exams. Psychological tests given to control subjects during exam-time showed increased scores for 'extraggression' (aggression towards others). When researchers tested those taking the fish oil, they found no such increase-- their levels of aggression during this highly demanding period were the same as those experienced whilst on holidays!(26) In another Japanese experiment, researchers randomly allocated medical students to receive either docosahexaenoic acid (DHA), one of the omega-3 fatty acids found in fish oil and an important component of brain tissue, or a placebo in a double-blind manner. The subjects took the pills for nine weeks, during which time they underwent more than twenty stressful final exams. In the group taking DHA, concentrations of norepinephrine were significantly reduced, suggesting that this fatty acid may help mitigate some of the hormonal effects of stress(27).

When Italian researchers gave fish oil to healthy subjects for 35 days, psychological profiling revealed significant favorable changes in vigor, anger, anxiety, confusion, depression, and fatigue. No such changes were observed during administration of an olive oil placebo(28).

Avoid recreational drugs, and keep alcohol consumption to a minimum.
Alcohol and illicit drugs are widely used in an effort to 'unwind', but as stress-relief agents their safety record is absolutely atrocious. While they may provide short-term escape, they do little to address the original source of stress and often create even more psychological turmoil by promoting addiction, social incohesion and ill health. In 1997, the Secretary of Health and Human Services, Donna E. Shalala, reported, *"About 14 million American--almost 10 percent of adults--meet diagnostic criteria for alcohol abuse and alcoholism"*(29). As we shall discuss in the next chapter, the potential health consequences of abusing 'socially-acceptable' drugs like alcohol are no laughing matter. If you truly value your health, you'll find a less toxic way to unwind.

Deal With It

Authorities have for far too long dumped the subject of stress into the too-hard basket, but don't you do the same. Psychological stress exerts a massive influence upon cardiovascular health, and no one who is even remotely serious about thwarting heart disease can afford to ignore its importance.

Chapter 30

"The first draught serveth for health, the second for pleasure, the third for shame, the fourth for madness."
Sir Walter Raleigh.

What About Alcohol?

Is drinking really good for your heart?

No discussion of diet and heart disease would be complete without addressing the subject of alcohol. For many, the claim that moderate drinking may lower the risk of heart disease sounds too good to be true. Is it?

Anything But Harmless

Before we proceed, it must be emphasized that alcohol is a substance bearing *enormous* destructive potential. In the United States, alcohol-related mortality is the third most common cause of death, claiming almost 110,000 lives every year--over four times the number of deaths from illicit drug use!(1,2) World-wide, alcohol is the fourth leading cause of disability, afflicting almost sixteen million people(3). Make no mistake; every year, alcohol unleashes an immeasurable amount of misery, ill health and premature death upon millions of its users around the globe.

What is a Safe Amount of Alcohol?

Governments and health agencies around the world have attempted to curb the frighteningly high morbidity and mortality arising from excessive alcohol intake by instituting guidelines for safe daily alcohol intake. Table 30a presents the recommended maximum daily alcohol intakes issued by the U.S. Department of Health and Human Services.

Are These Allowances Too Generous?

In a collaborative paper titled *Alcohol–Related Morbidity and Mortality*, American, Canadian, and Swedish researchers conducted a sweeping review of the literature in order to estimate the risk of various health disorders occurring at different levels of alcohol intake. The results of their search are presented in Table 30b. Apart from the few notable exceptions of CHD, stroke and diabetes, a mere one drink per day appears to increase the risk of every other major illness listed in the table, including various cancers, cirrhosis of the liver, epilepsy and, of course, alcohol use disorders. This increased risk applies for both males and females. In the case of breast cancer, the authors found that one

---

Table 30a. Recommended maximum daily alcohol intakes for the United States.

United States

Men: no more than two drinks* per day (i.e., no more than 24oz beer, three 1oz shots of whisky, two 5-oz glasses of wine).

Women: no more than one drink* per day (i.e., no more than 12oz beer, one and one-half 1oz shots of whisky, one 5-oz glass of wine).

Over 65: no more than one drink* per day

*Standard Drink Unit:
one 12 oz-beer (17g alcohol)
one 5-oz glass wine (16-20g alcohol)
one and 1/2 oz of 80-proof liquor (17g alcohol)

Source: *The Physicians' Guide to Helping Patients With Alcohol Problems*, U.S. Department of Health and Human Services, Public Health Service, National Institutes of Health, National Institute on Alcohol Abuse and Alcoholism, NIH Publication Number 95-3769, 1995.

---

alcoholic drink per day raises risk by fourteen percent while two and three drinks per day raise breast cancer risk by forty-one and fifty-nine percent, respectively.

Not surprisingly, the most dramatic risk increase was observed for cirrhosis of the liver, the workhorse organ responsible for breaking down the toxins in alcohol and removing them from the body. Compared to teetotalers, those averaging two alcoholic drinks per day experience an almost *ten-fold* risk of cirrhosis!(4)

Alcohol and Overall Mortality

Despite the increased risk of numerous diseases at even low levels of alcohol consumption, many studies have associated moderate drinking with lower overall mortality levels. This epidemiological association is accounted for primarily by a reduction in cardiovascular disease mortality, and it is this observation that has led to the belief that alcohol may protect against CHD. One sizable review of the literature concerning the relationship between alcohol consumption and all-cause mortality involved twenty large prospective studies, some of which followed participants for up to twenty-three years. Altogether, these studies involved more than 1.2 million participants and just over 135,000 deaths. The majority of these studies took place in the U.S., and among U.S. males, the level of alcohol consumption associated with the lowest all-cause mortality was sixty-nine grams per week--the equivalent of four standard drinks per week. In females, the corresponding figure was twenty-six grams of

Table 30b. Relative Risk for Major Diseases, by Gender & Average Drinking Category						
	Females			**Males**		
	Drinking Category*					
Disease	**I**	**II**	**III**	**I**	**II**	**III**
Mouth and oropharynx cancers	1.45	1.85	5.39	1.45	1.85	5.39
Esophagus cancer	1.80	2.38	4.36	1.80	2.38	4.36
Liver cancer	1.45	3.03	3.60	1.45	3.03	3.60
Breast cancer	1.14	1.41	1.59			
- Under 45 years	1.15	1.41	1.46			
- Over 45 years	1.14	1.38	1.62			
Other cancers	1.10	1.30	1.70	1.10	1.30	1.70
Diabetes mellitus	0.92	0.87	1.13	1.00	0.57	0.73
Neuropsychiatric conditions						
Epilepsy	1.34	7.22	7.52	1.23	7.52	6.83
Hypertensive disease	1.40	2.00	2.00	1.40	2.00	4.10
Cardiovascular diseases						
Coronary heart disease	0.82	0.83	1.12	0.82	0.83	1.00
Stroke						
- Ischemic stroke	0.52	0.64	1.06	0.94	1.33	1.65
- Hemorrhagic stroke	0.59	0.65	7.98	1.27	2.19	2.38
Other CVD causes	1.50	2.20	2.20	1.50	2.20	2.20
Digestive diseases						
Cirrhosis of the liver	1.26	9.54	9.54	1.26	9.54	9.54

*Definition of drinking categories:
Category I: for females, 0–19.99 g pure alcohol daily; for males, 0–39.99 g pure alcohol daily
Category II: for females, 20–39.99 g pure alcohol daily; for males, 40–59.99 g pure alcohol daily
Category III: for females, 40 g or more pure alcohol; for males, 60 g or more pure alcohol

Source: Rehm J, et al. Alcohol–Related Morbidity and Mortality. *Alcohol Research & Health*, 2003; (27) 1: 39.

alcohol--the equivalent of one-and-a-half standard drinks per week. In contrast, mortality risk began to rise (when compared to abstinence) at around 135 grams of alcohol (around eight drinks) per week(5).

A similar analysis conducted by Australian researchers a few years earlier reported that the relative risk of all-cause mortality in male drinkers was sixteen percent lower than teetotalers at an alcohol intake of ten to nineteen grams per day. At an intake of thirty to thirty-nine grams per day, the mortality risk in drinkers was the same as that of non-drinkers, while those who drank sixty grams and upwards of alcohol per day had a thirty-seven percent increase in mortality risk. In female drinkers the lowest relative risk (minus twelve percent) was seen at zero to nine grams of alcohol per day. At twenty to twenty-nine grams per day, the risk exceeded that in abstainers by thirteen percent; at sixty grams per day the relative risk was fifty-eight percent higher(6).

Before we discuss the validity of these findings, it should be pointed out that they apply only to people over fifty years of age. While the relationship between mortality and alcohol consumption in older folks travels a J-shaped curve, in young folks it points in only one direction--upwards! Mortality risk rises at even the lowest levels of alcohol consumption, and continues to rise in a linear fashion with increasing alcohol intakes(4-7). Alcohol is particularly hazardous in this age group because it greatly increases the risk of fatalities from accidental and violent causes. For example, in 2000, more than seventy-five percent of the fatalities from alcohol-related motor vehicle accidents in the U.S. occurred in people under fifty years of age(8).

Reduced Risk...or Misclassification?

Reports of reduced mortality from regular alcohol consumption, embraced by wine manufacturers, the public, and even many health authorities, may be based on a fatal research flaw. As a team of drug and alcohol researchers from the US, Canada and Australia recently pointed out, many studies failed to separate former drinkers (people who had consumed no drinks in the past year) from complete abstainers; in some instances, people who had not consumed alcohol for a mere 30 days were included as abstainers! Other studies failed to separate occasional drinkers (those who imbibed once a month or less) from complete abstainers. It is a well-documented observation that people often abstain or dramatically reduce their drinking frequency for health reasons. These could include a medical assessment pronouncing one to be at high risk of a certain ailment, the actual onset of a health condition, the disability and frailty often accompanying old age, and/or medication use. If such individuals are included as 'abstainers' in these studies, then these 'abstainers' will appear to be less healthy than light drinkers and at increased risk of premature death. Regular light drinking, in effect, may be a marker for good health among middle aged and older people, not a cause of it.

Indeed, when the researchers analyzed separately the studies that did not confuse abstainers with occasional drinkers and those who recently quit drinking, the protective association of light drinking with overall and heart disease mortality disappeared!(9) The researchers noted, *"As a consequence, estimates of the extent of the impact of cardiac benefits from light alcohol consumption on mortality risk may have been greatly over-estimated in previous meta-analyses"*. While light drinking may not be harmful, it may not be 'protective' either.

While uncertainty surrounds the alleged benefits of light drinking, there is little doubt about the increased risk associated with certain other drinking patterns.

Drinking Away From Meals

An aspect of drinking that has received scarce attention is the effect of drinking alcohol with, or away from, meals. Food significantly slows the absorption of alcohol, and may thus act to moderate the physiological effects of drinking.

A recent large Italian study found that those who drank wine away from meals exhibited higher death rates from all causes than those who drank wine with meals. This effect was especially pronounced in women. It must be noted that those who drank outside of meals tended to be older, had a higher average alcohol consumption, smoked more and had higher blood pressure, suggesting that those who consumed alcohol with meals did so as part of a more temperate lifestyle. However, when the researchers adjusted for these confounding factors, the relationship persisted(10).

Binge Drinking

Without question, binge drinking--the consumption of five or more drinks in one sitting--is a loser's game. Those who believe that their weekday temperance excuses their Saturday night excesses should know heavy drinking bouts significantly increase the risk of heart disease, even when one's usual alcohol intake is otherwise light or moderate(11-14).

Binge drinking has been linked to subsequent episodes of arrhythmia after holidays and long weekends, a potentially fatal phenomenon that researchers have nicknamed 'holiday heart syndrome'(15-17). Epidemiological evidence shows an association between heavy drinking and sudden cardiac death, and acute alcohol administration has been shown to facilitate the onset of arrhythmias in heavy drinkers(18).

Epidemiological studies suggest that heavy alcohol ingestion raises blood pressure, an effect that has been confirmed in controlled experiments with human volunteers(19, 20). In one of these, sixteen hypertensive men who regularly drank up to eighty grams of alcohol daily experienced significant drops in blood pressure when they stopped drinking for four days. Reintroduction of alcohol reversed this beneficial effect(21).

Paraoxonase 1 is an antioxidant enzyme that has been shown to inhibit LDL cholesterol oxidation. Scientists recently discovered that, while light drinking caused a twenty to twenty-five percent increase in paraoxonase 1 in both the blood and liver of rats, heavy drinking caused a twenty-five percent decrease in paraoxonase 1 activity. In humans, blood tests showed that light drinkers had a 395 percent higher paraoxonase 1 activity than non-drinkers, whereas heavy drinkers had a forty-five percent lower activity(22).

Needless to say, binge drinking has consequences that are not readily detected in studies tracking mortality rates. Excessive alcohol consumption dramatically increases the risk of sexual and physical assault, as any police officer, ambulance driver or nightclub doorman can readily attest. If you are the inebriated perpetrator of these acts, the legal repercussions can quite literally ruin your life. If you are the alcohol-impaired victim, violent injury and death are very real consequences. Alcohol also dramatically increases the likelihood that one will engage in sexual encounters that would be avoided in a sober state, raising the risk of unwanted pregnancy and the transmission of STDs.

Is Red Wine All it is Cracked Up to Be?

A review headed by Harvard researcher Eric B. Rimm found that while cross-country comparisons did indeed point to a protective association between red wine and CHD, case-control and prospective studies conducted among individuals residing within the same city, region or country did not support any notion that one type of drink was more heart-healthy than others. Of the ten prospective cohort studies Rimm and his team looked at, four found a significant protective association between heart disease and moderate wine drinking, four found such an association for beer, and four for spirits(23).

In an experimental study, researchers measured fibrinolytic activity (the ability to break down blood clots, which are believed to be a major instigating factor in many fatal coronary and cerebrovascular events) in subjects consuming different types of alcohol. The subjects consumed, on four separate days, the following beverages at dinner in the evening: carbonated mineral water, or beer (pilsner), red wine or spirits (Dutch gin). Compared to water, alcohol significantly increased fibrinolytic activity, but there was little difference in the anti-clotting effects of the different types of alcohol(24). In another study, researchers found that one drink of beer or stout delivered the same increase in blood antioxidant activity as a serving of red wine(25).

Red wine started to attract media attention after the medical mainstream began pushing it as the explanation for the so-called 'French Paradox'. Often when mainstream medicine cannot explain something, rather than consider the possibility that its hypothesis is untenable, it simply labels the contradiction a 'paradox'. In the case of the French, their high consumption of animal fats supposedly should have placed them at higher risk of heart disease. However, the French actually suffered very low rates of heart disease, an embarrassing and uncomfortable contradiction for those promoting the lipid hypothesis. Noting that red wine was consumed liberally in France, they quickly dubbed this as the explanation for the low rates of CHD among the French. However, the Italians also have a high consumption of red wine, but their rates of CHD are more in line with other Southern European countries who drink less wine.

If--and at this stage it is a very big 'if'--alcohol does impart any cardiovascular protection, then it appears that the bulk of this protection is due to plain old ethanol.

As such, public health messages pertaining to alcohol should focus on discouraging excessive drinking, binge drinking, and drink-driving. Those who get drunk on red wine, using the rationale that it is a heart-healthy thing to do, should be made aware that they are fooling no one but themselves.

Drink Driving

In the U.S., the legally mandated limit for blood alcohol concentration is 0.08. This figure gives many drivers the impression that drinking up to, but not beyond, the prescribed limit is OK.

Nothing could be further from the truth.

By the time you've reached the legal U.S. BAC limit, you have already multiplied your risk of being killed in a single-vehicle crash by eleven to fifty-two-fold, the level of risk varying with age. Even at BAC levels of 0.02 to 0.049, the risk of being killed in a single-vehicle crash increases three- to five-fold(26).

A recent review of 112 studies provides strong evidence that impairment in driving skills begins as soon as BAC departs from zero. The majority of these studies reported impairment at a BAC of 0.05 percent, while virtually all drivers tested exhibited impairment on some critical measure of driving performance by the time they reached a BAC of 0.08(27).

While it is unlikely that legislators will ever introduce zero-tolerance alcohol laws for motor-vehicle drivers, the only truly safe level of alcohol ingestion for drivers is just that--zero. Don't drink and drive, and don't accept a lift with someone who has been drinking--it might be the last ride you ever take.

Pregnancy

Alcohol consumption during pregnancy has been linked with a host of birth and developmental defects. Fortunately, many pregnant women are aware of the need to avoid alcohol during pregnancy.

Less well-recognized is the need for women who even have a chance of becoming pregnant to also avoid alcohol. After analyzing almost 25,000 pregnancies, Danish researchers found an increased risk of spontaneous abortion in the first trimester (seven to eleven weeks of gestation) for women consuming five or more drinks per week(28). Forty-five percent of all women participating in the 1988 National Maternal and Infant Health Survey reported consuming alcohol during the three months prior to finding out they were pregnant, with five percent reporting consumption of six or more drinks per week. Sixty percent of alcohol-consuming women did not know they were pregnant until after the fourth week of pregnancy, and many did not know until after the sixth week(29).

In other words, many women inadvertently expose the developing fetus to the harmful effects of alcohol without even realizing it.

To Drink or Not to Drink

If you do not currently drink but are considering doing so because of the reported association between lower CHD risk and alcohol use, realize that there are many other ways to lower your risk of cardiovascular and all-cause mortality that do not increase the risk of substance abuse, motor vehicle accidents, social incohesion, violence, and the increase in cancer, cardiovascular disease and liver dysfunction that can accompany alcohol use.

It should also be emphasized that science has not yet answered the question of whether individuals who are already exercising, following a healthy nutrient-dense diet, sleeping well and keeping a handle on chronic stress stand to gain from alcohol's alleged cardiovascular or overall mortality benefits, or whether alcohol may actually detract from the positive effect of these activities.

In Japan, where consumption of blood-thinning omega-3 fatty acids is higher and risk of CHD and ischemic stroke is lower than in the West, moderate drinking is not associated with any further reduction in CHD or stroke death, although it does increase the risk of hemorrhagic stroke(30,31). A seven-year follow-up study of over 19,000 Japanese men found a significantly lower all-cause mortality rate for moderate drinkers, but the authors noted that the *"background characteristics of moderate drinkers were healthier than either nondrinkers or heavy drinkers."*(32)

Given what we presently know about the effects of alcohol, drinking should not form one's front line defense against heart disease. That role should be relegated to the strategies recommended in this book: a nutrient-rich, low- to moderate-carbohydrate diet, daily nutritional supplementation, regular exercise, stress reduction, avoidance of high bodily iron stores, and sound sleeping habits.

Ultimately, the decision to drink alcohol is one that adult individuals will have to make for themselves using the available scientific evidence--and a good dose of common sense--as their guide. Because the main pattern of alcohol use among younger drinkers is binge drinking and because drinking during adolescence dramatically increases the likelihood of both short-term and long-term alcohol-related problems, adolescents should stay well away from the booze until their early twenties, when they are far more likely to have acquired the requisite maturity to make sensible drinking decisions(33,34).

If you are over fifty, only drink with meals, do not binge drink, never drink and drive and do not act like an anti-social boor after drinking, then based on the current available evidence, there appears to be no increased mortality risk if you drink lightly. If you are male, then one standard drink appears to be the amount associated with minimal risk. If you are female, the evidence indicates that one standard drink per day is too much. It *must* be remembered that these findings are derived, not from controlled clinical trials, but from confounder-prone epidemiological studies.

If you do binge drink, if you do consume *any* amount of alcohol prior to driving, if you do drink away from meals (in bars, parties, etc) or cannot refrain from acting in an obnoxious, aggressive and/or irritating manner after drinking, then you most certainly need to change your current drinking habits. Such patterns of alcohol use have clearly been shown to raise the risk of acute injury and death from violent and accidental causes and to also raise the risk of chronic illness and subsequent premature mortality.

Bottom Line on Booze

Guidelines for alcohol consumption are likely to remain the subject of heated debate for quite some time. Given the ethical and legal minefield awaiting any research team attempting to conduct a long-term, randomized clinical trial examining the effects of alcohol on mortality, it is unlikely that we will be able to draw upon such tightly controlled evidence anytime in the near future.

Despite the considerable ambiguities, there are several groups for whom alcohol is clearly best avoided. Pregnant women and women who even have a chance of becoming pregnant, adolescents, individuals with a personal or family history of alcohol abuse/dependence, psychiatric illness and those with liver disorders should not venture anywhere near alcohol. In those under fifty years of age, alcohol does not offer any mortality benefit whatsoever, but in fact increases mortality risk even at the lowest levels of consumption.

Section Three Summary

The 'Twelve Commandments' For a Healthy Heart

1. Do your best to keep a handle on stress; be especially conscious of avoiding stress during and after eating.
2. Exercise on a regular basis; at least thirty minutes on most days of the week.
3. Get to bed as soon as practical after darkness falls and sleep in the darkest, quietest possible surroundings.
4. Keep your blood sugar level well within the normal range. Eat a 'low glycemic load' diet; i.e., avoid high-carbohydrate intakes and the consumption of highly refined carbohydrates.
5. Maintain a healthy weight. If you are overweight, utilize a program incorporating increased activity and/or calorie restriction to reduce your bodyfat mass.
6. Avoid processed, packaged foods and eat fresh meats, vegetables, fruits, nuts and seeds regularly.
7. Consume omega-3 fats regularly.
8. Skip the low-fat fad: Enjoy animal and tropical fats but avoid omega-6-rich vegetable oils and trans-fat-rich margarines like the plague.
9. Take your supplements every day.
10. Avoid high bodily stores of iron.
11. Avoid cigarettes and passive smoke.
12. If you drink, consume no more than 1-2 glasses of alcohol per day. Only drink at mealtimes, and never binge drink.

"Unthinking respect for authority is the greatest enemy of truth."
Albert Einstein.

Epilogue

After hearing the case against the lipid hypothesis, most people I speak to have little trouble accepting that this theory is scientifically invalid. The question they then inevitably ask is: *"If the anti-cholesterol theory is wrong, why are we repeatedly told to eat low-fat diets and to take cholesterol-lowering drugs?"*

This question was largely, but not completely, answered in Chapter 12, where we examined the role of large vested interests in perpetuating the lipid hypothesis. The blame does not lie solely with powerful financial motivations; there are some extremely important psychosocial factors that have played a critical role in keeping the cholesterol theory alive. Foremost among these is the *herd mentality.*

In his sugar-damning book *Sweet and Dangerous*, Professor John Yudkin reflected: *"...one of the things that took me a long time to learn is that scientists as a group are no more, and no less, influenced by emotional and irrational reactions than other people are"*. In other words, researchers are only human. Like the rest of us, they are not immune to the powerful influence of currently accepted trends and paradigms. As in any other field, it is indeed a rare occurrence in science when some bold, gifted genius breaks out of the confines of current thinking and makes a truly revolutionary new discovery.

When one laboriously pores through the huge volume of research pertaining to cholesterol, one notices that the introduction to these papers almost always contains words similar to the following: *"It is widely acknowledged that elevated serum cholesterol is involved in the development of coronary heart disease, and cholesterol reduction has been shown to significantly reduce coronary mortality"*. Neither of these statements are even close to being true, but, as Malcolm Kendrick, M.D., Ph.D., explains, *"...medical papers are full of wild unsupported statements to which no-one seems to object. For example, you often read the phrase--'It is widely accepted that'. This is code for, 'we believe it, but we couldn't find any actual evidence.'"*

In 1956, professor Joseph A. Gengerelli, head of the Psychology Department of the University of California, Los Angeles, was quoted as saying that: *"We have a social force that selectively encourages and rewards the scientific hack. There is a great hustle and bustle, a rushing back and forth to scientific conferences, a great plethora of $50,000 grants for $100 ideas. I am suggesting that scientific, technical, and financial facilities are such in this country as to encourage a great number of mediocrities to go into science, and to seduce* *even those with creative talent and imagination to a mistaken view of the nature of the scientific enterprise."*(1)

Almost fifty years on, little has changed. Writing in a 2003 issue of the *Journal of American Physicians and Surgeons*, the late Cornell University Professor Emeritus Thomas Gold laments: *"In tribal society, what I call the 'herd instinct' presumably has some sociologic value. In science, however, we generally want diversity--many different avenues to be pursued. When people pursue the same avenue all together, they tend to shut out other approaches-- including what may be the right one.*

A flock of starlings may be able to change direction all at once, but this generally doesn't happen when one member of the herd decides to head in a different direction. If a scientist adopts a different viewpoint, there is no way to be sure that the others will follow. He may be left alone outside the herd. Moreover, he will be challenged to justify why he has departed. The others will never be asked why they stayed. The sheep in the interior of the field are well protected from the bite of the sheep dog."(2)

Because of the conformist mindset so prevalent amongst scientists and society in general, once proponents of the lipid hypothesis seized control of official CHD prevention policy in 1984, the rest was a breeze. The health organizations that handed out research grants were fully committed to the lipid hypothesis, as were the manufacturers of highly profitable lipid-lowering drugs, making funding for dissenting theories a highly unlikely proposition. After the lipid hypothesis became official policy, the question was no longer whether cholesterol caused heart disease, but how. Scientific investigation into heart disease over the last twenty years has accordingly centered around the lipid hypothesis, and a veritable mountain of research has been carried out examining every minute aspect of cholesterol metabolism. This preoccupation with blood lipids is no doubt a major reason why heart disease incidence has not declined, why it is still our number one killer, and why medical science has not even come close to establishing a cure for CHD.

As any propagandist worth his salt knows, the key to a successful campaign is repetition. Repeat something often enough--no matter how fallacious--via the media, literature, educational institutions and 'respected' organizations and authorities, and there is an outstanding chance that even the flimsiest lie will eventually become the perceived truth.

Once a belief has become deeply ingrained in our psyche, it takes on a whole new life of its own--it becomes part of the value structure and knowledge base from which we draw upon to navigate through an often chaotic and unpredictable world. It becomes, in effect, an integral part of our psychological make-up, a part of our very identity. Relinquishing such deeply embedded beliefs, regardless of their complete lack of scientific foundation, can be an extremely unsettling experience, one that often requires nothing less than Herculean discipline. The more one has built their life, career and social status around a false belief, the less likely one is to instigate such an effort. In fact, even in the face of highly compelling counter-evidence, many will do the exact opposite; they will stubbornly and often rabidly defend that which they have mistakenly come to accept as fact.

Tolstoy, commenting on this unfortunately universal syndrome, wrote: *"I know that most men, including those at ease with problems of the greatest complexity, can seldom accept even the simplest and most obvious truth, if it be such as would oblige them to admit the falsity of conclusions which they have delighted in explaining to colleagues, which they have proudly taught to others, and which they have woven, thread by thread, into the fabric of their lives."*

Perhaps Australia's Will Tõnisson, Ph.D., sums it up best when he writes: *"One of the negative attributes of human psychology is our tendency to fight to the death to defend our beliefs, performing amazing feats of mental gymnastics as we go. Many who have spent an entire career becoming an "authority", being a keynote speaker, publishing in learned journals, etc, on a paradigm that turns out to be fatally flawed will literally go to their grave defending what has essentially been their raison d'être. Their mind will be closed to counter arguments, regardless how "persuasive". The desire to be right may even spur them to greater efforts to "win the argument"--using fair or foul methods to preserve their ego. The ultimate consequence is the often painfully slow process of acceptance of new ideas."*

Instead of critically examining the edicts issued by authorities, most of us are all too often lulled into complacency, trusting those in charge of determining health guidelines and policy agendas to do the right thing. Many of our opinions are shaped by what we read, hear and see in the popular media, but most of the journalists compiling these stories have little knowledge of diet, metabolism or biochemistry. How many times have you read an article beginning with the words: *"According to experts, a new study shows that..."* or *"Leading authorities have stated that..."*? Instead of formulating their own conclusions through first-hand research, journalists often consult outside authorities for an 'expert' opinion. More often than not, these so-called 'experts' are either:

1) Researchers receiving funds from food or drug companies;
2) Spokespeople for health organizations receiving funds from food and/or drug companies;
3) Public relations spokespeople whose job is to disseminate information that casts the views and activities of those they represent in the most favorable possible light.

Scientists, doctors and the public alike frequently rely on advice from the health organizations they trust and respect, not realizing the recommendations proffered may well be the product of a hidden agenda. Such is the danger of relying on second-hand information--one must hope that the accuracy, honesty and objectivity of those supplying the information are of good merit.

At this point, skeptical readers may be asking: *"So why should we trust you, Colpo?"* My answer is--don't. Do your own research. Consult the references I have given, and if you have access to a medical or university library then be sure to read the study papers in full; this will often reveal a very different story to the one told in the more widely-read abstracts.

An independent, rational mind that is prepared to seek out information first-hand is a most powerful asset--by all means, use it!

Appendix A

The Myth of Vegetarianism

Some readers may object to my lavish praise for the healthful qualities of meat by pointing to studies that have shown vegetarians to enjoy lower rates of heart disease. While some studies have indeed found lower rates of CHD among vegetarians, there is not a shred of evidence to suggest that this phenomenon has anything to do with the avoidance of meat.

The studies most frequently cited in support of vegetarian diets have involved Seventh-day Adventists living in California. Scientific interest in this population was inspired by data from the early seventies showing that, as a group, Seventh-day Adventists enjoyed a significantly lower death rate from cancer than non-Adventists. Members of this religion are exhorted to abstain from alcohol and tobacco, and most also shun the use of pork products. In addition, approximately one-half of Seventh-Day Adventists follow a lacto-ovo vegetarian diet, using vegetables, fruits, whole grains and nuts abundantly while avoiding the use of tea and coffee.

A recent study of over 34,000 Californian Seventh-Day Adventists, published in 1999, found that vegetarians had lower risks of hypertension, diabetes, arthritis, colon cancer, prostate cancer, fatal CHD in males, and death from all causes. Again, vegetarians displayed a number of healthful dietary habits unrelated to meat intake that were not shared by their omnivorous brethren. Vegetarians consumed more tomatoes, nuts, and fruit, but less coffee and donuts than non-vegetarians. Non-vegetarian Seventh-Day Adventists also consumed alcoholic beverages twenty times more frequently than their vegetarian counterparts(1). As an earlier study of Adventists published in 1975, these observations clearly showed that those who shunned meat also adopted other dietary measures that protected their health(2).

Reinforcing this notion was the fact that, along with many of the aforementioned disorders, obesity increased as meat consumption increased. Obesity is well known to confer an increased risk of heart disease and cancer. Meat consumption, however, has nothing whatsoever to do with the accumulation of excess body fat; several clinical trials have in fact shown that replacing dietary carbohydrates with high protein foods like beef and poultry often dramatically boosts weight loss (3,4). A year-long Finnish study that compared weight loss on lactovegetarian and omnivorous diets also failed to support the contention that vegetarian diets possess superior fat-burning capabilities. In fact, the omnivorous diet produced slightly greater weight loss than the vegetarian diet (10.4kg versus 9.2kg, respectively)(5). The greater meat consumption of obese Seventh-Day Adventists was simply one of numerous characteristics present with greater frequency among those living less healthy lifestyles. Why single out meat when so many other possible culprits were present?

What do other studies show?

What about other large-scale studies, involving populations other than Seventh-Day Adventists, that recruited vegetarians and non-vegetarians and compared their subsequent mortality rates?

Three such studies have been conducted, all from the UK: the Health Food Shoppers Study, the Oxford Vegetarian Study and the EPIC-Oxford Study. The Health Food Shoppers Study, involving almost 10,000 health food store patrons in England, found a similar all-cause death rate among vegetarians and omnivores after seventeen years (6).

The Oxford Vegetarian Study compared over 6,800 vegetarians and non-vegetarians and found a twenty percent reduction in overall mortality among the former after twelve years(7). More recent follow-up by the Oxford authors, however, found that the reduction in overall mortality had disappeared. In fact, the only significant difference remaining for any cause of death was seen for mental and neurological diseases, which were 2.5 times higher among vegetarians(8).

The EPIC-Oxford Study, involving 56,000 subjects, also found no difference in overall mortality between vegetarians and omnivores after 5.9 years. Vegetarians displayed slightly higher mortality from all cancers and stroke(9).

Contrary to popular claims, the above studies show that vegetarianism offered no protection from stroke, breast cancer, colorectal cancer, lung cancer, stomach cancer, or prostate cancer. Vegetarians did enjoy a non-significant reduction in coronary heart disease mortality, but avoidance of meat is unlikely to explain the difference. In the Health Food Shoppers and Oxford studies, the proportion of smokers was lower among vegetarians than non-vegetarians. In the Oxford study, vegetarians weighed less, drank less alcohol and exercised more. Information about exercise habits was not available for EPIC-Oxford, but vegetarians in this study were less likely to be heavy smokers or overweight. Similar to the situation observed with Seventh-Day Adventists, these results are confounded by the fact that vegetarians tend to be a health-conscious group who smoke less cigarettes, drink less alcohol and engage in regular physical activity.

The importance of non-dietary factors in the reduction of heart disease among vegetarians is further emphasized by the results of a large study by researchers at the German Cancer Research Center. In 1978 they began following 1,904 vegetarians, 225 of whom died over the next eleven years. Because 470 deaths would have been expected in a sample of typical Germans, this study has frequently been cited in support of vegetarianism. This study, however, could not even begin to be used by any rational commentator as evidence that meat avoidance is beneficial. For starters, when the researchers compared death rates among strict vegetarians who never ate meat and 'moderate' vegetarians who occasionally ate meat or fish, they found similar cancer, cardiovascular disease and all-cause mortality rates among the two groups.

Furthermore, only four percent of males and three percent of females in the study were smokers; the corresponding figures for the rest of Germany were forty-one and twenty-six percent, respectively. The vegetarians in the study were generally better educated and were more likely to be employed in professional jobs than the general population. They were also far less likely to be overweight(10). Little surprise, then, that this group experienced lower mortality than the general population!

When the authors examined the effect of various confounding factors, they found that the strongest predictor by far of reduced all-cause and cardiovascular mortality was a higher level of physical activity(11).

The German study merely adds to the considerable volume of evidence showing that being physically active, avoiding overweight and eschewing cigarettes all increase longevity. The claim that shunning a nutrient-packed food like meat contributes to an increase in life span, through some bizarre twist of biochemistry, is a shameless exercise in junk science.

It should also be pointed out that studies examining meat-eaters who follow healthier-than-usual lifestyles have revealed mortality rates similar to or superior to those seen in the aforementioned vegetarian studies. An eight-year follow-up of over 5,200 Californian Mormon high priests found fifty-three percent lower cancer mortality, a forty-eight percent reduction in cardiovascular deaths, and fifty-three percent lower all-cause mortality than the rest of the white California population. For middle-aged high priests adhering to the three important health practices of never smoking cigarettes, engaging in regular physical activity and getting proper sleep, the reductions were even more impressive; cancer, cardiovascular and total deaths were reduced by sixty-six, eighty-six and seventy-eight percent, respectively!(12)

In another Californian study, this time involving residents of Alameda County, ten years of follow-up revealed that the strongest predictors of survival were: 1) never smoking cigarettes; 2) regular physical activity; 3) moderate or no use of alcohol; 4) attaining seven to eight hours of sleep per day, and; 5) maintaining proper weight(13).

Despite the vociferous claims of vegetarian activists, who have shown themselves to be in no way averse to bending the truth when it suits their agenda, the fact remains that vegetarianism has *not* been demonstrated to offer any reduction in cancer or all-cause mortality--even when using the garbage-laden modern Western diet as the reference standard! There also exists no reliable evidence to implicate meat in the causation of heart disease. To the contrary, meat is the richest dietary source of several nutrients that are essential for optimal cardiovascular function, including carnitine, taurine, proline, carnosine, the B group of vitamins and, in the case of organ meats, CoQ10 (brain, kidney, liver) and omega-3 fats (brain).

Appendix B

The Low Fat 'Gurus': Dean Ornish and Nathan Pritikin

Dean Ornish

One low fat proponent who has received quite a bit of media attention is Dean Ornish, MD, an individual with some rather interesting views on what constitutes the ideal diet. In the early 1970's, Ornish met Swami Satchidananda, the late Indian yoga guru who sung the praises not only of yoga and meditation, but also a low-fat vegetarian diet. Ornish described the experience as *"life-changing"* and became a devoted disciple of the late swami.

Converting to vegetarianism because of a *"life-changing"* meeting with a yoga guru, as opposed to a meticulous review of the medical and anthropological literature, is hardly what one would consider an objective and scientific approach to formulating an optimal dietary regimen.

Ornish, however, has been able to attain an air of credibility among many of his conservative medical colleagues because of a small intervention trial he has conducted, one that allegedly demonstrates the benefits of following a low-fat vegetarian diet. The fact that the results of this trial have been reported in respected journals like *The Lancet* and the *Journal of the American Medical Association* has helped him win the ear of medical professionals, media outlets and even a sizable segment of the general population.

If the members of these groups scrutinized Ornish's published papers a little more closely, they would quickly realize Ornish's research fails to support most of his very public claims.

The Lifestyle Heart Trial

In a 1990 issue of *The Lancet*, Ornish and several of his colleagues published the one-year results of the Lifestyle Heart Trial, which initially involved forty-eight patients with coronary artery disease (as determined by quantitative coronary arteriography)(1). Twenty-eight of these patients had been randomized to follow a multi-faceted intervention program that included:

- A minimum of three hours' exercise per week.
- Stress management tactics for at least one hour every day. These included stretching, breathing techniques, meditation, progressive relaxation, and imagery.
- A vegetarian diet that contained around 10% of calories as fat, 15-20% protein, and 70-75% carbohydrates. The diet included fruits, vegetables,

grains, legumes, and soybean products without caloric restriction. The only animal products allowed were egg whites and one cup of non-fat milk or yogurt.

- Twice weekly group support sessions.

Those in the control group were not asked to make any diet or lifestyle changes, although they were free to do so if they wished.

At the start of the study and after 12 months, each patient underwent a coronary arteriogram to determine whether advanced arterial plaques had progressed, regressed or remained unchanged.

After one year, the researchers reported that eighty-two percent of those in the experimental group had experienced regression of arterial plaque, compared to only forty-two percent of those in the control group. The experimental group subjects also experienced significantly less chest pain.

Ornish has repeatedly inferred that these improvements underscore the value of a low-fat, vegetarian diet.

In reality, they do no such thing.

Control Your Variables

One of the most basic rules of science is to control all possible variables. The experimental group in the Lifestyle Heart Trial underwent multiple interventions; exercise, stress management and a multitude of dietary modifications. Average bodyweight also decreased in the treatment group during the study, but remained unchanged in the control group.

Thus, the treatment group therefore differed in several ways to the control group.

Ornish is justified in claiming that his collective assortment of treatments reduced chest pain and increased the incidence of arteriographically-determined coronary plaque regression. However, he can in no way claim that fat restriction or the avoidance of meat was a contributing factor--such a claim is precluded by the multi-faceted nature of his intervention program.

Ornish claims that the beneficial changes seen in the treatment group were correlated with reduction in dietary fat intake. So what; mathematical correlation does not equate to physiological causation! The association may well have arisen simply because those who adhered most strictly to the prescribed fat guidelines also adhered more strictly to the remaining dietary and lifestyle guidelines.

Did Ornish measure serum antioxidant levels in his subjects? Measures of glycemic control? Iron status? Blood or tissue trans fatty acid levels? Inflammatory markers? If he did, he never presented the data in his published papers. All these things can impact upon cardiovascular health, and are influenced by a multitude of factors other than total fat intake.

Exercise, stress management, weight loss and plant-based antioxidants have all been shown to significantly improve arterial function and/or structure. Any of these factors, either alone or in combination with each other, could easily account for the changes observed(2-6). In contrast, no properly controlled study has ever shown that drastically reducing fat intake or eliminating meat consumption will bring about such improvements.

Before Ornish proclaims to the world that restricting fat and avoiding meat will reduce the incidence of heart disease, he--or preferably some more neutral party--should conduct properly-controlled trials that actually demonstrate this contention. In other words, trials in which;

- Two groups eat a diet identical in every respect except that one derives its protein content primarily from meat, the other from plant foods;
- Both groups eat a diet identical in every respect except that one is much lower in fat (especially animal fat) than the other.

Until such trials are conducted, Ornish and his like-minded vegetarian colleagues should refrain from slandering meat and animal fat. To do so without any tightly controlled evidence to fall back on is to show a complete disregard for the scientific method.

Do Ornish's Interventions Actually Save Lives?

When all is said and done, the most telling data in any intervention study is the survival rate of the control and treatment groups. It's all well and good to lavish praise on a treatment's ability to lower chest pain, improve angiogram results, and even reduce the incidence of cardiac events, but these are all outcomes whose diagnosis is open to a substantial amount of subjective interpretation. Doctors can argue about the interpretation of test results and the necessity of surgery until the cows come home, but death is final and indisputable.

So while I am not real keen on the whole idea of dying, I have to admit that death is a great yardstick by which to judge the efficacy of an intervention--especially one that is highly-touted for its alleged life-saving qualities.

In 1998, the *Journal of the American Medical Association* published the five-year follow-up data for the Lifestyle Heart Trial(7). While the experimental group experienced a significantly reduced overall incidence of cardiac events (a classification that included angioplasty, bypass surgery, heart attack, and hospitalization for any cardiac cause), the treatment group actually experienced one more death than the control group (two people in the intervention group died compared to one person in the control group).

According to Ornish, one of the treatment group deaths was in a participant who had stopped following the intervention. Another intervention subject reportedly got a little too enthusiastic whilst exercising, exceeding his prescribed target heart rate with fatal consequences.

The unfavorable mortality outcome in the small Lifestyle Heart Trial appears to have been due largely to unfortunate circumstances, and gives little useful insight into how Ornish's interventions may affect survival among CHD patients. Let us instead look to a larger study by Ornish and his colleagues to see if his treatment program has demonstrated any ability to actually save lives.

The Multicenter Lifestyle Demonstration Project

The Multicenter Lifestyle Demonstration Project sought to apply the intervention in Ornish's original trial to a larger group of patients recruited from clinics across the U.S.(8). Practitioners from eight medical centers around the country were trained in all aspects of the Lifestyle program, which they proceeded to administer to patients with coronary artery disease. The study was not a randomized, controlled trial; instead, outcomes in the 194 patients who completed the intervention were compared with 139 patients who did not take part in the Lifestyle program.

After three years, there were no significant differences in cardiac event rates nor mortality between patients in the intervention and control groups. The number of cardiac events per patient year of follow-up when comparing the experimental group with the control group was as follows: 0.012 versus 0.012 for myocardial infarction, 0.014 versus 0.006 for stroke, 0.006 versus 0.012 for non-cardiac deaths, and 0.014 versus 0.012 for cardiac deaths (none of the differences were statistically significant).

To be fair, there is always the possibility that the treatment group fell prey to unfavorable confounding factors. The treatment subjects reportedly had a higher incidence of previous myocardial infarction and a longer history of coronary disease, although the angiographic severity of artery disease was similar between the two groups. Patients in the experimental group were required not to have undergone coronary artery bypass grafting (CABG) within six weeks or percutaneous transluminal coronary angioplasty (PTCA) within six months of the start of the study, while all the control subjects had recently undergone either of these procedures. While some might argue that the higher incidence of surgery may have favorably affected survival in the control group, the longevity benefits of revascularization procedures are highly questionable; controlled clinical trials have found that, for most patients, CABG or PTCA offer no mortality advantage whatsoever to standard medical therapy. The latter, in fact, shows a trend towards increased mortality (see Appendix C).

In their favor, the intervention participants lost weight and improved their exercise tolerance. No corresponding data were given for the control group, but given the absence of the intense counseling afforded to the intervention group, it is unlikely that the former would have experienced such changes--a contention supported by the original Lifestyle trial.

Whether confounding factors acted in favor of the treatment group, the controls, or neither, is nigh impossible to ascertain with any certainty. Regardless, the fact remains that there currently does not exist any hard published data to show that Ornish's Lifestyle program--touted as *"The Only System Scientifically Proven to Reverse Heart Disease Without Drugs or Surgery"*(9)--can actually save even a single life.

As we learnt in Chapter 8, trials involving subjects following omnivorous diets who were instructed to exercise, take fish oil supplements, or consume more fish and/or fruits and vegetables, have produced marked reductions in cardiac and overall mortality. The Lyon Diet Heart Study, for example, produced a whopping eighty-one percent reduction in coronary mortality and a sixty percent decrease in overall mortality(10).

The results of trials such as the Lyon Diet Heart Study should be kept firmly in mind when assessing the exuberant but unfounded claims of outspoken vegetarian advocates like Ornish.

Interestingly, despite his virulent denunciation of meat eating and his apparent emphasis on whole food consumption, Ornish has no qualms about accepting handsome promotional and consulting fees from processed food manufacturers like McDonald's, PepsiCo and ConAgra Foods(11).

Nathan Pritikin

Nathan Pritikin was a hugely influential low fat proponent during the late 1970s and early 1980s. In 1957, Pritikin discovered he had a serious heart condition, but was told by his doctor that little could be done to improve his condition.

A dissatisfied Pritikin took matters into his own hands and began researching heart disease in the hope of finding a remedy. He read about primitive cultures who avoided heart disease, and concluded that it was a low fat diet, high in unrefined cereal grains that kept them healthy (his reading material obviously failed to mention cultures that thrived on high fat, grain-free diets like the Masai, Samburus, Pacific Islanders and Eskimos).

Pritikin was also aware that during World War II, death rates from CHD decreased in a number of European countries, even though their residents were living in a state of heightened fear and anxiety from the fighting and bombing going on around them. Pritikin discovered that fat consumption had decreased during the war years, further reinforcing his conclusion that a low fat diet was conducive to cardiovascular health. Fat consumption did indeed go down during the war years, but so did consumption of sugar and refined cereal grains, a point that was lost in his rush to vilify fat.

Pritikin also discovered that in studies where dogs had their arteries deliberately blocked, exercise stimulated the growth of tiny new blood vessels, improving circulation. Pritikin embarked on a low fat diet devoid of processed foods, began exercising regularly, and gradually his condition began to improve. The formerly sick and weakly Pritikin eventually achieved a high level of fitness, eliminating all symptoms of CHD.

Pritikin achieved widespread media acclaim as a spokesperson for the low fat movement, and went on to become a best-selling author. He opened the Pritikin Longevity Center in Santa Barbara, California, where patients were treated with both exercise and a low-fat diet devoid of processed foods.

Increasing physical activity and eliminating refined foods were a huge step in the right direction, but Pritikin's views on fat could not be described as anything but fanatical. He initially advocated the complete elimination of dietary fat, believing the minimal amount that occurred naturally in low fat vegetable foods to be sufficient. When those who were able to adhere to his extreme recommendations began suffering from essential fatty acid deficiencies, he revised his recommendations to allow a meager ten percent of daily calories from fat. Whilst Nathan Pritikin conquered heart disease, he still died before his time, committing suicide while hospitalized for leukemia complications in 1985 at the age of sixty-nine.

The experiences of nutritionist Ann Louise Gittleman provide a revealing insight into the problems caused by Pritikin's extreme low-fat recommendations. A former Director of Nutrition at the Pritikin Longevity Center, Gittleman explains in her book *Beyond Pritikin* that while many patients did indeed experience positive improvements during their initial stay at the center, follow-up visits were often an entirely different story. Patients frequently complained about weight gain and continual hunger that could not be satisfied no matter how much food was eaten. Symptoms resembling those of gluten sensitivity became increasingly common, as patients began consuming unprecedented amounts of whole grains, an inevitable byproduct of Pritikin's edict to consume eighty percent of calories as complex carbohydrates.

Gittleman began to have her doubts about the Pritikin regimen, and whilst pursuing her own research became aware of certain facts that Pritikin had overlooked. One of these was the importance of essential fatty acids. Gittleman realized that many of the symptoms experienced by Pritikin Longevity Center patients were due not only to excessive carbohydrate consumption, but to a deficiency of crucial fats. *"Pritikin said fat was the problem. I was beginning to see fat as the solution"*, wrote Gittleman, who left the center in 1982(12). Gittleman went onto become a popular author and well-known nutritionist, recommending a low carbohydrate 'Fat Flush' diet for weight loss and a more moderate carbohydrate 'maintenance' diet for general health.

Conclusion

There is every reason in the world to encourage people to exercise frequently, stop smoking, eat minimally processed foods, and find ways to get a handle on the stresses of modern life. The evidence for low-fat diets, on the other hand, is based on a mixture of erroneous assumptions, half-truths and downright lies.

Appendix C

Coronary Intervention: Lifesaver, or Waste of Time?

The Less-Than-Flattering Facts About Bypass Surgery and Angioplasty.

"Miraculous" and *"lifesaving"* are among the glowing adjectives often used to describe coronary artery bypass surgery and balloon angioplasty. Repeatedly hailed as being among modern medicine's most wondrous achievements, the majority of us simply take for granted that these procedures have been documented to significantly extend the life expectancy of CHD patients. Of course, most of us have never examined the published results of randomized trials that tested these procedures...

Bypassing the Hype

Coronary bypass surgery involves sawing open the sternum and spreading the ribs apart so that a cardiac surgeon can access the heart. The surgeon then attaches a grafted section of vein or artery (usually taken from the chest or legs) to a blocked or narrowed coronary artery. The graft is attached above and below the blocked section of artery, creating a 'bypass' that will hopefully allow blood to flow freely to the heart. Several blockages can be bypassed during the procedure.

The first recorded bypass operation was performed by Dr. Rene Favoloro at the Cleveland Clinic in Ohio. Within a couple of years of Favoloro's landmark operation, the use of bypass surgery began to climb rapidly. By 1975, there were 60,000 bypass operations being performed annually in the United States; this figure rose to 230,000 by 1987. Currently, over 500,000 bypass surgeries are performed each year(1). Coronary bypass surgery is now the most commonly performed operation in the U.S., and an extremely lucrative endeavor for its practitioners. With the average procedure costing $61,000, coronary heart surgery is a $32 billion-a-year enterprise in the U.S. alone.

One of the most striking aspects of bypass surgery's rise to prominence was the fact that it occurred long before the procedure was subjected to the most fundamental of tests: the randomized, controlled clinical trial. New drugs are not allowed onto the market until their clinical efficacy and side effects have been examined in controlled trials. Bypass surgery quite literally hit the ground running, becoming a mainstay of coronary care despite not ever having been subject to controlled clinical investigation.

It was not until September of 1975 that the results of the first randomized trial of bypass surgery were published in the prestigious *New England Journal of Medicine*. A total of 596 patients from thirteen Veterans Administration hospitals had been entered into the study. Ninety-five percent of the patients had moderate or severe angina, and almost two-thirds had suffered a previous heart attack. Two groups were created, one of which was randomized to undergo bypass surgery. The other group was managed with standard non-surgical medical therapy, which involved the use of nitrates, beta-blockers, and antiarrhythmic medication.

The results were dismal. After three years, there was no difference in the survival rate of the two groups; eighty-seven percent of the medical group were still alive, compared to eighty eight percent of the surgical group(2).

For the first time, the 'lifesaving' work of bypass surgeons had been put to the test, and the disappointing results directly challenged the validity of the procedure upon which they had built their lucrative and esteemed careers. Not surprisingly, this group comprised the most vocal critics of the Veterans Administration trial.

Some complained that the trial did not extend long enough (wishful thinking as it turns out; a 22-year follow-up published in 1998 found that the survival rates were twenty-five percent and twenty percent in the medical and surgical groups, respectively(3)). Others complained that the trial patients were somehow atypical. The most prominent criticism was reserved for the seemingly high operative death rate; 5.6 percent of the surgical group died due to complications arising from the operation itself.

Defenders of bypass surgery clamored for a new trial, one involving the crème de la crème of bypass surgeons. They got their wish when the NHLBI sponsored the Coronary Artery Surgery Study (CASS), which recruited patients with coronary artery disease exhibiting either mild stable angina or who had no angina after suffering a heart attack. The medical centers involved in this new study included some of the most important names in the cardiology and heart surgery arena: Harvard, Yale, Stanford, Duke, the University of Washington, and the University of Alabama at Birmingham. Surely, such a trial, involving the best surgeons in the field, would return a lower operative mortality rate and demonstrate the true value of open-heart surgery.

When the eagerly awaited CASS results were finally published in 1984, they did indeed show a far lower operative mortality rate (1.4 percent) than that seen in the Veterans study. Nonetheless, this improvement still failed to impart any overall mortality advantage to the patients assigned to surgery. After six years, seventy-nine and eighty percent of the medical and surgical groups were alive and free of myocardial infarction, respectively(4). A further report published after ten years' follow-up also reported no difference in overall mortality or non-fatal heart attack between the two groups(5).

While the CASS trial was underway in the U.S., European researchers were conducting a randomized trial of their own. The European Coronary Surgery Study Group followed 768 men with mild to moderate angina and fifty percent or greater blockage of at least two major coronary arteries. Unlike the American studies, the European researchers observed a significant benefit from surgery at the five-year mark, with survival rates of ninety-two and eighty-three percent in the surgical and medical groups, respectively(6). During the subsequent seven years, however, the percentage of patients who survived decreased more rapidly in the surgically treated group than in the medically treated group (seventy-one versus sixty-seven percent alive after twelve years, respectively)(7).

All the aforementioned trials were instigated at least thirty years ago; one may wonder whether the passing of time has bought with it improved surgical techniques and accompanying increases in survival for bypass patients?

In 2004, the *Journal of the American College of Cardiology* presented the one-year results of MASS-II, a randomized trial that compared three different therapeutic strategies for stable angina patients with greater than seventy percent blockage of multiple coronary arteries. A total of 611 patients were assigned to bypass surgery, medical therapy, or angioplasty.

After twelve months, the survival rates were 98.5 percent for medical therapy patients, 96 percent for bypass patients, and 95.6 percent for those who underwent angioplasty(8). An earlier trial by the MASS investigators, involving 214 patients followed for an average of three years, observed no deaths in the medical therapy group but one death each in the bypass and angioplasty groups(9).

A similar study by Danish researchers compared an invasive strategy of either angioplasty or bypass surgery with that of conservative medical therapy in recent myocardial infarction patients. The 505 patients were followed up from one to 4.5 years. At a median 2.4 years' follow-up, the survival rate was 96.4 percent in the invasive treatment group and 95.6 percent in the conservative treatment group, a non-significant difference (the researchers did not report separate figures for bypass surgery and angioplasty). Invasive treatment was, however, associated with a significantly lower incidence of reinfarction (5.6 versus 10.5 percent)(10).

While the mortality benefit of bypass surgery is at best negligible, and in most instances non-existent, there do appear to be certain groups in whom the procedure may produce significant survival improvements. The Veterans

Administration and European Coronary Surgery studies, along with a number of non-randomized studies, found that patients with blockages of the left main artery--which is one of two major coronary arteries arising from the aorta-- enjoyed a markedly improved survival outlook(6,11). The European Coronary Surgery Study Group also found that survival was improved substantially in patients with blockages in three arteries (patients with two-vessel disease did not experience any improvement in mortality outcomes), severe exercise-induced ischemia (ST-segment depression of greater than 1.5mm), or with peripheral arterial disease. Ten years of follow-up in the CASS study found that bypass surgery also significantly improved the survival prospects of patients with left ventricular dysfunction(5).

For such high-risk categories, bypass surgery may indeed constitute a life-saving option. For most other stable coronary artery disease patients, there exists virtually no evidence to show that this procedure can in any way extend life span.

The Ballooning Popularity of Angioplasty

Angioplasty is considered a less invasive, traumatic and expensive procedure than bypass surgery. It involves steering a guide-wire with a small balloon attached into a section of coronary artery that has been narrowed by atherosclerotic plaque. The cardiologist places the balloon in the narrowed section of artery and then inflates it in an attempt to push the plaque aside and increase the size of the artery.

After the above procedure (known as balloon angioplasty) is completed, the cardiologist may also place a hollow metal mesh tube, called a 'stent', inside the artery. The idea is that the stent will hopefully prevent the artery from narrowing again. About seventy to ninety percent of angioplasties performed nowadays involve placement of a stent.

The first human coronary balloon angioplasty was performed in 1977, while stenting was introduced in 1987. Similar to bypass surgery, the use of angioplasty experienced explosive growth long before its efficacy was scrutinized in tightly controlled trials. The rapid growth of balloon angioplasty has even outpaced that of bypass surgery, with over 570,000 procedures performed in 2001 at an average cost of $29,000 each(1).

Balloon Angioplasty on Trial

Of the numerous trials conducted so far that have compared balloon angioplasty with standard medical therapy, none have showed any mortality benefit for patients receiving the former option(8-10,12-14). In fact, a collective analysis of all the angioplasty versus medical therapy trials reveals a trend towards higher mortality with the former!(15)

Why Bother?

While clinical trials have shown that coronary bypass surgery does not extend the lives of most of its recipients, they have consistently shown that surgery is far more likely to provide significant relief from angina symptoms than standard medical therapy. The same applies for balloon angioplasty. So while these procedures may not extend life, they will indeed improve the quality of life for many of their recipients.

Neither procedure is without its risks. With an average in-hospital mortality rate of 2.4 percent, over 12,000 of the bypass procedures performed in the U.S. each year will result in the death of the patient. Furthermore, approximately twelve percent of vein grafts fail within one year of surgery, with the failure rate climbing as high as forty-five percent twelve years after surgery(16-18). As such, many patients will undergo repeat surgery.

The current in-hospital mortality rate for patients undergoing angioplasty is 0.9 percent(1). Around 1.5 percent of all angioplasty patients require bypass surgery within twenty-four hours because of operative complications(19). During stent angioplasty--which now constitutes the majority of balloon angioplasty procedures--difficulties in placing the stent, severe coronary spasm or dislodging of the stent can cause complications requiring further surgery. Re-occlusion after balloon angioplasty occurs in thirty to sixty percent of cases(20).

Shunning Surgery

Obviously, any strategy that could significantly relieve angina pain without imparting the risk, expense, and highly invasive nature of bypass surgery and angioplasty would be eagerly welcomed by angina patients around the world. Well, there is such a strategy, one that is surprisingly simple, affordable and readily available.

It is called *exercise*.

In the March 2004 issue of *Circulation,* German researchers reported on a study in which 101 male patients with stable coronary artery disease were randomized to either undergo stent angioplasty or to participate in an exercise-training program. For the first two weeks, those in the exercise group trained in the hospital six times a day, ten minutes at a time, on a stationary bicycle at seventy percent of their symptom-limited heart rate (the symptom-limited heart is the heart rate at which evidence of ischemia becomes apparent during an exercise test; needless to say, this should be ascertained during a professionally supervised session).

After this initial two-week period, the exercising patients took their stationary bikes home with them. They were asked to cycle at the prescribed heart rate for twenty minutes per day, and to participate in one sixty-minute group aerobic exercise session each week.

The aim of the study was to see which strategy produced the most favorable effect on clinical outcomes--including heart attack, stroke, hospitalization for worsening angina, surgery or further angioplasty--during a twelve-month follow-up period. Thankfully, none of the patients died, but when the final data was tallied, it was observed that twenty-one of the fifty patients who underwent PCI had a subsequent coronary event, as compared to only six of the fifty-one exercising patients--a highly significant difference.

The exercisers also experienced far greater improvements in maximal exercise tolerance, and were thirty-two percent less likely to experience progression of atherosclerosis. Furthermore, the superior results seen in the exercise group were achieved at half the cost necessitated by the PCI procedure(21).

One need not be a rocket scientist to work out why exercise is superior to sticking metal tubes in one's arteries or unleashing a power saw on someone's sternum: neither bypass surgery nor stenting address the actual cause of coronary artery disease. Exercise, on the other hand, provides a stimulus for arterial remodeling. In the same way that pumping iron makes your muscles shapelier and stronger, exercise induces improvements in arterial function and structure.

The Gravy Train Continues Along its Merry Way...

Clearly, the benefits of bypass surgery and balloon angioplasty have been wildly overblown, and many patients have no business undergoing these procedures. Even a 1989 *Journal of the American Medical Association* article stated that forty-four percent of all bypass surgeries were of questionable necessity(22). Needless to say, their warning has done little to stop the runaway growth of bypass surgery and angioplasty. Not at all surprising when one considers the staggering amount of money and prestige attached to the performance of these procedures...

Appendix D

Testing Your CHD Risk

If cholesterol measurements provide little insight into one's true CHD risk, what medical tests can one use to attain a clearer picture of one's cardiovascular health? Table D1 lists a number of simple tests that measure markers of blood glucose metabolism, iron status, blood clotting tendency and inflammatory activity.

Please note that the list in Table A1 is not meant to be an exhaustive one; rather, it is a compilation of easily administered tests that can be ordered by a regular physician. If your doctor will not order the tests you are after, a non-profit organization known as the Life Extension Foundation can arrange blood tests at competitive rates for people just about anywhere in the U.S. Phone 1-800-544-4440, or visit their web site at http://www.lef.org/

Table D1: CHD risk testing

Test	Purpose	Relevance	Current normal range	Suggested range	Notes
Fasting Glucose	Measures glucose concentration in serum during fasted state	Elevated blood glucose, even at upper end of normal range, greatly increases CVD & all-cause mortality.	< 100 mg/dl	< 89 mg/dl.	Lowest all-cause mortality associated with fasting glucose range of 80-89 mg/dl (Chapter 18).
Fasting Insulin	Measures insulin concentration in serum during fasted state	Elevated insulin may increase risk of cardiovascular mortality via several mechanisms.	< 27 mcIU/mL	Under 5 mcIU/mL	
Hemoglobin A1c (HbA1c)	Measures serum concentrations of glycated, or glycosylated hemoglobin	Used as marker of blood glucose control during previous two to three months	4%-6%	< 5%	Recent study of >10,000 people found increasing mortality with rising HbA1c. HbA1c less than 5% conferred lowest CVD & mortality(1).
2-hour post-load glucose	Measures blood glucose levels for up to 2 hours after ingestion of glucose.	Can be used in conjunction with fasting glucose measurements to improve detection of impaired glycemic control	<140 mg/dl	Linear increase in CHD risk with increasing post-load glucose values.	In over 45s, 2-hour test may detect significant portion of individuals with impaired glycemic control who would otherwise be missed if relying on fasting blood glucose test only(2).
Serum ferritin	Measures iron content in blood. Accurate reflector of bodily iron stores.	High bodily iron stores may increase risk of CVD, diabetes, liver disease, and cancer.	15-300mcg/L	See notes	Ideal level unknown. Based on available research, levels below 55mcg/l may be optimal for reducing CVD and mortality (Chapter 22).
White blood cell count	Measures leukocyte (white blood cell) levels.	Leukocyte count is a marker for inflammation.	Between 4,300 and 10,800 cmm (4.3 - 10.8x109/L)	< 6,000 cmm (6.0x109/L)	Elevated WBC is a consistent, independent predictor of CVD events in those initially free of CHD & those with CHD. Leukocyte count test is common, inexpensive & reliable(4,5).
hsCRP	Used as marker of inflammatory activity.	Causal role for CRP in CHD yet to be established, but CRP serves as marker for inflammation. Higher CRP levels associated with increased CHD risk(3).	< 3.0mg/l	< 0.05mg/l	CRP levels may be temporarily elevated during acute illness & infection. When used in CHD risk assessment, CRP tests should be administered when one has recovered from the aforementioned conditions.
Fibrinogen	Measures fibrinogen concentration in serum	Fibrinogen is a protein that promotes blood clot formation.	200-400 mg/dl	200-300 mg/dl	
Homo-cysteine (HcY)	Measures serum levels of homocysteine	HcY is a potentially atherogenic amino acid.	<12 mmol/L	<9 mmol/L; available evidence suggests the lower the better.	See Appendix E for discussion of homocysteine.

Appendix E

What About Homocysteine?

It was in 1968, a full seven years after the American Heart Association officially embraced the lipid hypothesis, that a Harvard-trained researcher by the name of Kilmer McCully began investigating a substance known as *homocysteine.* McCully's interest in this little-known compound arose after he became aware of two very unusual case studies in the medical literature. The unfortunate young subjects of these reports died from a rare genetic disorder known as *homocysteinuria,* a condition characterized by abnormally high levels of homocysteine in the blood and urine.

What struck McCully about these two case reports was that both patients--the first aged eight and the second only two months old--were found to have extensive atherosclerosis at autopsy. The eight-year old victim had died because the arteries to his brain were narrowed and blocked by a blood clot, causing a stroke. McCully wondered whether homocysteine was causing cardiovascular disease in people with less pronounced elevations of homocysteine, by directly damaging the cells and tissues of the arteries. After unearthing animal studies that showed that deficiencies of vitamins B6, B12 and folic acid caused arterial disease, McCully could barely contain himself-- these vitamins, after all, were involved in keeping homocysteine levels under control!

The excited researcher, suspecting he was onto something momentous, started conducting his own homocysteine experiments. He started to paint an increasingly detailed picture of just how homocysteine might promote atherosclerosis, and in the early seventies he began publishing his findings in the medical literature.

You and I might regard pioneering scientists like Kilmer McCully--whose landmark findings hold the potential to save millions of lives--as heroic. Orthodoxy, however, regards such researchers as a menace. McCully's theory completely contradicted the reigning cholesterol theory, the very theory that the medical hierarchy had already hailed as the official explanation for heart disease. McCully's research, in effect, posed a direct threat to the many lucrative careers that had been built on the back of the lipid hypothesis.

Back in 1970, McCully's research on homocysteine and artery disease had been praised by a special Scientific Advisory Committee at his place of employ, Harvard's Massachusetts General Hospital. By 1977, McCully's laboratory at the same institution had been taken away, and he lost staff support for his research. McCully was told shortly after this that his position would not be renewed in 1979. He was further informed that, unless he was unable to obtain another NIH grant, his salary would be cut to almost nothing by January 1978. Obtaining grant support with no lab and no position was virtually impossible, and after McCully's requests for more time were denied by top officials at Harvard and Mass General, the highly decorated researcher was left jobless.

During the next two years, McCully--with his Harvard degrees and fourteen years' professorship at the same hallowed institution--was turned down by over fifty potential employers across the country. He was repeatedly told to abandon his research and to accept a lower-level position as a pathologist. When he began to hear rumors of defamatory phone calls emanating from Harvard, portraying his habits and character in a very unflattering light, McCully decided enough was enough. He enlisted a prominent Boston lawyer to represent him in a case against his former employers at Harvard and Mass General. It was only after taking this step that he finally received a job offer, albeit at a far less prestigious institution, the V.A. Hospital in Providence, Rhode Island (1).

Why All the Fuss?

Homocysteine is formed when the body converts an amino acid called methionine, which we obtain from our diet via protein-containing foods, into another amino acid known as cysteine. Once synthesized, homocysteine itself is usually converted back to either cysteine or methionine. This recycling of homocysteine is made possible by two processes: *re-methylation* or *trans-sulphuration*. The former requires vitamin B12 and folic acid to take place, while the latter requires vitamin B6.

The cysteine that is produced as a result of trans-sulphuration is used to create glutathione, one of the body's most important antioxidants. In fact, the synthesis of glutathione is dependent on the trans-sulphuration of homocysteine. A failure to efficiently convert homocysteine into cysteine, due to a lack of vitamins B6, B12 and/or folic acid, may result in sub-optimal levels of glutathione. This in turn, will leave our organs and tissues--including those of the cardiovascular system--increasingly susceptible to free radical attack. This contention is supported by research showing marked increases in free radical activity in individuals whose blood homocysteine levels rose after ingesting a large dose of methionine(2).

In addition to stimulating free radical damage, homocysteine itself may be directly toxic to arteries. In laboratory and animal experiments, homocysteine promotes blood clotting, inflammation, impaired arterial function and accelerated formation of atherosclerotic lesions(3).

In individuals with inherited defects in homocysteine metabolism, blood concentrations of this amino acid can skyrocket, reaching levels of up to 400 mmol/L---way higher than the typical range of 5-15 mmol/L! Not insignificantly, these individuals suffer a far greater prevalence of premature CHD than normal folks(4).

Epidemiological evidence shows that it is not just those with off-the-chart homocysteine readings that are at higher risk of CHD. Even within the normal range, CHD risk rises in step with increasing homocysteine concentrations; individuals at the upper end of the normal range are at much greater risk of experiencing CHD or stroke than those at the lower end(5). Numerous studies have also found that homocysteine concentrations increase as blood levels of folic acid and vitamins B6 and B12 decrease(6,7).

The first large-scale prospective study on the homocysteine-CHD relationship involved almost 15,000 male physicians aged forty to eighty-four, with no prior history of CHD or stroke, who provided blood samples at the study's commencement. After five years, the blood samples of the men who had suffered a heart attack during the study were thawed out and each compared to a control sample from a participant who had not experienced a coronary event. Compared to the men with the lowest homocysteine concentrations, those with the highest levels had a 3.5-fold increased risk of experiencing a non-fatal or fatal heart attack(8). A subsequent twenty-four-year follow-up study of over 1,300 Swedish women with no previous history of heart attack, found a five-fold greater risk of fatal heart attack among those in the upper fifth of homocysteine levels, compared to those in the lowest fifth(9).

By now readers are no doubt asking if elevated homocysteine directly promotes CHD, or, similar to cholesterol, is simply guilty by association. The evidence so far tentatively supports the former proposition. So far, only a handful of clinical trials have examined the effects of homocysteine-lowering therapies in cardiovascular disease. These trials involved patients with pre-existing CHD or stroke, or individuals with end-stage kidney disease, a group that is at high risk of cardiovascular disease. Most of these studies used only folic acid, which by itself did not produce any significant difference in non-fatal or fatal outcomes in the short trial periods involved (one to two years)(10-12).

As of this writing, the results of three studies that examined the effect of folic acid *and* vitamins B6 and B12 have been reported. The first of these was a one-year, double-blind, placebo-controlled Swiss trial, which found a significant reduction in recurrent cardiovascular events among coronary angioplasty patients who were randomized to receive these vitamins. Only 15.4 percent of patients receiving the three B-vitamins died, had a non-fatal heart attack, or required a repeat angioplasty procedure, compared to 22.8 percent of those receiving placebo(13).

However, the more recent and much larger Norwegian Vitamin Trial (NORVIT), involving 3,749 patients and spanning 3.5 years, found no beneficial effect of B-vitamins upon CVD outcomes. In fact, a group receiving a folic-acid/vitamin-B6 combination reportedly experienced a slight increase in heart attack, stroke, cancer and overall mortality compared to those receiving folic-acid-only, vitamin-B6 only, or placebo. This disappointing outcome was not due to a lack of homocysteine reduction; the combination of vitamin B6 and folic acid, as well as folic acid alone, effectively lowered homocysteine levels by twenty-eight percent(14).

The NORVIT results have been reported in the popular media, but, as of this book's first publication, have not yet been peer-reviewed and presented in the scientific literature; until the full report is available, it's hard to make any intelligent commentary on the conduct and outcome of this trial. Until further light is shed on the worrying results of the NORVIT trial, high dosages of isolated B-vitamins may be best avoided. A daily multi-vitamin/mineral formulation with high potencies of the entire B-complex may be a much wiser option (see Chapter 27).

The Vitamin Intervention for Stroke Prevention (VISP) trial aimed to determine whether daily treatment with high-dose folate (25 mg) B6 (25mg) and B12 (400 mcg) would significantly reduce stroke and the combined end point of stroke, death, and myocardial infarction compared with lower doses of the same vitamin trio (20 mcg folate, 200 mcg B6, 6 mcg B12). The difference in outcomes between the two groups were so small that the study was stopped prematurely because of futility(15).

Reflecting on these disappointing results, the VISP researchers decided to take a closer look at several factors that may have affected their results and camouflaged any positive effect of high-dose B-vitamin therapy. They pinpointed several factors, including folate fortification of grain products, which began in the U.S. in 1998, the same year the VISP trial began; inclusion of the recommended daily intake for B12 in the low-dose group; treatment with injectable B12 in patients with low serum B12 levels in both study groups; a dose of B12 too low for patients suffering B12 malabsorption; supplementation with non-study vitamins; and the inclusion of patients with significant renal impairment, who tend to respond poorly to vitamin therapy. The authors decided to reanalyze their data, this time excluding subjects who fell into most of the above categories. Among the remaining 2,155 patients, thirty-seven percent of whom were female, there was a twenty-one percent risk reduction in the combined end point of ischemic stroke, coronary disease, or death in the high-dose group compared with the low-dose group. This was despite a significantly greater percentage of smokers in the high-dose vitamin group.

Patients with above average baseline B12 status randomized to high-dose vitamin had the best overall outcome, and those with blood B12 levels less than the median assigned to low-dose B-vitamins had the worst outcome. The authors emphasized that some elderly patients may need 1000mcg of B12, instead of the more commonly studied 400mcg dose, to achieve optimal blood levels of this vitamin. The authors also found no significant relationship between the magnitude of reduction of homocysteine between baseline and one month and subsequent cardiovascular events, suggesting that high-dose B-vitamin supplementation exerts positive cardiovascular effects independent of homocysteine lowering (more on this later)(16).

The only thing certain at present about homocysteine is that its exact role in the initiation and progression of cardiovascular disease is still uncertain. Perhaps the inconsistent and less-than-striking results obtained with B-vitamin therapy in trials of patients with established cardiovascular disease are examples of the *"too little, too late"* phenomenon. Is it possible that optimal B-vitamin intakes from an earlier age would provide greater reductions in CHD? Or perhaps greater dosages of these vitamins may provide greater benefits, a possibility supported by the finding that 1000mcg of B12 is the minimum amount required by many older folks to achieve satisfactory blood B12 levels?

Animal studies lend support to the contention that homocysteine is directly involved in the instigation and progression of CHD. Atherosclerosis-prone strains of mice develop larger and more numerous atherosclerotic plaques when fed diets that induce high blood homocysteine levels. So too do mice bred to display defects in homocysteine metabolism(17,18).

While science is yet to paint the full picture, the available evidence strongly suggests that lowering elevated homocysteine levels is a worthwhile CHD-prevention measure. Reducing homocysteine levels requires no expensive or potentially toxic drugs, nor does it necessitate any bizarre dietary changes; both B-vitamin supplementation and increased fruit and vegetable consumption have been repeatedly demonstrated to lower homocysteine levels.

What is an effective dose of homocysteine-lowering B-vitamins? Well, in the successful Swiss intervention trial discussed earlier, researchers used a daily dose of one milligram (1000 micrograms) of folic acid, four hundred micrograms of vitamin B12, and ten milligrams of vitamin B6. Dutch researchers examined the effect of the same vitamins in individuals with homocysteine levels above 16 mmol/L, and found that a combination of five milligrams of folic acid, four hundred micrograms of B12, and fifty mg of B6, reduced homocysteine levels to 16 mmol/L or under in twenty-six of thirty individuals, compared with only seven of thirty receiving a placebo. In subjects whose levels were already under 16 mmol/L, vitamin supplementation reduced homocysteine levels by an average of thirty percent!(19)

In a study with patients on a waiting list for coronary intervention, four hundred micrograms of folic acid, two milligrams of vitamin B6, and six micrograms of vitamin B12 more than halved homocysteine levels, which dropped from an average of 23.4 to 11.3 mmol/l. In addition, certain measures of arterial function showed marked improvement in the vitamin-treated group, as did their cardiac response to exercise testing. In contrast, another group of patients receiving a placebo did not experience any such positive changes(20).

High doses of the nutrient *betaine* can help lower elevated homocysteine levels even in patients unresponsive to vitamin B6 therapy(21). Effective dosages are three to six grams as *betaine glycine*, also known as trimethylglycine (TMG).

Dietary changes can also lower homocysteine levels. Don't worry about cutting dietary methionine; while multi-gram dosages of isolated methionine supplements raise homocysteine levels in humans, controlled research shows dietary methionine to have no such effect(22). In fact, the best way to increase one's dietary intake of B6 and B12 is to eat methionine-rich protein foods like meat! Animal foods are the only source of bioavailable B12; compared to meat-eating omnivores, vegetarians consistently exhibit higher blood levels of homocysteine, with the highest concentrations found in vegans (those who shun all animal products, including eggs and dairy)(23-25). A 6-month randomized, controlled clinical trial found that those assigned to a high protein diet experienced a twenty-one percent drop in homocysteine levels, but no decrease was observed among those assigned to a low protein diet or control subjects following their usual diet(26).

In addition to being a good source of B6 and B12, organ meats (but not muscle meat) are also a good source of folate, along with fruits and vegetables. Intervention trials in which subjects increased their fruit and vegetable intake have repeatedly shown homocysteine reductions, albeit of a smaller magnitude than B-vitamin supplementation(27,28). In subjects normally consuming 162 grams of fruits and vegetables each day, four weeks of eating 500 grams daily of these folate-rich foods lowered homocysteine levels by eleven percent.

Beyond Homocysteine

The benefits of plentiful B-vitamin intake do not stop at homocysteine reduction. Research indicates that B6 may reduce blood clotting, and that even mildly deficient levels of this vitamin may impair the activity of *lysyl oxidase*, an enzyme important for healthy connective tissue formation(29,30). Researchers have also linked lowered blood levels of vitamin B6 with increased blood levels of fibrinogen and C-reactive protein (indicating increased clotting and inflammatory activity), independent of homocysteine levels(31,32).

To lower homocysteine and maintain optimal B-vitamin status:

- Take your vitamins--in the form of a daily multi with high potencies of the B-complex. If high homocysteine levels persist in spite of high-dose B-vitamin use, consider supplementation with three to six grams of betaine glycine.
- Aim to eat around 400-500 grams of vegetables and fruits each day;
- Do as the cavemen did by regularly enjoying vitamin B6-, B12-, and folic acid-rich meats.

Appendix F

Copper Deficiency versus Copper Overload

Dietary surveys indicate that copper intake from food in the U.S. is relatively low (average copper intake is 1.4 milligrams and 1.1 milligrams per day for males and females, respectively(1)), and animal and human experiments indicate that sub-optimal intakes of this mineral can promote cardiovascular disease(2-17). However, food is only one of many avenues by which humans can ingest copper; some other common sources include water that is rich in copper (due to naturally high copper levels and/or copper plumbing), copper intra-uterine devices, copper-containing dental fillings, and exposure to copper-containing pesticides. Birth control pills, estrogen replacement therapy, low protein diets, beer drinking, and a low zinc intake may also increase bodily stores of copper. As such, many individuals may need to be more concerned about getting too much copper than not getting enough.

A study involving healthy men whose diets were supplemented with seven milligrams of copper per day for five months detected changes suggestive of increased inflammation and free radical activity. Compared to control subjects, the copper-supplemented subjects also showed reduced antibody responses after immunization with influenza vaccines, indicating impaired immune function(18). Nutritionist Ann Louise Gittleman has extensively studied the phenomenon of copper overload, after discovering that high bodily stores of copper explained both her own and many of her clients' persistent tiredness.

When it comes to copper, the most prudent course of action may be the consumption of filtered, copper-free water and avoidance of copper-containing supplements. Individuals who follow the dietary guidelines recommended in Chapter 26 should have little trouble with copper deficiency, especially if they regularly consume foods like nuts, seafood or liver. For more information on the subject of copper overload, I would highly recommend Gittleman's book *Why Am I Always So Tired?* (HarperSanFrancisco).

Appendix G

Is Vitamin E a Heart-Saver?

In 1996, British researchers published the results of the 1.4-year double-blind Cambridge Heart Antioxidant Study (CHAOS), which showed a whopping seventy-seven percent reduction of non-fatal heart attacks in those randomized to take 400-800 international units (IU) of vitamin E daily. Before you drop this book and sprint frantically to the nearest health food store, be aware that this decrease in non-fatal events was accompanied by a slight increase of fatal cardiovascular deaths. When the overall death figures were tallied up, they showed that 3.5 percent of the vitamin E users had died from cardiovascular causes, compared to 2.7 percent of the placebo subjects. However, when one compares the mortality rate according to the vitamin E dosage, one learns that those taking 400 IU daily enjoyed fifteen percent lower cardiovascular mortality, while those taking 800 IU suffered a twenty-nine percent increase, as compared to the placebo group(1).

The question that begs to be asked, of course, is: If the low dose lowered mortality, why did the higher dose increase it?

While vitamin E is famous for its antioxidant actions, laboratory studies have shown that, at high doses, it may have pro-oxidant effects(2,3). High doses of vitamin E may displace other fat-soluble antioxidants, such as gamma-tocopherol (see below), and may possibly inhibit glutathione S-transferase, a family of enzymes exerting an important role in the detoxification of drugs, carcinogens and products of free radical damage(4,5). So while moderate amounts of supplemental vitamin E may be beneficial, larger amounts (over 400 IU) may cause harm by disrupting the body's natural antioxidant balance.

The huge Italian GISSI trial, which found significant mortality benefits for fish oil in CHD patients, also recorded a twenty percent risk reduction in cardiovascular deaths among those taking 300 IU of vitamin E daily(6).

In the Women's Health Study, women assigned to take 600 IU of vitamin E every other day for ten years experienced a twenty-four percent reduction in cardiovascular mortality, but no reduction in the incidence of heart attack or overall mortality(7).

These observed mortality reductions with vitamin E supplements have not been replicated by other researchers; several other controlled trials, up to 6.3 years in length and using daily vitamin E dosages from fifty to 600 IU, have failed to produce any reduction in cardiovascular or all-cause mortality(8).

The fleeting nature of positive trial results seen with vitamin E may be due in no small part to the type of vitamin E employed. All of the aforementioned clinical studies used *alpha-tocopherol*, which is only one of the numerous tocopherols and tocotrienols that make up vitamin E in real foods. Alpha-tocopherol is also the vitamin E isomer used in the overwhelming majority of commercially available supplements.

Laboratory and animal research suggests that more consistent and robust reductions in cardiovascular disease could be achieved if other forms of vitamin E were employed. An important vitamin E isomer known as *gamma-tocopherol* has been shown to inhibit the formation of proinflammatory eicosanoids and subsequent inflammation-induced damage in rats. This beneficial effect was not seen in rats given alpha-tocopherol(9). Other rodent studies have shown both alpha- and gamma-tocopherol to decrease blood clot formation, inhibit the generation of free radicals, and to reduce LDL oxidation. Gamma-tocopherol, however, was significantly more potent than alpha-tocopherol in exerting these effects(10). Laboratory researchers recently observed that a mixed-tocopherol preparation (containing gamma-, delta-, and alpha-tocopherol) was far more effective in protecting red blood cell lipids from oxidative damage than alpha-tocopherol alone(11).

In humans, researchers have reported that blood levels of gamma-tocopherol, but not alpha-tocopherol, were reduced in CHD patients(12,13). Seven years' follow-up of over 34,000 postmenopausal women found that the intake of dietary vitamin E, which contains a significant portion of gamma-tocopherol, but not supplements, which consist predominantly of alpha-tocopherol, was inversely correlated with CHD death. Those with the highest dietary intake of vitamin E enjoyed a sixty-two percent reduction in CHD mortality risk, a figure that intervention trial participants receiving alpha-tocopherol could only dream of(14).

In an experimental study, researchers randomly assigned subjects to one of three groups--alpha-tocopherol, mixed tocopherols, or a control group--and proceeded to administer compounds that encouraged blood platelet aggregation. In the mixed tocopherol group, platelet aggregation decreased significantly, but no such benefit was noted in the alpha-tocopherol and control groups(15). In kidney dialysis patients, fourteen-days' supplementation with gamma-enriched tocopherols significantly lowered blood C-reactive protein levels, an indicator of inflammatory activity in the body. An alpha-tocopherol-enriched mixture did not achieve the same benefit(16).

In addition, a number of trials have shown that alpha-tocopherol supplements produce marked reductions in blood gamma-tocopherol concentrations, a finding with potentially ominous long-term implications(17-21).

Anyone taking vitamin E supplements would be wise to include a mixed tocopherol and tocotrienol formula, or to emphasize gamma-tocopherol-rich foods. By far and away, the best dietary sources of gamma-tocopherol are sesame seeds, pecans, walnuts, pistachios and pumpkin seeds, while pine nuts, brazils, and cashews also contain relatively high amounts.

Sesame seeds, in particular, are especially effective for raising blood levels of gamma-tocopherol, and they may also exert another highly beneficial action-- the achievement of a more favorable omega-6:omega-3 ratio. When rats were fed omega-6-rich oils, those given phytochemicals from sesame seeds known as *lignans* showed higher levels of omega-3 and lower levels of omega-6 fats in their livers than those not receiving sesame lignans(22-24).

Based on the results of research conducted thus far, the use of alpha-tocopherol supplements in amounts over 400 IU per day may be best avoided.

Appendix H

Familial Hypercholesterolemia: No Indictment of Cholesterol

Familial hypercholesterolemia (FH) is a rare genetic aberration that occurs with a frequency of approximately one in 500 people. FH individuals lack the receptors necessary for removing cholesterol from the bloodstream and therefore exhibit much higher blood cholesterol concentrations than average. Some studies have reported a higher incidence of heart disease among FH individuals, a finding triumphantly cited as 'proof' of the atherogenicity of cholesterol. Like every other argument used in support of the lipid hypothesis, the FH dogma quickly loses credibility when examined closely.

FH: Exaggerated Risk?

During the period 1980-1989, the UK's Scientific Steering Committee followed 282 men and 244 women aged 20-74 with FH. The mortality rate in this group was compared with that of the general population in England and Wales. During the follow-up period, twenty-four of the subjects died; fifteen of these deaths were due to coronary heart disease, almost four times the number expected from an identically sized sample in the general population. But the increased CHD mortality was not uniform among all age groups; most of the increased risk was borne by FH patients aged 20-39 years. Those aged 30-49 also had a significantly higher death rate than average. The 60-74 age category, however, suffered no excess mortality. In fact, they enjoyed a fifty-six percent relative risk reduction in coronary death and a thirty-one percent reduction in overall mortality(1).

If elevated cholesterol caused heart disease, then an increased risk should have been evident across all age groups in FH individuals. But it wasn't; the lack of association between FH and CHD in those over 60 mirrored the lack of association between cholesterol and CHD seen in older members of the general population.

Furthermore, the subjects in the Steering Committee study were not a random selection of healthy FH individuals. Many were recruited for the study after screening instigated by personal or family histories of heart disease revealed their FH status. In the general population, many FH individuals remain healthy and therefore unrecognized. The CHD risk observed among the FH subjects in the UK study, therefore, may have been largely due to the increased risk that accompanies a family and/or personal history of CHD. Supporting this possibility is the fact that younger members of the study, who suffered the highest death rates, were more likely to have a family history of heart disease.

Nonetheless, the increased risk among FH individuals was so high that family history alone was unlikely to fully explain the extra deaths. It appears that the younger FH subjects suffered a heightened vulnerability to environmental factor/s that encouraged the onset of coronary heart disease.

The potential role of environmental factors is further underscored by the findings of Dutch researchers, who took three FH individuals and traced their family tree right back to a single pair of ancestors in the 19th century. The researchers traced a total of 412 descendants spanning eight generations. Between 1830-1989 there were sixty deaths among those with a 100 percent probability of carrying the FH mutation. In the period 1830-1869 those with definite FH were less than half as likely to die as the general population. Their death rate rose to 2.3 times that of the general population between 1935-1964, before declining to 1.8 times the average rate in the period 1965-1989.

The mortality rate among descendants of one of the screened FH individuals was virtually identical to the national average. The death rate among ancestors of the second screenee was 1.7 times that of the first, while the death rate among ancestors of the third screenee—whose FH status was revealed after suffering a heart attack at the age of 51—was 3.3 times higher. Summarizing their findings the researchers wrote: *"In the 19th century, mortality seemed lower than in the general population. It rose after 1915, reached a maximum during the 1950s, and decreased thereafter. During the decades with excess mortality, survival in the branches of the pedigree differed significantly, ranging from normal life expectancy to severe excess mortality. This large variation of risk suggests that previous studies, with families based on selected patients, may have overestimated mortality. Moreover, such large variation in mortality in two directions (over time and within generations) in a pedigree indicates that the disorder has strong interactions with environmental factors."*(2) That researchers from Utah and Finland also found FH compatible with normal life span in earlier generations living under different environmental conditions suggests that environmental factors play a pivotal role in determining any excess mortality risk in FH individuals(3,4).

During the last century, several environmental factors that increase heart disease risk have become far more widespread, including (but not limited to) physical inactivity, psychosocial stress, consumption of refined polyunsaturate-rich vegetable oils, trans fat-laden margarines, refined carbohydrates, and nutrient-depleted packaged foods.

Irrelevant Extrapolation

In most people, LDL receptors assist in removing cholesterol from the bloodstream into cells where it is needed. In people with familial hypercholesterolemia, the absence of these receptors allows blood cholesterol levels to reach levels far higher than normal. Similar to what is seen in experiments with herbivorous animals fed cholesterol-raising diets, familial hypercholesterolemics often develop cholesterol deposits in areas far away from the coronary arteries, including the eyes and tendons of the feet and hands. In herbivorous animals and familial hypercholesterolemics, simple blood cholesterol elevations can indeed result in 'fatty deposits' (more correctly referred to as *xanthomas*) throughout the circulatory system. But in non-FH humans, who comprise 99.8 percent of the population, this is not the case; instead of merely being crystallized cholesterol deposits like the xanthomas of FH patients, atherosclerotic plaques are often complex mixtures of white blood cells, smooth muscle tissue, calcium, connective tissue, fatty acids, and cholesterol. And in the general population, advanced atherosclerosis has been observed in patients with very low cholesterol levels, as low as 111 mg/dl (see Chapter 4).

As explained in Chapter 13, the traditional theory that blood cholesterol and fats clog our arteries like mud inside a pipe is useless as an explanation for the vast majority of human coronary disease. The use of FH, a rare genetic anomaly found in 0.2 percent of the population, as support for this simplistic paradigm is equally disingenuous.

To Treat or Not to Treat

Due to their very high cholesterol levels, people with FH tend to be the subject of inordinate pressure from doctors to begin lipid-lowering therapy. The belief that FH individuals will benefit greatly from aggressive cholesterol reduction is an ingrained tenet of modern medical practice.

A recent review in *Expert Opinion on Drug Safety* articulates the current drug-centric view of modern medicine towards FH individuals: *"Life expectancy of FH patients is reduced by 15 - 30 years unless they are adequately treated with lipid-lowering therapy. Patients with this disorder need long-term drug therapy..."*(5).

A 1993 article published in the *American Journal of Cardiology* claimed that: *"...20 mg of lovastatin per day is estimated to save lives and save money in all men ages 35-44 years with hFH and in women ages 35-44 years with hFH and any other risk factor."*(6) This "estimate" is not based on factual clinical trial data, as lovastatin has *never* been shown to save lives, be it in FH or normal individuals. The only long-term studies examining the effect of lovastatin have shown either unchanged or increased mortality (see Table 23a, Chapter 23).

In fact, no cholesterol-lowering drug has ever been shown to lower mortality in FH individuals. While the literature is replete with statin studies showing significant cholesterol reductions in FH subjects, virtually all long-term trials that actually examined mortality have excluded FH individuals. Therefore, the claim that these individuals will experience mortality benefits from cholesterol-lowering drug therapy is currently based, not on clinical evidence, but on wishful thinking.

Shunning Drugs, Embracing Health

Sydney businessman Frank Cooper is a familial hypercholesterolemic who has authored a book titled *Cholesterol and the French Paradox*. When blood work at the age of twenty-nine revealed a cholesterol reading of 510 mg/dl, Cooper's doctor immediately recommended lipid-lowering drugs and told him he had a *"50/50 chance"* of surviving to fifty without them.

Cooper was prescribed clofibrate but *"after a month of not feeling myself"* he stopped the drug. Still worried about his high cholesterol and wondering whether he should resume clofibrate, Cooper began researching. After learning of the serious side effect profile and the poor mortality record of clofibrate, Cooper had little trouble deciding clofibrate would not be a part of his future. Over the ensuing years, Cooper experimented with nicotinic acid, cholestyramine, and various statin drugs. He abandoned every one of these cholesterol-lowering agents within a short period of time due to side effects. Cooper is hardly the only FH patient to experience side effects from cholesterol-lowering treatments; a study of twenty-two professional athletes with FH found that only six could tolerate statin drugs. The remaining sixteen had to discontinue the drugs due to side effects(7).

During his studies, Cooper became particularly fascinated by the research dealing with the French and their very low rate of heart disease. Here was a population with a high saturated fat intake and average cholesterol levels similar to those in the UK and USA, but with only one-third of the heart disease mortality rate. Cooper discovered that while cholesterol levels were similar between these nations, the French ate far more fresh vegetables, had a higher intake of antioxidants, but ate less sugars and far less polyunsaturated vegetable oils than the residents of the US and UK. In 1997, Cooper decided to eschew drugs completely and resolved to base his CHD-prevention strategy on healthy eating and living, instead of toxic drugs. It is a decision he has never regretted. His cholesterol level has stabilized at 387 mg/dl, and Cooper recently passed the age of fifty with no hint of heart disease, nor any other health problems. In fact, when Cooper recently underwent a CT scan of his arteries, it revealed a low level of calcification in his blood vessels. Cooper derives further affirmation of his decision from the fact that his mother lived an active life until 85, despite also having FH and a cholesterol level of 348 mg/dl(8).

References

Chapter 1

1. American Heart Association, Inc. Financial Statements, June 30, 2005. Available online: http://www.americanheart.org/downloadable/heartsmart/1132768869358American%20Heart%20Association%20-%206-30-2005%20Final.pdf (accessed November 26, 2005).
2. Index of Non-Profit Organizations Receiving Corporate Funding. Center for Science in the Public Interest Integrity in Science web site. Available online: http://www.cspinet.org/integrity/nonprofits/american_heart_association.html (accessed June 8, 2004).
3. American Heart Association, Statement 19 for fiscal year 2005, Form 990, p. 4, Pt. 5.
4. Herrick JB. Clinical features of sudden obstruction of the coronary arteries. *Journal of the American Medical Association*, 1912; 59: 2015-2020.
5. Harper AE. Coronary heart disease - an epidemic related to diet? *American Journal of Clinical Nutrition*, 1983; 37: 669-681.
6. Stallones RA. The rise and fall of ischemic heart disease. *Scientific American*, Nov, 1980; 243 (5): 43-49.
7. Rosamond WD, et al. Trends in the Incidence of Myocardial Infarction and in Mortality Due to Coronary Heart Disease, 1987 to 1994. *New England Journal of Medicine*, Sep 24, 1998; 339 (13): 861-867.
8. Center for Disease Control. Hospitalization Rates for Ischemic Heart Disease - United States, 1970-1986. *MMWR Weekly*, Apr 28, 1989; 38 (16); 275-276, 281-284.
9. Lampe FC, et al. Trends in rates of different forms of diagnosed coronary heart disease, 1978 to 2000: prospective, population based study of British men. *British Medical Journal*, May 7, 2005; 330: 1046.
10. Sytkowski PA, et al. Changes in risk factors and the decline in mortality from cardiovascular disease. The Framingham Study. *New England Journal of Medicine*, Jun 7, 1990; 322 (23): 1635-1641.
11. McGovern PG, et al. Trends in acute coronary heart disease mortality, morbidity, and medical care from 1985 through 1997: The Minnesota Heart Survey. *Circulation*, Jul, 2001; 104: 19-24.
12. Hayashi T, et al. Recent decline in hospital mortality among patients with acute myocardial infarction. *Circulation Journal*, 2005; 69 (4): 420-426.
13. Gottlieb S, et al. Mortality trends in men and women with acute myocardial infarction in coronary care units in Israel. A comparison between 1981–1983 and 1992–1994. *European Heart Journal*, 2000 21: 284-295.
14. Rea TD, et al. Temporal patterns in long-term survival after resuscitation from out-of-hospital cardiac arrest. *Circulation*, Sept 9, 2003; 108 (10): 1196-1201.
15. Bishop JE. Deaths from heart disease are occurring later in life. *Wall Street Journal*, Nov. 13, 1996.
16. Weiss W. Cigarette smoking and lung cancer trends: A light at the end of the tunnel? *Chest*, 1997; 111: 1414-1416.
17. USDA U.S. Food Supply database. Available online: http://www.cnpp.usda.gov/nutrient_content.html (accessed September 8, 2005).
18. Antar MA, et al. Changes in retail market food supplies in the United States in the last seventy years in relation to the incidence of coronary heart disease, with special reference to dietary carbohydrates and essential fatty acids. *American Journal of Clinical Nutrition*, Mar, 1964; 14: 169-178.

Chapter 2

1. Mensink RF, Katan MB. Effect of dietary fatty acids on serum lipids and lipoproteins: A meta-analysis of 27 trials. *Arteriosclerosis and Thrombosis*, 1992; Vol. 12: 911-919.

2. Nelson GJ, et al. Low-fat diets do not lower plasma cholesterol levels in healthy men compared to high-fat diets with similar fatty acid composition at constant caloric intake. *Lipids,* Nov, 1995; 30 (11): 969-976.

3. Yudkin J. Diet and coronary thrombosis. Hypothesis and fact. *Lancet,* July 27, 1957; II: 155-162.

4. Kannel WB, et al. Cholesterol in the prediction of atherosclerotic disease. New perspectives based on the Framingham Study. *Annals of Internal Medicine,* 1979; 90: 85-91.

5. Anderson KM, et al. Cholesterol and mortality. 30 years of follow-up from the Framingham study. *Journal of the American Medical Association,* 1987; 257: 2176–2180.

6. Scientific steering committee on behalf of the Simon Broome Register group. Risk of fatal coronary heart disease in familial hypercholesterolaemia. *British Medical Journal,* 1991; 303: 893–896.

7. Forette F, et al. The prognostic significance of isolated systolic hypertension in the elderly. Results of a ten year longitudinal survey. *Clinical and Experimental Hypertension. Part A, Theory and Practice,* 1982; 4: 1177–1191.

8. Siegel D, et al. Predictors of cardiovascular events and mortality in the Systolic Hypertension in the Elderly Program pilot project. *American Journal of Epidemiology,* 1987; 126: 385–389.

9. Nissinen A, et al. Risk factors for cardiovascular disease among 55 to 74 year-old Finnish men: a 10-year follow-up. *Annals of Medicine,* 1989; 21: 239–240.

10. Krumholz HM, et al. Lack of association between cholesterol and coronary heart disease mortality and morbidity and all-cause mortality in persons older than 70 years. *Journal of the American Medical Association,* 1994; 272: 1335–1340.

11. Weijenberg MP, et al. Serum total cholesterol and systolic blood pressure as risk factors for mortality from ischemic heart disease among elderly men and women. *Journal of Clinical Epidemiology,* 1994; 47: 197–205.

12. Simons LA, et al. Diabetes, mortality and coronary heart disease in the prospective Dubbo study of Australian elderly. *Australian and New Zealand Journal of Medicine,* 1996; 26:66–74.

13. Weijenberg MP, et al. Total and high density lipoprotein cholesterol as risk factors for coronary heart disease in elderly men during 5 years of follow-up. The Zutphen Elderly Study. *American Journal of Epidemiology,* 1996; 143: 151–158.

14. Simons LA, et al. Cholesterol and other lipids predict coronary heart disease and ischaemic stroke in the elderly, but only in those below 70 years. *Atherosclerosis,* 2001; 159: 201–208.

15. Abbott RD, et al. Age-related changes in risk factor effects on the incidence of coronary heart disease. *Annals of Epidemiology,* 2002; 12: 173–181.

16. Zimetbaum P, et al. Plasma lipids and lipoproteins and the incidence of cardiovascular disease in the very elderly. The Bronx aging study. *Arteriosclerosis Thrombosis and Vascular Biology,* 1992; 12: 416–423.

17. Fried LP, et al. Risk factors for 5-year mortality in older adults: the Cardiovascular Health Study. *Journal of the American Medical Association,* 1998; 279: 585–592.

18. Chyou PH, Eaker ED. Serum cholesterol concentrations and all-cause mortality in older people. *Age and Ageing,* 2000; 29: 69–74.

19. Menotti A, et al. Cardiovascular risk factors and 10-year all-cause mortality in elderly European male populations; the FINE study. *European Heart Journal,* 2001; 22: 573–579.

20. Räihä I, et al. Effect of serum lipids, lipoproteins, and apolipoproteins on vascular and nonvascular mortality in the elderly. *Arteriosclerosis Thrombosis and Vascular Biology,* 1997; 17: 1224–1232.

21. Brescianini S, et al. Low total cholesterol and increased risk of dying: are low levels clinical warning signs in the elderly? Results from the Italian Longitudinal Study on Aging. *Journal of the American Geriatrics Society*, Jul, 2003; 51 (7): 991-996.
22. Forette B, et al. Cholesterol as risk factor for mortality in elderly women. *Lancet*, 1989; 1: 868–870.
23. Jonsson A, et al. Total cholesterol and mortality after age 80 years. *Lancet*, 1997; 350: 1778–1779.
24. Weverling-Rijnsburger AW, et al. Total cholesterol and risk of mortality in the oldest old. *Lancet*, 1997; 350: 1119–1123.
25. Gotto AM, et al. The cholesterol facts. A summary of the evidence relating dietary fats, serum cholesterol and coronary heart disease. A joint statement by the American Heart Association and the National Heart, Lung and Blood Institute. *Circulation*, 81: 1721-1733. 1994.
26. Schatz IJ, et al. Cholesterol and all-cause mortality in elderly people from the Honolulu Heart Program: a cohort study. *Lancet*, Aug 4, 2001; 358 (9279): 351-355.
27. Iso H, et al. Serum total cholesterol and mortality in a Japanese population. *Journal of Clinical Epidemiology*, 1994 Sep; 47 (9): 961-969.
28. Matsuzaki M, et al. Large scale cohort study of the relationship between serum cholesterol concentration and coronary events with low-dose simvastatin therapy in Japanese patients with hypercholesterolemia. *Circulation Journal*, Dec, 2002; 66 (12): 1087-1095.
29. Stamler J, et al. Is relationship between serum cholesterol and risk from coronary heart disease continuous and graded? Findings in 356 222 primary screenees of the Multiple Risk Factor Intervention Trial (MRFIT). *Journal of the American Medical Association*, Nov 28, 1986; 256 (20): 2823-2828.
30. Iso H, et al. Serum cholesterol levels and six-year mortality from stroke in 350,977 men screened for the Multiple Risk Factor Intervention Trial. *New England Journal of Medicine*, Apr, 1989; 320 (14): 904-910.
31. Kircher T, et al. The autopsy as a measure of accuracy of the death certificate. *New England Journal of Medicine*, Nov 14, 1985; 313: 1263-1269.
32. Jordan JM, Bass MJ. Errors in death certificate completion in a teaching hospital. *Clinical and Investigative Medicine*, 1993; 16: 249-255.
33. Davis BR, et al. Standardized physician preparation of death certificates. *Controlled Clinical Trials*, 1987; 8: 110-120.
34. Lloyd-Jones D, et al. Accuracy of Death Certificates for Coding Coronary Heart Disease as the Cause of Death. *Annals of Internal Medicine*, Dec 15, 1998; 129 (12): 1020-1026.
35. Messite J, Stellman SD. Accuracy of death certificate completion: the need formalized physician training. *Journal of the American Medical Association*, 1996; 275: 794-796.
36. Multiple Risk Factor Intervention Trial Research Group. Multiple risk factor intervention trial. Risk factor changes and mortality results. *Journal of the American Medical Association*, 1982 Sep 24;248(12):1465-1477.
37. Strandberg TE, et al. Low cholesterol, mortality, and quality of life in old age during a 39-year follow-up. *Journal of the American College of Cardiology*, Sept 1, 2004; 44 (5): 1002-1008.
38. Jacobs D, et al. Report of the Conference on Low Blood Cholesterol: Mortality Associations. *Circulation*, 1992; 86: 1046-1060.
39. Ulmer H, et al. Why Eve is not Adam: prospective follow-up in 149650 women and men of cholesterol and other risk factors related to cardiovascular and all-cause mortality. *Journal of Womens Health*, Jan-Feb, 2004; 13 (1): 41-53.

336

Chapter 3

1. Jacobs D, et al. Report of the Conference on Low Blood Cholesterol: Mortality Associations. *Circulation,* 1992; 86: 1046-1060.
2. Zureik M, et al. Decline in serum total cholesterol and the risk of death from cancer. *Epidemiology,* Mar, 1997; 8 (2): 137-143.
3. Horwich TB, et al. Low serum total cholesterol is associated with marked increase in mortality in advanced heart failure. *Journal of Cardiac Failure,* 2002; 8 (4): 216-224.
4. Sharp SJ, Pocock SJ. Time trends in serum cholesterol before cancer death. *Epidemiology,* Mar, 1997; 8 (2): 132-136.
5. Muldoon MF, et al. Lowering cholesterol concentrations and mortality: a quantitative review of primary prevention trials. *British Medical Journal,* 1990; 301; 309-314. Note: A 2001 analysis by the same authors found that the association between violent death and cholesterol-lowering has not been observed in more recent trials involving women, those who have already suffered a heart attack, and those using statin drugs. The association outside these groups still holds, however. See: Muldoon MF, et al. Cholesterol reduction and non-illness mortality: meta-analysis of randomised clinical trials. *British Medical Journal,* Jan 6, 2001; 322 (7277): 11-15.
6. Golomb BA, et al. Severe irritability associated with statin cholesterol-lowering drugs. *Quarterly Journal of Medicine,* 2004; 97: 229-235.
7. Hyyppa MT, et al. Does simvastatin affect mood and steroid hormone levels in hypercholesterolemic men? A randomized double-blind trial. *Psychoneuroendocrinology,* Feb, 2003; 28 (2): 181-194.
8. Wells AS, et al. Alterations in mood after changing to a low-fat diet. *British Journal of Nutrition,* Jan, 1998; 79 (1): 23-30.
9. Kaplan JR, et al. The effects of fat and cholesterol on social behavior in monkeys. *Psychosomatic Medicine,* Nov-Dec, 1991; 53 (6): 634-642.
10. Steegmans PHA, et al. Higher Prevalence of Depressive Symptoms in Middle-Aged Men With Low Serum Cholesterol Levels. *Psychosomatic Medicine,* Mar 1, 2000; 62 (2): 205-211.
11. Morgan RE, et al. Plasma cholesterol and depressive symptoms in older men. *Lancet,* 1993; 341: 75–9.
12. Ellison LF, Morrison HI. Low serum cholesterol concentration and risk of suicide. *Epidemiology,* Mar 2001; 12 (2): 168-172.
13. Horrobin DF. Lowering cholesterol concentrations and mortality. *British Medical Journal,* 1990; 301: 554.
14. Zhang J, et al. Serum cholesterol concentrations are associated with visuomotor speed in men: findings from the third National Health and Nutrition Examination Survey, 1988–1994. *American Journal of Clinical Nutrition,* Aug, 2004; 80: 291-298.
15. Muldoon MF, et al. Serum cholesterol and intellectual performance. *Psychosomatic Medicine,* Jul-Aug, 1997; 59 (4): 382-387.
16. Benton D. Do low cholesterol levels slow mental processing? *Psychosomatic Medicine,* Jan-Feb, 1995; 57 (1): 50-53.
17. Swan GE, et al. Decline in cognitive performance in aging twins. Heritability and biobehavioral predictors from the National Heart, Lung, and Blood Institute Twin Study. *Archives of Neurology,* May, 1992; 49 (5): 476-481.
18. Kuusisto J, et al. Association between features of the insulin resistance syndrome and alzheimer's disease independently of apolipoprotein e4 phenotype: cross sectional population based study. *British Medical Journal,* Oct, 1997; 315: 1045-1049.
19. Wardle J, et al. Randomized trial of the effects of cholesterol-lowering dietary treatment on psychological function. *American Journal of Medicine,* May, 2000; 108 (7): 547-553.
20. Roth T, et al. Comparative effects of pravastatin and lovastatin on nighttime sleep and daytime performance. *Clinical Cardiology,* 1992; 15: 426-432.

21. Muldoon MF, et al. Effects of lovastatin on cognitive function and psychological well-being. *American Journal of Medicine,* 2000; 108: 538-546.
22. Muldoon MF, et al. Randomized trial of the effects of simvastatin on cognitive functioning in hypercholesterolemic adults. *American Journal of Medicine,* Dec 1, 2004; 117: 823-829.

Chapter 4

1. Landé K. E., Sperry W. M. Human atherosclerosis in relation to the cholesterol content of the blood. *Archives of Pathology,* 1936; 22:301-312.
2. Mathur KS, et al. Serum cholesterol and atherosclerosis in man. *Circulation,* 1961; 23; 847-852.
3. Paterson JC, et al. Serum lipid levels and the severity of coronary and cerebral atherosclerosis in adequately nourished men, 60 to 69 years of age. *Circulation,* 1963; 27; 229-236.
4. McGee CT . *Heart Frauds: Uncovering the Biggest Health Scam in History.* Piccadilly Books, Apr, 2001: 82.
5. Marek Z, et al. Atherosclerosis and levels of serum cholestrol in postmortem investigations. *American Heart Journal,* 1962; 63; 768-774.
6. Méndez J, Tejada C. Relationship between serum lipids and aortic atherosclerotic lesions in sudden accidental deaths in Guatemala City. *American Journal of Clinical Nutrition,* 1967; 20; 1113-1117.
7. Cabin HS, Roberts WC. Relation of serum total cholesterol and triglyceride levels to the amount and extent of coronary arterial narrowing by atherosclerotic plaque in coronary heart disease. *American Journal of Medicine,* 1982; 73: 227-234.
8. Feinleib M, et al. The relation of antemortem characteristics to cardiovascular findings at necropsy. The Framingham Study. *Atherosclerosis,* 34: 145-157. 1979.
9. Solberg LA, et al. Stenoses in the coronary arteries. Relation to atherosclerotic lesions, coronary heart disease, and risk factors. The Oslo Study. *Laboratory Investigation,* 1985; 53 (6): 648-655.
10. Okumiya N, et al. Coronary atherosclerosis and antecedent risk factors: Pathologic and epidemologic study in Hisayama, Japan. *American Journal of Cardiology,* Jul 1, 1985; 56: 62-66.
11. Rhoads, GG, et al. Coronary risk factors and autopsy findings in Japanese-American men. *Laboratory Investigation,* 1978; 38 (3): 304-311.
12. Kritchevsky D. Dietary Protein, cholesterol and atherosclerosis: A review of the early history. *Journal of Nutrition,* 1995; 125: 589S-593S.
13. Steiner A, Kendall FE. Atherosclerosis and arteriosclerosis in dogs following ingestion of cholesterol and thiouracil. *Archives of Pathology,* 42: 433-444. 1946.
14. Duff L. Experimental cholesterol arteriosclerosis and its relationship to human arteriosclerosis. *Archives of Pathology,* 1935; 20: 81-123, 259-304.
15. McNamara DJ., The Impact of Egg Limitations on Coronary Heart Disease Risk: Do the Numbers Add Up? *Journal of the American College of Nutrition,* 2000; 19 (90005): 540S-548S.
16. Rudel LL, et al. Compared with dietary monounsaturated and saturated fat, polyunsaturated fat protects African green monkeys from coronary artery atherosclerosis. *Arteriosclerosis, Thrombosis, and Vascular Biology,* Dec, 1995; 15 (12): 2101-2110.
17. Rudel LL, et al. Dietary polyunsaturated fat modifies low-density lipoproteins and reduces atherosclerosis of nonhuman primates with high and low diet responsiveness. *American Journal of Clinical Nutrition,* Aug, 1995; 62 (2): 463S-470S.
18. Wolfe MS, et al. Dietary polyunsaturated fat decreases coronary artery atherosclerosis in a pediatric-aged population of African green monkeys. *Arteriosclerosis and Thrombosis,* Apr, 1994; 14 (4): 587-597.

19. Eggen DA, et al. Regression of experimental atherosclerotic lesions in rhesus monkeys consuming a high saturated fat diet. *Arteriosclerosis*, Mar-Apr, 1987; 7 (2): 125-134.
20. Kannel WB, Gordon T. The search for an optimum serum cholesterol. *Lancet*, Aug 14, 1982: 374-375.
21. Stare F. The AMA' campaign against cholesterol. *Journal of the American Medical Association*, Jun 9, 1989; 261 (22): 3240-3241.

Chapter 5
1. Keys A. Atherosclerosis: a problem in new public health. *Journal of Mount Sinai Hospital*, 1953; 20: 118-139.
2. Yerushalmey J, Hilleboe HE. Fat in the diet and mortality from heart disease. A methodological note. *New York State Journal of Medicine,* 1957; 57: 2343-2354.
3. Yudkin J. Diet and coronary thrombosis. Hypothesis and fact. *Lancet,* Jul 27, 1957; II: 155-162.
4. Marmot MG, et al. Changing social-class distribution of heart disease. *British Medical Journal*, Oct 21, 1978; 2 (6145): 1109-1112.
5. Epstein FH. The relationship of lifestyle to international trends in CHD. *International Journal of Epidemiology*, 1989; 18 (3, Suppl 1): S203-S209.
6. Keys, A. Coronary heart disease in seven countries. *Circulation,* 1970; 41 (Suppl 1): 1-211.
7. Page IH, et al., Dietary fat and its relation to heart attacks and strokes. *Circulation,* 1961; 23:133-136.
8. Kendricks M. Comments made during The International Network of Cholesterol Skeptics online discussion. Available online: www.thincs.org/discuss.cavemen.htm (accessed Sept 8, 2005).
9. No author listed. Health Revolutionary: The Life and Work of Ancel Keys. Available online: http://www.asph.org/movies/keys.pdf (accessed Sept 8, 2005).
10. No author listed. Introduction to the 2003 Conference on the Mediterranean Diet, Jan 12-14, 2003, Boston, Massachusetts. Available online: www.e-guana.net/organizations/org/intromed10book.pdf (accessed Sept 8, 2005).

Chapter 6
1. Food intake data from Food and Agriculture Organization of the United Nations, Statistical Database, 2000, available online at http://apps.fao.org. CHD mortality data from *World Health Statistics Annual, Volume 1, 1966* (figures for Italy are from 1961 edition) and *1997-1999 World Health Statistics Annual,* available online at http://www.who.int/research/en/ (accessed Sept 8, 2005).
2. Mann GV, et al. Cardiovascular disease in the Masai. *Journal of Atherosclerosis Research,* 1964; 4; 289-312.
3. Mann GV, et al. Physical fitness and immunity to heart-disease in Masai. *Lancet,* Dec 25, 1965; 2 (7426): 1308-1310.
4. Day J, et al. Anthropometric, physiological and biochemical differences between urban and rural Masai. *Atherosclerosis,* 1976; 23: 357-361.
5. Mann GV, et al. Atherosclerosis in the Masai. *American Journal of Epidemiology,* Jan, 1972; 95 (1): 26-37.
6. Mann G. *Coronary Heart Disease: The Dietary Sense and Nonsense.* Veritas Society, London. 1993.
7. Biss K, et al. Some unique biological characteristics of the Masai of east Africa. *New England Journal of Medicine,* Apr 1, 1971; 284 (13): 694-699.
8. Shaper, AG. Cardiovascular studies in the Samburu tribe of Northern Kenya. *American Heart Journal*, 1962; 63 (4); 437-442.

9. Temple NJ. Coronary heart disease - dietary lipids or refined carbohydrates? *Medical Hypotheses*, 1983; 10: 425-435.

10. Prior IA, et al. Cholesterol, coconuts, and diet on Polynesian atolls: a natural experiment: the Pukapuka and Tokelau island studies. *American Journal of Clinical Nutrition*, 1981 Aug; 34 (8): 1552-1561

11. Stanhope JM, et al. The Tokelau Island Migrant Study: serum lipid concentration in two environments. *Journal of Chronic Disease*, 1981; 34 (2-3): 45-55.

12. Joseph JG, et al. Elevation of systolic and diastolic blood pressure associated with migration: the Tokelau island migrant study. *Journal of Chronic Disease*, 1983; 36 (7): 507-516.

13. Ostbye T, et al. Type 2 (non-insulin-dependent) diabetes mellitus, migration and westernisation: the Tokelau Island Migrant Study. *Diabetologia*, Aug, 1989; 32 (8): 585-590.

14. Prior IA, et al. Migration and gout: the Tokelau Island migrant study. *British Medical Journal (Clinical Research Edition)*, Aug 22, 1987; 295 (6596): 457-461.

15. Malhotra SL. Epidemiology of ischaemic heart disease in India with special reference to causation. *British Heart Journal*, 1967; 29: 895-905.

16. Marmot MG, et al. Epidemiologic studies of coronary heart disease and stroke in Japanese men living in Japan, Hawaii and California: prevalence of coronary and hypertensive heart disease and associated risk factors. *American Journal of Epidemiology*, 1975; 102: 514-525

17. Marmot MG, Syme SL. Acculturation and coronary heart disease in Japanese-Americans. *American Journal of Epidemiology*, 1976; 104: 225-247.

18. Longevity statistics from: Population Division of the United Nations Secretariat, *World Population Prospects: The 2000 Revision, Volume I: Comprehensive Tables, Demographic Yearbook 1999*, and Population and Vital Statistics Report, Statistical papers, Series A Vol. LIV, No.1. Food intake data from: Food and Agriculture Organization of the United Nations, Statistical Database, 2000, available online at http://apps.fao.org

19. Tanaka H, et al. Secular trends in mortality for cerebrovascular disease in Japan, 1960-1979. *Stroke*, 1982; 13: 574-581.

20. Nakayama C, et al. A 15.5-Year Follow-up Study of Stroke in a Japanese Provincial City: The Shibata Study. *Stroke*, 1997; 28 (1): 45-52.

21. Sauvaget C, et al. Animal Protein, Animal Fat, and Cholesterol Intakes and Risk of Cerebral Infarction Mortality in the Adult Health Study. *Stroke*, 2004; 35: 1531.

22. Sauvaget C, et al. Intake of animal products and stroke mortality in the Hiroshima/Nagasaki Life Span Study. *International Journal of Epidemiology*, Aug 1, 2003; 32 (4): 536-543.

23. Iso H, et al. Fat and protein intakes and risk of intraparenchymal hemorrhage among middle-aged Japanese. *American Journal of Epidemiology*, Jan 1, 2003; 157 (1): 32-39.

24. Castelli WP, Concerning the Possibility of a Nut... *Archives of Internal Medicine*, Jul, 1992; 152: 1371-1372.

25. Gordon T, et al. Diet and its relation to coronary heart disease in three populations. *Circulation*, Mar, 1981; 63; 500-515.

26. No authors listed. Ecological analysis of the association between mortality and major risk factors of cardiovascular disease. The World Health Organization MONICA Project. *International Journal of Epidemiology*, Jun, 1994; 23 (3): 505-516.

27. Ginter E. Cardiovascular disease prevention in eastern Europe. *Nutrition*, May, 1998; 14 (5): 452-457.

28. Blackburn H. Ancel Keys. Available online: http://mbbnet.umn.edu/firsts/blackburn_h.html (accessed Sept 8, 2005).
29. Yusuf S, et al. Effect of potentially modifiable risk factors associated with myocardial infarction in 52 countries (the INTERHEART study): case-control study. *Lancet*, Sep 11, 2004; 364 (9438): 937-9352.
30. Walldius G, et al. High apolipoprotein B, low apolipoprotein A-I, and improvement in the prediction of fatal myocardial infarction (AMORIS study): a prospective study. *Lancet*, 2001; 358: 2026–2033.
31. Connor SL, et al. Diets lower in folic acid and carotenoids are associated with the coronary disease epidemic in Central and Eastern Europe. *Journal of the American Dietetic Association*, 2004; 104: 1793-1799.

Chapter 7

1. Paul O, et al. A longitudinal study of coronary heart disease. *Circulation*, Jul 1963; 28: 20-31.
2. Gordon T. The Framingham Diet Study: diet and the regulation of serum cholesterol. In: *The Framingham Study: An Epidemiological Investigation of Cardiovascular Disease, Section 24*. U.S. Government Printing Office, Washington, D.C., 1970.
3. Medalie JH, et al. Five-year myocardial infarction incidence. II. Association of single variables to age and birthplace. *Journal of Chronic Diseases*, Jun, 1973; 26 (6): 325-349.
4. Morris JN, et al. Diet and heart: a postscript. *British Medical Journal*, 1977; 2: 1307-1314.
5. Yano K, et al. Dietary intake and the risk of coronary heart disease in Japanese men living in Hawaii. *American Journal of Clinical Nutrition*, Jul, 1978; 31: 1270-1279.
6. Garcia-Palmieri MR, et al. Relationship of dietary intake to subsequent coronary heart disease incidence: The Puerto Rico Heart Health Program. *American Journal of Clinical Nutrition*, Aug, 1980; 33 (8): 1818-1827.
7. Gordon T, et al. Diet and its relation to coronary heart disease in three populations. *Circulation*, Mar, 1981; 63; 500-515.
8. Shekelle RB, et al. Diet, serum cholesterol, and death from coronary heart disease: the Western Electric Study. *New England Journal of Medicine*, 1981; 304: 65-70.
9. McGee DL, et al. Ten-year incidence of coronary heart disease in the Honolulu Heart Program: relationship to nutrient intake. *American Journal of Epidemiology*, 1984; 119: 667-676.
10. Kromhout D, de Lezenne Coulander C. Diet, prevalence and 10-year mortality from coronary heart disease in 871 middle-aged men: the Zutphen Study. *American Journal of Epidemiology*, 1984; 119: 733-741.
11. Kushi LH, et al. Diet and 20-year mortality from coronary heart disease: the Ireland-Boston Diet-Heart Study. *New England Journal of Medicine*, 1985; 312: 811-818.
12. Lapidus L, et al. Dietary habits in relation to incidence of cardiovascular disease and death in women: a 12-year follow-up of participants in the population study of women in Gothenburg, Sweden. *American Journal of Clinical Nutrition*, 1986; 44 (4): 444-448.
13. Khaw KT, Barrett-Connor E. Dietary fiber and reduced ischemic heart disease mortality rates in men and women: a 12-year prospective study. *American Journal of Epidemiology*, Dec, 1987; 126 (6): 1093-1102.
14. Farchi G, et al. Diet and 20-y mortality in two rural population groups of middle-aged men in Italy. *American Journal of Clinical Nutrition*, Nov, 1989; 50 (5): 1095-1103.
15. Posner BM, et al. Dietary lipid predictors of coronary heart disease in men: the Framingham Study. *Archives of Internal Medicine*, 1991; 151: 1181-1187.
16. Dolecek TA. Epidemiological evidence of relationships between dietary polyunsaturated fatty acids and mortality in the multiple risk factor intervention trial. *Proceedings of the Society for Experimental Biology and Medicine*, Jun, 1992; 200 (2): 177-182.

17. Fehily AM, et al. Diet and incident ischaemic heart disease: the Caerphilly Study. *British Journal of Nutrition,* 1993; 69: 303-314.
18. Goldbourt U, et al. Factors predictive of long-term coronary heart disease mortality among 10,059 male Israeli civil servants and municipal employees: a 23-year mortality follow-up in the Israeli Ischemic Heart Disease Study. *Cardiology*, 1993; 82: 100-121.
19. Esrey KL, et al. Relationship between dietary intake and coronary heart disease mortality: Lipid Research Clinics Prevalence Follow-Up Study. *Journal of Clinical Epidemiology,* Feb, 1996; 49 (2): 211-216.
20. Ascherio A, et al. Dietary fat and risk of coronary heart disease in men: cohort follow up study in the United States. *British Medical Journal,* 1996; 313: 84-90.
21. Pietinen P, et al. Intake of fatty acids and risk of coronary heart disease in a cohort of Finnish men: the Alpha-Tocopherol, Beta-Carotene Cancer Prevention Study. *American Journal of Epidemiology*, 1997; 145: 876-887.
22. Hu FB, et al. Dietary fat intake and the risk of coronary heart disease in women. *New England Journal of Medicine,* 1997; 337 (21): 1491-1499.
23. Tanasescu M, et al. Dietary fat and cholesterol and the risk of cardiovascular disease among women with type 2 diabetes. *American Journal of Clinical Nutrition,* Jun, 2004; 79: 999-1005.

Note: The Hu et al and Tanasescu et al papers are worthy of further mention. Both of these reported on the Nurses' Health Study, with Hu et al including 80,082 women who were 34 to 59 years of age and had no known coronary disease, stroke, cancer, 'hypercholesterolemia', or diabetes in 1980 were followed for 14 years. Hu and his colleagues claimed that each 5% increase of calories from saturated fat, as compared with an equivalent energy intake from carbohydrates, was associated with a 17 percent increase in the risk of coronary disease. Reduced risks were also detected for monounsaturated and polyunsaturated fats, leading the authors to conclude that *"replacing saturated and trans unsaturated fats with unhydrogenated monounsaturated and polyunsaturated fats is more effective in preventing coronary heart disease in women than reducing overall fat intake".*

The authors' claim that replacement of saturates with carbohydrates and unsaturated fats lowers CHD risk is totally contradicted by decades of non-supportive clinical research (see Chapter 8). Furthermore, after the authors adjusted for potential confounders like age, smoking, total energy intake, and percentage of calories obtained from protein and specific types of fat, neither blood cholesterol, animal fats nor saturated fat were associated with any noteworthy increase in the risk of CHD. In fact, each five percent increase of energy from animal fats was associated with a 2% decrease in CHD risk. While this risk reduction was statistically insignificant, it hardly supports any contention that animal fats--the main source of saturates--are harmful!

The 2004 paper by Tanasescu examined the relationship between various types of dietary fat and cardiovascular disease in 5,674 diabetic women from the Nurses' Health Study. They claimed higher intake of saturated fat and low dietary ratio of polyunsaturated:saturated fat was associated with a higher risk of CVD. However, their own data show that after adjusting for such confounders as age, various dietary and lifestyle factors, and intake of unsaturated and trans fats, neither animal fat or saturated fat were significantly associated with CVD.

24. Laaksonen DE, et al. Prediction of cardiovascular mortality in middle-aged men by dietary and serum linoleic and polyunsaturated fatty acids. *Archives of Internal Medicine,* 2005; 165: 193-199.
25. Tucker KL, et al. The Combination of High Fruit and Vegetable and Low Saturated Fat Intakes Is More Protective against Mortality in Aging Men than Is Either Alone: The Baltimore Longitudinal Study of Aging. *Journal of Nutrition*, Mar, 2005; 135: 556-561.

26. Leosdottir M, et al. Dietary fat intake and early mortality patterns--data from The Malmo Diet and Cancer Study. *Journal of Internal Medicine*, 2005; 258: 153-165.

27. Reed DM, et al. Predictors of atherosclerosis in the Honolulu Heart Program. I. Biologic, dietary, and lifestyle characteristics. *American Journal of Epidemiology*, Aug, 1987; 126 (2): 214-225.

28. Reed DM, et al. A prospective study of cerebral artery atherosclerosis. *Stroke*, Jul, 1988; 19 (7): 820-825.

29. Moore MC, et al. Dietary-atherosclerosis study on deceased persons. Relation of selected dietary components to raised coronary lesions. *Journal of the American Dietetic Association*, Mar, 1976; 68 (3): 216-223.

30. He K, et al. Dietary fat intake and risk of stroke in male US healthcare professionals: 14 year prospective cohort study. *British Medical Journal*, 2003; 327 (7418): 777-782.

31. Iso H, et al. Prospective study of fat and protein intake and risk of intraparenchymal hemorrhage in women. *Circulation*, Feb 13, 2001; 103 (6): 856-863.

32. Iso H, et al. Fat and protein intakes and risk of intraparenchymal hemorrhage among middle-aged Japanese. *American Journal of Epidemiology*, Jan 1, 2003; 157 (1): 32-39.

33. Sauvaget C, et al. Intake of animal products and stroke mortality in the Hiroshima/Nagasaki Life Span Study. *International Journal of Epidemiology*, Aug 1, 2003; 32 (4): 536-543.

34. Gillman MW, et al. Inverse association of dietary fat with development of ischemic stroke in men. *Journal of the American Medical Association*, 1997; 278: 2145-2150.

35. Tzonou A, et al. Diet and coronary heart disease: a case-control study in Athens, Greece. *Epidemiology*, Nov, 1993; 4 (6): 511-516.

36. Suh I, et al. Moderate dietary fat consumption as a risk factor for ischemic heart disease in a population with a low fat intake: a case-control study in Korean men. *American Journal of Clinical Nutrition,* Apr, 2001; 73 (4): 722-727.

37. Zukel WJ, et al. A short-term community study of the epidemiology of coronary heart disease. A preliminary report on the North Dakota study. *American Journal of Public Health*, Dec, 1959; 49: 1630-1639.

38. Papp OA, et al. Dietary intake in patients with and without myocardial infarction. *Lancet*, Aug 7, 1965; 19: 259-261.

39. Little JA, et al. Diet and serum-lipids in male survivors of myocardial infarction. *Lancet*, May 1, 1965; 62: 933-935.

40. Finegan A, et al. Diet and coronary heart disease. Dietary analysis on fifty females. *American Journal of Clinical Nutrition,* Jan, 1969; 22 (1): 8-9.

41. Bassett DR, et al. Coronary heart disease in Hawaii: dietary intake, depot fat, "stress", smoking, and energy balance in Hawaiian and Japanese men. *American Journal of Clinical Nutrition,* Nov, 1969; 22: 1483-1503.

Chapter 8

1. Cornfield J, Mitchell S. Selected risk factors in coronary disease. *Archives of Environmental Health*, Sept, 1969; 19: 382-394.

2. Morrison LM. A nutritional program for prolongation of life in coronary atherosclerosis. *Journal of the American Medical Association*, Dec 10, 1955; 159 (15): 1425-1428.

3. Hu FB, et al. Dietary protein and risk of ischemic heart disease in women. *American Journal of Clinical Nutrition*, Aug, 1999; 70 (2): 221-227.

4. Schnyder G, et al. Effect of homocysteine-lowering therapy with folic acid, vitamin B12, and vitamin B6 on clinical outcome after percutaneous coronary intervention: the Swiss Heart study: a randomized controlled trial. *Journal of the American Medical Association*, Aug 28, 2002; 288 (8): 973-979.

5. Korpela H, et al. Effect of selenium supplementation after acute myocardial infarction. *Research Communications in Chemical Pathology and Pharmacology*, Aug, 1989; 65 (2): 249-252.
6. Rose GA, et al. Corn oil in treatment of ischaemic heart disease. *British Medical Journal*, 1965; 1: 1531-1533.
7. Ball KP, et al. Low-fat diet in myocardial infarction: a controlled trial. *Lancet*, 1965; 2: 501-504.
8. Hood B, et al. Long-term prognosis in essential hypercholesterolemia: the effect of strict diet. *Acta Medica Scandanavica*, Aug. 1965; 178 (2): 161-173.
9. Christakis G, et al. Effect of the Anti-Coronary Club on coronary heart disease risk factor status. *Journal of the American Medical Association*, Nov. 7, 1966; 198 (6): 597-604.
10. Bierenbaum ML, et al. Modified fat dietary management of the young male with coronary disease. A five year-report. *Journal of the American Medical Association*, Dec. 25, 1967; 202 (13): 1119-1123.
11. National Diet Heart Study. Final report. *Circulation*, 1968, 37. 1-428.
12. Medical Research Council. Controlled trial of soya-bean oil in myocardial infarction. *Lancet*, 1968; 2: 693-699.
13. Dayton S, et al. A controlled clinical trial of a diet high in unsaturated fat in preventing complications of atherosclerosis. *Circulation*, 1969; 40 (Suppl. II): 1-63.
14. Nitenberg A, et al. Acetylcholine-induced coronary vasoconstriction in young, heavy smokers with normal coronary arteriographic findings. *American Journal of Medicine*, 1993; 95: 71–77.
15. C Ip, et al. Requirement of essential fatty acid for mammary tumorigenesis in the rat. *Cancer Research*, 1985; Vol. 45, Issue 5: 1997-2001.
16. Leren P. The effect of plasma cholesterol lowering diet in male survivors of myocardial infarction. A controlled clinical trial. *Acta Medica Scandanavica Supplement*, 1966; 466: 1-92.
17. Leren P. The Oslo Diet-Heart Study: Eleven Year Report. *Circulation*, Nov 1970; Vol. 42: 935-942.
18. Miettinen M, et al. Effect of cholesterol-lowering diet on mortality from coronary heart-disease and other causes. A twelve-year clinical trial in men and women. *Lancet*, Oct 21, 1972, 2(7782).835-8.
19. Halperin M, et al. Effect of diet on coronary-heart-disease mortality. *Lancet*, Aug 25, 1973; 2 (7826): 438-439.
20. Smith RL, Pinckney ER. *The Cholesterol Conspiracy*. Warren H. Green, Inc., St. Louis, Missouri, 1993.
21. Woodhill JM, et al. Low fat, low cholesterol diet in secondary prevention of coronary heart disease. *Advances in Experimental Medicine and Biology*, 1978; 109: 317-330.
22. Frantz Jr ID, et al. Test of effect of lipid lowering by diet on cardiovascular risk. The Minnesota coronary survey. *Arteriosclerosis*, 1989; 9: 129-135
23. Burr ML, et al. Effects of changes in fat, fish, and fibre intakes on death and myocardial reinfarction: diet and reinfarction trial (DART). *Lancet*, 1989; 2: 757-761.
24. Watts GF, et al. Effects on coronary artery disease of lipid-lowering diet, or diet plus cholestyramine, in the St Thomas' atherosclerosis regression study (STARS). *Lancet*, 1992; 339: 563-569.
25. Watts GF, et al. Dietary fatty acids and progression of coronary artery disease in men. *American Journal of Clinical Nutrition*, 1996; 64: 202-209.
26. Connor WE. The decisive influence of diet on the progression and reversibility of coronary heart disease. *American Journal of Clinical Nutrition*, 1996; 64: 253-254.
27. Ornish D, et al. Can lifestyle changes reverse coronary heart disease? The Lifestyle Heart Trial. *Lancet*, 1990; 336: 129-133.

28. Schuler G, et al. Regular physical exercise and low fat diet. Effects of coronary heart disease. *Circulation*, 1992; 86: 1-11.
29. De Lorgeril M, et al. Mediterranean alpha-linolenic acid-rich diet in secondary prevention of coronary heart disease. *Lancet*, 1994; 343: 1454-1459.
30. Lemaitre RN, et al. n-3 Polyunsaturated fatty acids, fatal ischemic heart disease, and nonfatal myocardial infarction in older adults: the Cardiovascular Health Study. *American Journal of Clinical Nutrition,* 2003; 77: 319-325.
31. Baylin A, et al. Adipose tissue alpha-linolenic acid and nonfatal acute myocardial infarction in Costa Rica. *Circulation*, Apr 1, 2003; 107 (12): 1586-1591.
32. Yli-Jama P, et al. Serum free fatty acid pattern and risk of myocardial infarction: a case-control study. *Journal of Internal Medicine*, Jan, 2002; 251 (1): 19-28.
33. Marchioli R, et al. Early protection against sudden death by n-3 polyunsaturated fatty acids after myocardial infarction: time-course analysis of the results of the Gruppo Italiano per lo Studio della Sopravvivenza nell'Infarto Miocardico (GISSI)-Prevenzione. *Circulation*, 2002; 105: 1897–1903.
34. Simini B. Serge Renaud: from French paradox to Cretan miracle. *Lancet*, 2000: 355: 48.
35. Howard BV, et al. Low-Fat Dietary Pattern and Risk of Cardiovascular Disease: The Women's Health Initiative Randomized Controlled Dietary Modification Trial. *Journal of the American Medical Association*, Feb 8, 2006; 295: 655-666.
36. Prentice RL, et al. Low-Fat Dietary Pattern and Risk of Invasive Breast Cancer: The Women's Health Initiative Randomized Controlled Dietary Modification Trial. *Journal of the American Medical Association*, Feb 8, 2006; 295: 629-642.
37. Beresford SAA, et al. Low-Fat Dietary Pattern and Risk of Colorectal Cancer: The Women's Health Initiative Randomized Controlled Dietary Modification Trial. *Journal of the American Medical Association*, Feb 8, 2006; 295: 643-654.
38. Multiple Risk Factor Intervention Trial Research Group. Multiple risk factor intervention trial. Risk factor changes and mortality results. *Journal of the American Medical Association,* Sep 24, 1982; 248 (12): 1465-1477.
39. Strandberg TE, et al. Long-term mortality after 5-years multifactorial primary prevention of cardiovascular diseases in middle-aged men. *Journal of the American Medical Association*, 1991; 266: 1225-1229.
40. Wilhelmsen L, et al. The multifactor primary prevention trial in Goteburg, Sweden. *European Heart Journal*, Apr, 1986; 7 (4): 279-288.
41. European collaborative trial of multifactorial prevention of coronary heart disease: final report on the 6-year results. World Health Organisation European Collaborative Group. *Lancet*, Apr 19, 1986; 1 (8486): 869-872.
Note: Three dietary intervention trials reported by a Dr Ram B. Singh of Morabad, India have been intentionally omitted from this chapter. All three trials allegedly found significant cardiovascular and overall mortality reductions among subjects assigned to omega-3 and/or fruit- and vegetable-enriched diets. Serious concerns, however, have been raised over Singh's credibilty and the validity of his research data. See: White C. Suspected research fraud: difficulties of getting at the truth. *British Medical Journal*, 2005; 331: 281-288.

Chapter 9

1. Corr LA, Oliver MF. The low fat/low cholesterol diet is ineffective. *European Heart Journal*, 1997; 18: 18-22.
2. Pfizer Inc. Annual Report 2004. Available online: http://www.pfizer.com/pfizer/annualreport/2004/financial/financial2004.pdf (accessed September 8, 2005).
3. Top 500 Prescription Drugs. *Med Ad News,* May 2005. Available online: http://www.pharmalive.com/special_reports/sample.cfm?reportID=191 (accessed September 8, 2005).

4. Shepherd J, et al. Prevention of Coronary Heart Disease with Pravastatin in Men with Hypercholesterolemia. *New England Journal of Medicine*, Nov. 16, 1995; 333 (20): 1301-1308.
5. Sacks FM, et al. The Effect of Pravastatin on Coronary Events after Myocardial Infarction in Patients with Average Cholesterol Levels. *New England Journal of Medicine*, Oct 3, 1996; 335 (14): 1001-1009.
6. Sacks FM, et al. Relationship Between Plasma LDL Concentrations During Treatment With Pravastatin and Recurrent Coronary Events in the Cholesterol and Recurrent Events Trial. *Circulation*, 1998; 97: 1446-1452.
7. The Long-Term Intervention with Pravastatin In ischaemic Disease (LIPID) Study Group. Prevention of cardiovascular events and death with pravastatin in patients with coronary heart disease and a broad range of initial cholesterol levels. *New England Journal of Medicine*, 1998. Vol. 339: 1349-1357.
8. Downs JR, et al. Primary prevention of acute coronary events with lovastatin in men and women with average cholesterol levels. *Journal of the American Medical Association*, 1998; 279: 1615-1622.
9. Heart Protection Study Collaborative Group. MRC/BHF Heart Protection Study of cholesterol lowering with simvastatin in 20 536 high risk individuals: a randomised placebo-controlled trial. *Lancet*, 2002; 360: 7-22M.
10. Ravnskov U. Implications of 4S evidence on baseline lipid levels. *Lancet*, Jul 15, 1995; 346 (8968): 181.
11. Shepherd J, et al. Pravastatin in elderly individuals at risk of vascular disease (PROSPER): a randomised controlled trial. *Lancet*, 2002; 360 (9346): 1623-1630.
12. Matsuzaki M, et al. Large scale cohort study of the relationship between serum cholesterol concentration and coronary events with low-dose simvastatin therapy in Japanese patients with hypercholesterolemia. *Circulation Journal*, Dec, 2002; 66 (12): 1087-1095.
13. Kano H, et al. A HMG-CoA reductase inhibitor improved regression of atherosclerosis in the rabbit aorta without affecting serum lipid levels: possible relevance of up-regulation of endothelial NO synthase mRNA. *Biochemical and Biophysical Research Communications*, 1999; 259: 414-419.
14. Soma MR, et al. HMG CoA reductase inhibitors. In vivo effects on carotid intimal thickening in normocholesterolemic rabbits. *Arteriosclerosis, Thrombosis, and Vascular Biology*, 1993; 13 (4): 571-578.
15. Tsunekawa T, et al. Cerivastatin, a hydroxymethylglutaryl coenzyme a reductase inhibitor, improves endothelial function in elderly diabetic patients within 3 days. *Circulation*, 2001; 104: 376.
16. Laufs U, et al. Rapid effects on vascular function after initiation and withdrawal of atorvastatin in healthy, noncholesterolemic men. *American Journal of Cardiology*, 2001; 88: 1306–1307.
17. O'Driscoll G, et al. Simvastatin, an hmg-coenzyme a reductase inhibitor, improves endothelial function within 1 month. *Circulation*, 1997; 95: 1126-1131.
18. Schror K. Platelet reactivity and arachidonic acid metabolism in type II hyperlipoproteinaemia and its modification by cholesterol-lowering agents. *Eicosanoids*, 1990; 3 (2): 67-73.
19. Puccetti L, et al. Time-dependent effect of statins on platelet function in hypercholesterolaemia. *European Journal of Clinical Investigation*, 2002; 32 (12): 901-908.
20. Puccetti L, et al. Atorvastatin reduces platelet-oxidized-LDL receptor expression in hypercholesterolaemic patients. *European Journal of Clinical Investigation*, 2005; 35 (1): 47-51.

21. Sparrow CP, et al. Simvastatin Has Anti-Inflammatory and Antiatherosclerotic Activities Independent of Plasma Cholesterol Lowering. *Arteriosclerosis, Thrombosis, and Vascular Biology*, 2001; 21: 115-121.

22. Ridker PM, et al. Long-term effects of pravastatin on plasma concentration of C-reactive protein. *Circulation*, 1999; 100: 230-235.

23. Albert MA, et al. Effect of statin therapy on C-reactive protein levels: The Pravastatin Inflammation/CRP Evaluation (PRINCE): a randomized trial and cohort study. *Journal of the American Medical Association*, 2001; 286: 64-70.

24. Jialal I, et al. Effect of hydroxymethyl glutaryl coenzyme A reductase inhibitor therapy on high sensitive C-reactive protein levels. *Circulation*, 2001; 103: 1933-1935.

25. Plenge JK, et al. Simvastatin lowers C-reactive protein within 14 days: an effect independent of low-density lipoprotein cholesterol reduction. *Circulation*, 2002; 106: 1447-1452.

26. Blake GJ, Ridker PM. Novel clinical markers of vascular wall inflammation. *Circulation Research*, 2001; 89:763-771.

27. Weitz-Schmidt G, Welzenbach K, Brinkmann V, et al. Statins selectively inhibit leukocyte function antigen-1 by binding to a novel regulatory integrin site. *Nature Medicine*, 2001; 7 (6): 687-692.

28. Wilson SH, et al. Simvastatin preserves coronary endothelial function in hypercholesterolemia in the absence of lipid lowering. *Arteriosclerosis, Thrombosis, and Vascular Biology*, 2001; 21: 546–554.

29. Rikitake Y, et al. Anti-oxidative properties of fluvastatin, an HMG-CoA reductase inhibitor, contribute to prevention of atherosclerosis in cholesterol-fed rabbits. *Atherosclerosis*, 2001; 154 (1): 87-96.

30. Inami S, et al. Effects of statins on circulating oxidized low-density lipoprotein in patients with hypercholesterolemia. *Japanese Heart Journal*, 2004; 45 (6): 969-975.

31. Yasunari K, et al. HMG-CoA reductase inhibitors prevent migration of human coronary smooth muscle cells through suppression of increase in oxidative stress. *Arteriosclerosis, Thrombosis, and Vascular Biology*, 2001; 21 (6): 937-942.

32. Hidaka Y, et al. Inhibition of cultured vascular smooth muscle cell migration by simvastatin (MK-733). *Atherosclerosis*, 1992; 95 (1): 87-94.

33. Raiteri M, et al. Pharmacological control of the mevalonate pathway: effect on arterial smooth muscle cell proliferation. *Journal of Pharmacology and Experimental Therapeutics*, 1997; 281: 1144–1153.

34. Axel DI, et al. Effects of cerivastatin on human arterial smooth muscle cell proliferation and migration in transfilter cocultures. *Journal of Cardiovascular Pharmacology*, 2000; 35: 619–629.

35. Corsini A, et al. Relationship between mevalonate pathway and arterial myocyte proliferation: in vitro studies with inhibitors of HMG-CoA reductase. *Atherosclerosis*, 1993;101: 117–125.

36. Shah PK. Plaque disruption and coronary thrombosis: new insight into pathogenesis and prevention. *Clinical Cardiology*, 1997; 20 (11, Suppl 2): II-38-44.

37. Crisby M, et al. Pravastatin treatment increases collagen content and decreases lipid content, inflammation, metalloproteinases, and cell death in human carotid plaques: implications for plaque stabilization. *Circulation*, 2001; 103: 926–933.

38. Bea F, et al. Simvastatin promotes atherosclerotic plaque stability in apoe-deficient mice independently of lipid lowering. *Arteriosclerosis, Thrombosis, and Vascular Biology*, 2002; 22 (11): 1832-1837.

39. Sukhova GK, et al. Statins reduce inflammation in atheroma of nonhuman primates independent of effects on serum cholesterol. *Arteriosclerosis, Thrombosis, and Vascular Biology*, 2002; 22 (9): 1452-1458.

40. Takemoto M, et al. Statins as antioxidant therapy for preventing cardiac myocyte hypertrophy. *Journal of Clinical Investigation*, 2001, 108 (10): 1429-1437.
41. Nadruz W, et al. Simvastatin Prevents Load-Induced Protein Tyrosine Nitration in Overloaded Hearts. *Hypertension*, 2004; 43 (5): 1060-1066.
42. Wolfrum S, et al. Acute reduction of myocardial infarct size by a hydroxymethyl glutaryl coenzyme A reductase inhibitor is mediated by endothelial nitric oxide synthase. *Journal of Cardiovascular Pharmacology*, Mar, 2003; 41 (3): 474-480.
43. Cannon CP, et al. Intensive versus moderate lipid lowering with statins after acute coronary syndromes. *New England Journal of Medicine*, 2004; 350 (15): 1495-1504.
44. Schaefer EJ, et al. Effects of *atorvastatin* versus other statins on fasting and postprandial C-Reactive Protein and Lipoprotein-Associated Phospholipase A2 in patients with coronary heart disease versus control subjects. *American Journal of Cardiology*, 2005; 95:1025–1032.
45. Grundy SM, et al. Implications of Recent Clinical Trials for the National Cholesterol Education Program Adult Treatment Panel III Guidelines. *Circulation*, 2004; 110: 227-239.
46. Ricks D, Rabin R. Panel's ties to drugmakers not cited in new. cholesterol guidelines. *Newsday.com*, Jul 15, 2004. Available online: http://www.citizens.org/docUploads/Panel's%20ties%20to%20drugmakers%20not%20ci ted%20in%20new%20cholesterol%20guidelines.pdf (accessed September 8, 2005).
47. de Lemos JA, et al. Early intensive vs a delayed conservative simvastatin strategy in patients with acute coronary syndromes: Phase Z of the A to Z Trial. *Journal of the American Medical Association*, Sep 15, 2004; 292: 1307-1316.
48. LaRosa JC, et al. Intensive lipid lowering with atorvastatin in patients with stable coronary disease. *New England Journal of Medicine*, Mar 8, 2005; 352 (14): 1425-1435.
49. O'Riordan M. Treating to New Targets: A new era in the treatment of established coronary heart disease. *TheHeart.org*, 9 Mar 2005. Available online: http://www.theheart.org/viewArticle.do?primaryKey=400939 (accessed September 8, 2005).
50. Ridker PM, et al. C-Reactive Protein Levels and Outcomes after Statin Therapy. *New England Journal of Medicine*, Jan 6, 2005; 352: 20-28.
51. Nissen SE, et al. Statin Therapy, LDL Cholesterol, C-Reactive Protein, and Coronary Artery Disease. *New England Journal of Medicine*, Jan 6, 2005; 352: 29-38.
52. Ridker PM, et al. Inflammation, pravastatin, and the risk of coronary events after myocardial infarction in patients with average cholesterol levels. Cholesterol and recurrent events (CARE) Investigators. *Circulation*, 1998; 98: 839-884.
53. Heeschen C, et al. Withdrawal of statins increases event rates in patients with acute coronary syndromes. *Circulation*, 2002; 105: 1446-1452.
54. Jenkins DJ, et al. Effects of a dietary portfolio of cholesterol-lowering foods vs lovastatin on serum lipids and C-reactive protein. *Journal of the American Medical Association*, Jul 23, 2003; 290(4): 502-510.
55. Pereira MA, et al. Effects of a low-glycemic load diet on resting energy expenditure and heart disease risk factors during weight loss. *Journal of the American Medical Association*, Nov 24, 2004; 292 (20): 2482-90.
56. Esposito K, et al. Effect of weight loss and lifestyle changes on vascular inflammatory markers in obese women: a randomized trial. *Journal of the American Medical Association*, Apr 9, 2003; 289 (14): 1799-1804.
57. Okita K, et al. Can exercise training with weight loss lower serum C-reactive protein levels? *Arteriosclerosis, Thrombosis, and Vascular Biology*, 2004; 24 (10): 1868-1873.
58. Sharman MJ, Volek JS. Weight loss leads to reductions in inflammatory biomarkers after a very-low-carbohydrate diet and a low-fat diet in overweight men. *Clinical Science*, Oct, 2004; 107 (4): 365-369.

59. Seshadri P, et al. A randomized study comparing the effects of a low-carbohydrate diet and a conventional diet on lipoprotein subfractions and C-reactive protein levels in patients with severe obesity. *American Journal of Medicine*, 2004; 117 (6): 398-405.

60. Ciubotaru I, et al. Dietary fish oil decreases C-reactive protein, interleukin-6, and triacylglycerol to HDL-cholesterol ratio in postmenopausal women on HRT. *Journal of Nutritional Biochemistry*, Sep, 2003; 14 (9): 513-521.

61. Hulten E, et al. The Effect of Early, Intensive Statin Therapy on Acute Coronary Syndrome: A Meta-analysis of Randomized Controlled Trials. *Archives of Internal Medicine*, 2006; 166: 1814-1821.

62. Hayward RA, et al. Narrative Review: Lack of Evidence for Recommended Low-Density Lipoprotein Treatment Targets: A Solvable Problem. *Annals of Internal Medicine*, Oct 3, 2006; 145 (7): 520-530.

63. For examples, see: the DIT (Drug Information Technologies) Message Board, which had 3,764 posts on statin drugs as of August 14, 2004 (http://forum.ditonline.com/index.php); the Lipitor board at www.rxlist.com, which had 3,676 posts as of September 8, 2005 (http://www.rxlist.com/rxboard/lipitor.pl).

64. Jackevicius CA, et al. Adherence with statin therapy in elderly patients with and without acute coronary syndromes. *Journal of the American Medical Association*, Jul 24-31, 2002; 288 (4): 462-467.

65. Avorn J, et al. Persistence of use of lipid-lowering medications: a cross-national study. *Journal of the American Medical Association*, May 13, 1998; 279 (18): 1458-1462.

66. Cohen JS. *Over Dose: The Case Against the Drug Companies: Prescription Drugs, Side Effects, and Your Health*. Penguin USA. 2001.

67. MRC/BHF Heart Protection Study Collaborative Group. Heart protection study of cholesterol lowering therapy and antioxidant vitamin supplementation in a wide range of patients at increased risk of coronary heart disease death: early safety and efficacy experience. *European Heart Journal*, 1999; 20: 7254.

68. The ALLHAT Officers and Coordinators for the ALLHAT Collaborative Research Group. Major outcomes in moderately hypercholesterolemic, hypertensive patients randomized to pravastatin vs usual care: The Antihypertensive and Lipid-Lowering Treatment to Prevent Heart Attack Trial (ALLHAT-LLT). *Journal of the American Medical Association,* Dec. 18, 2002; 288:2998-3007.

69. Barnett, BP. RE: Notice of request for participation by consumer and interested persons in public hearing June 28, June 29, 2000 [Docket No. 00N-1256]. Available online: http://www.fda.gov/ohrms/dockets/dailys/00/jun00/060200/ape0042.rtf. (accessed September 8, 2005).

70. See: No listed author. Pulled drug may be linked to 52 deaths. *USA Today*, Aug. 13, 2001 (http://www.usatoday.com/news/health/2001-08-13-cholesterol-drug.htm), and: 1 Stop Baycol Lawyer web site (http://www.1-stop-baycol-lawyer.com/) Both URLs accessed September 8, 2005.

71. Omar MA, Wilson JP. FDA adverse event reports on statin-associated rhabdomyolysis. *Annals of Pharmacotherapy,* Feb, 2002; 36 (2): 288-295.

72. Philips, PS et al. Statin-associated myopathy with normal creatine kinase levels. *Annals of Internal Medicine,* Oct. 1, 2002; 137: 581-585.

73. Draeger A, et al. Statin therapy induces ultrastructural damage in skeletal muscle in patients without myalgia. *Journal of Pathology*, 2006; 210: 94–102.

74. Hughes S. PRINCESS supports early use of statins after MI. *TheHeart.org*, Aug. 31, 2004.

75. Langsjoen PH, Langsjoen AM. The clinical use of HMG CoA-reductase inhibitors and the associated depletion of coenzyme Q10. A review of animal and human publications. *Biofactors*, 2003; 18 (1-4): 101-111.

76. National Heart, Lung, and Blood Institute, National Institutes of Health Data Fact Sheet. *Congestive Heart Failure in the United States: A New Epidemic.* Available online: http://www.medhelp.org/NIHlib/GF-241.html (accessed September 8, 2005).

77. Langsjoen PH. Statin-induced cardiomyopathy. Introduction to the citizens petition on statins. Available online: http://www.redflagsweekly.com/features/2002_july08P.html (accessed September 8, 2005).

78. Silver MA, et al. Effect of Atorvastatin on Left Ventricular Diastolic Function and Ability of Coenzyme Q10 to Reverse That Dysfunction. *American Journal of Cardiology*, 2004; 94: 1306-1310.

79. Banerjee P, et al. Diastolic heart failure: a difficult problem in the elderly. *American Journal of Geriatric Cardiology*, Jan-Feb. 2004; 13 (1):16-21.

80. Patent applications 4,933,165 (filed January 18, 1989) and 4,929,437 (filed February 2, 1989) can be viewed by visiting http://patft.uspto.gov/netahtml/srchnum.htm and entering the patent numbers in the 'query' box, then clicking on the 'search' tab (accessed September 8, 2005).

81. Jula A, et al. Effects of diet and simvastatin on serum lipids, insulin, and antioxidants in hypercholesterolemic men: a randomized controlled trial. *Journal of the American Medical Association,* Feb 6, 2002; 287 (5): 598-605.

82. Wagstaff LR, et al. Statin-Associated Memory Loss: Analysis of 60 Case Reports and Review of the Literature. *Pharmacotherapy*, 2003; 23 (7): 871-880.

83. Roth T, et al. Comparative effects of pravastatin and lovastatin on nighttime sleep and daytime performance. *Clinical Cardiology*, 1992; 15: 426-432.

84. Muldoon MF, Barger SD, Ryan CM, et al. Effects of lovastatin on cognitive function and psychological well-being. *American Journal of Medicine*, 2000; 108: 538-546.

85. Barres BA, Smith SJ. Cholesterol--making or breaking the synapse. *Science*, Nov 9, 2001; 294 (5545): 1296-1297.

86. Graveline D. *Lipitor: Thief of Memory.* Infinity Publishing, Haverford, PA, Jan. 2004.

87. Newman TB, Hulley SB. Carcinogenicity of lipid-lowering drugs. *Journal of the American Medical Association,* Jan 3, 1996; 275: 55-60.

88. Dalen J, Dalton W. Does Lowering Cholesterol Cause Cancer? *Journal of the American Medical Association*, Jan 3, 1996; 275: 67-69.

89. Bradford RH et al. Expanded Clinical Evaluation of Lovastatin (EXCEL) study results. I. Efficacy in modifying plasma lipoproteins and adverse event profile in 8245 patients with moderate hypercholesterolemia. *Archives of Internal Medicine*, Jan, 1991; 151 (1): 43-49.

90. Strandberg TE, et al. Mortality and incidence of cancer during 10-year follow-up of the Scandinavian Simvastatin Survival Study (4S). *Lancet*, Aug 28, 2004; 364: 771-777.

91. Ravnskov U. Evidence that statin treatment causes cancer, and Ravnskov U, et al. Evidence from the simvastatin trials that cancer is a probable long-term side effect. Unpublished letter to the editor of *Lancet*, available online: http://www.thincs.org/unpublic.htm (accessed March 27, 2003).

92. Kwak B, et al. Statins as a newly recognized type of immunomodulator. *Nature Medicine*, Dec, 2000; 6 (12): 1399-1402.

93. Iwata H, et al. Use of hydroxy-methyl-glutaryl coenzyme A reductase inhibitors is associated with risk of lymphoid malignancies. *Cancer Science*, Feb, 2006; 97 (2): 133-138.

94. Edison RJ, Muenke M. Central nervous system and limb anomalies in case reports of first-trimester statin exposure. *New England Journal of Medicine*, Apr 8, 2004; 350 (15): 1579-1582. See also erratum for this report: Edison RJ, Muenke M. Gestational exposure to lovastatin followed by cardiac malformation misclassified as holoprosencephaly. *New England Journal of Medicine*, Jun 30, 2005; 352 (26): 2759.

95. Gordon S. Cholesterol Drugs Tied to Birth Defects: U.S. study finds high number of abnormalities in babies of women taking statins. *HON News*, Apr 7, 2004. Available online: http://www.hon.ch/News/HSN/518293.html (accessed Feb 10, 2006).
96. Kenis I, et al. Simvastatin has deleterious effects on human first trimester placental explants. *Human Reproduction*, 2005; 20: 2866-2872.
97. Rizvi K, et al. Do lipid-lowering drugs cause erectile dysfunction? A systematic review. *Family Practice*, Feb 2002; 19: 95-98.
98. de Graaf L, et al. Is decreased libido associated with the use of HMG-CoA-reductase inhibitors? *British Journal of Clinical Pharmacology*, 2004; 58 (3): 326-328.
99. Carvajal A, et al. HMG CoA Reductase Inhibitors and Impotence: Two Case Series from the Spanish and French Drug Monitoring Systems. *Drug Safety*, 2006; 29 (2): 143-149.

Chapter 10
1. Page IH, et al., Atherosclerosis and the fat content of the diet. *Circulation,* 1957; 16: 164-178.
2. Page IH, et al., Dietary fat and its relation to heart attacks and strokes. *Circulation,* 1961; 23:133-136.
3. Alton Blakeslee and Jeremiah Stamler, M.D. *Your Heart Has Nine Lives. Nine ways to protect yourself against coronary heart disease.* 1963 Prentice Hall.
4. Stare FJ. Practical guidelines to calorie needs. *Los Angeles Times*, October 23, 1969.
5. Smith, RL. *The Cholesterol Conspiracy*. Warren H. Green, Inc. 1993.
6. De Bakey M, et al. Serum Cholesterol Values in Patients Treated Surgically for Atherosclerosis. *Journal of the American Medical Association,* 1964, 189:9:655-659.
7. Status of Articles Offered to the General Public for the Control or Reduction of Blood Cholesterol and for the Prevention and Treatment of Heart and Artery Disease Under the Federal Food, Drug, and Cosmetic Act. *Federal Register*, Dec 12, 1959.
8. Oils, Fats, and Fatty Acids in Dietary Management: Proposal to Require Label Statements. *Federal Register*, May 18, 1965.
9. Taubes G. The Soft Science of Dietary Fat. *Science,* Mar 30, 2001; 291: 2536-2545.
10. No listed author. The Lipid Research Clinics Coronary Primary Prevention Trial results. I. Reduction in incidence of coronary heart disease. *Journal of the American Medical Association,* Jan 20, 1984; 251 (3): 351-364.
11. No listed author. The Lipid Research Clinics Program. The Coronary Primary Prevention Trial: Design and implementation. *Journal of Chronic Diseases*, 1979; 32: 609-631.

Chapter 11
1. Lowering Blood Cholesterol To Prevent Heart Disease. National Institutes of Health Consensus Development Conference Statement, December 10-12, 1984. Available online: http://consensus.nih.gov/cons/047/047_statement.htm (accessed September 8, 2005).
2. Moore, Thomas J, *Heart Failure,* Random House, 1989.
3. National Cholesterol Education Program, Program Description. Available online: http://www.nhlbi.nih.gov/about/ncep/ncep_pd.htm (accessed September 8, 2005)

Chapter 12
1. Center for Science in the Public Interest. Lift the Veil report: Professional associations, charities, and industry front groups. Available online: http://www.cspinet.org/new/pdf/lift_the_veil_guts_fnl.pdf (accessed September 8, 2005).
2. American Heart Association. Current Heart-Check mark products. Available online: http://216.185.112.90/productlist.aspx (accessed August 18, 2004).
3. Angell M. Is academic medicine for sale? *New England Journal of Medicine,* May 18, 2000; 342 (20): 1516-1518.

4. Norton JW. Is academic medicine for sale? *New England Journal of Medicine,* August 17, 2000; 343 (7): 508.
5. Bodenheimer T. Uneasy alliance - clinical investigators and the pharmaceutical industry. *New England Journal of Medicine,* May 18, 2000; 342 (20): 1539-1544.
6. Bekelman JE, et al. Scope and impact of financial conflicts of interest in biomedical research: a systematic review. *Journal of the American Medical Association,* Jan 22-29, 2003; 289 (4): 454-65.
7. Henry DA, et al. Medical specialists and pharmaceutical industry-sponsored research: a survey of the Australian experience. *Medical Journal of Australia,* 2005; 182 (11): 557-560.
8. Willman D. The National Institutes of Health: Public Servant or Private Marketer? *Los Angeles Times,* Dec 22, 2004. Available online: http://www.latimes.com/news/nationworld/nation/la-na-nih22dec22,0,7519657.story?coll=la-home-headlines (accessed September 8, 2005).
9. Willman D. U.S. Scientists' Deals With Drug Firms Under Review. *Los Angeles Times,* Dec 29, 2003.
10. Willman D. NIH Directors No Longer Drug Firm Consultants. *Los Angeles Times,* Jan 23, 2004.
11. Willman D. NIH Seeks Outside Inquiry of Scientist. *Los Angeles Times,* Jan 28, 2005.
12. Willman D. NIH to Ban Deals With Drug Firms. *Los Angeles Times,* Feb 1, 2005.
13. Weiss R. NIH Workers angered by new ethics rules restrictions on outside income meet with derision at meeting. *Washington Post,* Thurs, Feb 3, 2005: A25. Available online: http://www.washingtonpost.com/wp-dyn/articles/A58845-2005Feb2.html?sub=AR (accessed September 8, 2005).
14. Connolly C. Director of NIH Agrees To Loosen Ethics Rules. *Washington Post,* Fri, Aug 26, 2005: A19. Available online: http://www.washingtonpost.com/wp-dyn/content/article/2005/08/25/AR2005082501664.html (accessed October 30, 2005).
15. Cauchon D. FDA Advisers Tied to Industry. *USA Today,* Sept. 25, 2000.
16. Ravnskov U. Cholesterol lowering trials in coronary heart disease: frequency of citation and outcome. *British Medical Journal,* Jul 4, 1992; 305: 15-19. See also: Frequency of citation and outcome of cholesterol-lowering trials, *British Medical Journal,* Aug 15, 1992; 305: 420-422, for commentary on Ravnskov's article and Ravnskov's subsequent reply.
17. Ravnskov U. Quotation bias in reviews of the diet-heart idea. *Journal of Clinical Epidemiology,* May, 1995; 48 (5): 713-719.
18. From the Executive Summary of the Third Report of the National Cholesterol Education Program (NCEP) Expert Panel on Detection, Evaluation, and Treatment of High Blood Cholesterol in Adults (Adult Treatment Panel III). *Journal of the American Medical Association,* May 16, 2001; 285 (19): 2486-2497: *"Dr Grundy has received honoraria from Merck, Pfizer, Sankyo, Bayer, and Bristol-Myers Squibb. Dr Hunninghake has current grants from Merck, Pfizer, Kos Pharmaceuticals, Schering Plough, Wyeth Ayerst, Sankyo, Bayer, AstraZeneca, Bristol-Myers Squibb, and G. D. Searle; he has also received consulting honoraria from Merck, Pfizer, Kos Pharmaceuticals, Sankyo, AstraZeneca, and Bayer. Dr McBride has received grants and/or research support from Pfizer, Merck, Parke-Davis, and AstraZeneca; has served as a consultant for Kos Pharmaceuticals, Abbott, and Merck; and has received honoraria from Abbott, Bristol-Myers Squibb, Novartis, Merck, Kos Pharmaceuticals, Parke-Davis, Pfizer, and DuPont. Dr Pasternak has served as a consultant for and received honoraria from Merck, Pfizer, and Kos Pharmaceuticals, and has received grants from Merck and Pfizer. Dr Stone has served as a consultant and/or received honoraria for lectures from Abbott, Bayer, Bristol-Myers Squibb, Kos Pharmaceuticals, Merck, Novartis, Parke-Davis/Pfizer, and*

352

Sankyo. Dr Schwartz has served as a consultant for and/or conducted research funded by Bristol-Myers Squibb, AstraZeneca, Merck, Johnson & Johnson-Merck, and Pfizer."

19. Grundy SM, et al. Implications of Recent Clinical Trials for the National Cholesterol Education Program Adult Treatment Panel III Guidelines. *Circulation*, 2004; 110: 227-239.
20. Lenzer J. Scandals have eroded US public's confidence in drug industry. *British Medical Journal*, Jul 31, 2004; 329: 247.
21. Kassirer JP. Physicians' Ties With the Pharmaceutical Industry: A Critical Element of a Wildly Successful Marketing Network. Available online: http://www.theomnivore.com/Kassirer_Physicians_Big_Pharma.html (accessed September 8, 2005).
22. Simons J. The $10 Billion Pill. *Forbes*, Jan. 6, 2003.
23. Neergaard L. Documents Show Vioxx Sales Tactics. *Yahoo! News*, Fri, May 6. Available online: http://news.yahoo.com/news?tmpl=story&u=/ap/20050506/ap_on_bi_ge/vioxx (accessed May 12, 2005).
24. Wazana A. Physicians and the pharmaceutical industry. Is a gift ever just a gift? *Journal of the American Medical Association,* January 19, 2000; 283 (3): 373-380.
25. Prosser H, et al. Influences on GPs' decision to prescribe new drugs-the importance of who says what. *Family Practice*, Jan, 2003; 20: 61-68.
26. Tuffs A. Only 6% of drug advertising material is supported by evidence. *British Medical Journal*, Feb 28, 2004; 328: 485.
27. See: http://www.heartsavers.org/phil_sokolof.htm (accessed 16 January 2003; site not operational on September 8, 2005).
28. Lindeberg S, Lundh B. Apparent absence of stroke and ischaemic heart disease in a traditional Melanesian island: a clinical study in Kitava. *Journal of Internal Medicine,* Mar, 1993; 233 (3): 269-275.
29. Prior IA, et al. Cholesterol, coconuts, and diet on Polynesian atolls: a natural experiment: the Pukapuka and Tokelau island studies. *American Journal of Clinical Nutrition,* Aug, 1981; 34 (8): 1552-1561.
30. Müller H, et al. A Diet Rich in Coconut Oil Reduces Diurnal Postprandial Variations in Circulating Tissue Plasminogen Activator Antigen and Fasting Lipoprotein (a) Compared with a Diet Rich in Unsaturated Fat in Women. *Journal of Nutrition,* 2003; 133: 3422-3427.

Chapter 13
1. Ross R. Atherosclerosis - an inflammatory disease. *New England Journal of Medicine*, Jan 14, 1999; 340 (2): 115-126.
2. Allison MA, et al. Patterns and Risk Factors for Systemic Calcified Atherosclerosis. *Arteriosclerosis, Thrombosis, and Vascular Biology*, 2004; 24: 331.
3. Stary HC, et al. A definition of initial, fatty streak, and intermediate lesions of atherosclerosis. A report from the Committee on Vascular Lesions of the Council on Arteriosclerosis, American Heart Association. *Arteriosclerosis and Thrombosis*, 1994; 14: 840-856.

Chapter 14
1. Marmot MG, et al. Epidemiologic studies of coronary heart disease and stroke in Japanese men living in Japan, Hawaii and California: prevalence of coronary and hypertensive heart disease and associated risk factors. *American Journal of Epidemiology*, 1975; 102: 514-525.
2. Marmot MG, Syme SL. Acculturation and coronary heart disease in Japanese-Americans. *American Journal of Epidemiology,* 1976; 104: 225-247.

3. Wolf S. Predictors of myocardial infarction over a span of 30 years in Roseto, Pennsylvania. *Integrative Physiological and Behavioral Science*, Jul-Sep, 1992; 27 (3): 246-257.

4. Marmot MG, et al. Employment grade and coronary heart disease in British civil servants. *Journal of Epidemiology and Community Health*, Dec 1978; 32 (4): 244-249.

5. Kuper H, Marmot M. Job strain, job demands, decision latitude, and risk of coronary heart disease within the Whitehall II study. *Journal of Epidemiology and Community Health*, Feb 2003; 57 (2): 147-153.

6. Bosma H, et al. Low job control and risk of coronary heart disease in Whitehall II (prospective cohort) study. *British Medical Journal*, Feb 22, 1997; 314 (7080): 558-565.

7. Theorell T, et al. Decision latitude, job strain, and myocardial infarction: a study of working men in Stockholm. The SHEEP Study Group. Stockholm Heart epidemiology Program. *American Journal of Public Health*, 1998; 88 (3): 382-388.

8. Ala-Mursula L, et al. Employee control over working times: associations with subjective health and sickness absences. *Journal of Epidemiology and Community Health*, Apr 1, 2002; 56 (4): 272-278.

9. Malinauskiene V, et al. Low job control and myocardial infarction risk in the occupational categories of Kaunas men, Lithuania. *Journal of Epidemiology and Community Health*, Feb 1, 2004; 58 (2): 131-135.

10. Cheng Y, et al. Association between psychological work characteristics and health functioning in American women: prospective study. *British Medical Journal*, 2000; 320: 1432-1436.

11. Peter R, et al. Does a stressful psychosocial work environment mediate the effects of shift work on cardiovascular risk factors? *Scandinavian Journal of Work Environment & Health*, Aug, 1999; 25 (4): 376-381.

12. Quinlan M, et al. The global expansion of precarious employment, work disorganization, and consequences for occupational health: a review of recent research. *International Journal of Health Services*, 2001; 31: 335-414.

13. Vahtera J, et al. Organisational downsizing, sickness absence, and mortality: 10-town prospective cohort study. *British Medical Journal*, Mar 6, 2004; 328: 555.

14. Kivimaki M, et al. Work stress and risk of cardiovascular mortality: prospective cohort study of industrial employees. *British Medical Journal*, Oct 19, 2002; 325 (7369): 857-857.

15. National Sleep Foundation Sleep in America 2001 poll. National Sleep Foundation polls can be accessed at: http://www.sleepfoundation.org/hottopics/index.php?secid=16 (accessed September 8, 2005).

16. Geary LH. I quit! *CNN/Money*, Dec 30, 2003. Available online: http://money.cnn.com/2003/11/11/pf/q_iquit/?cnn=yes (accessed September 8, 2005).

17. Liu Y, et al. Overtime work, insufficient sleep, and risk of non-fatal acute myocardial infarction in Japanese men. *Occupational and Environmental Medicine*, Jul 2002; 59 (7): 447-451.

18. Sokejima S, Kagamimori S. Working hours as a risk factor for acute myocardial infarction in Japan: case-control study. *British Medical Journal*, Sep, 1998; 317: 775-780.

19. Falger PR, Schouten EG. Exhaustion, psychological stressors in the work environment, and acute myocardial infarction in adult men. *Journal of Psychosomatic Research*, Dec, 1992; 36 (8): 777-786.

20. Theorell T, Rahe RH. Behavior and life satisfactions characteristics of Swedish subjects with myocardial infarction. *Journal of Chronic Diseases*, Mar, 1972; 25 (3): 139-147.

21. Uehata T. Long working hours and occupational stress-related cardiovascular attacks among middle-aged workers in Japan. *Journal of Human Ergology*, 1991; 20: 147-153.
22. Netterstrom B, et al. Relation between job strain and myocardial infarction: a case-control study. *Occupational and Environmental Medicine*, May, 1999; 56 (5): 339-342.
23. Tennant C. Experimental stress and cardiac function. *Journal of Psychosomatic Research*, Jun. 1996; 40 (6): 569-583.
24. Steptoe A, et al. Influence of socioeconomic status and job control on plasma fibrinogen responses to acute mental stress. *Psychosomatic Medicine*, Jan-Feb, 2003; 65 (1): 137-144.
25. Schiffer F, et al. Evidence for emotionally-induced coronary arterial spasm in patients with angina pectoris. *British Heart Journal*, 1980; 44: 62-66.
26. Mansour VM, et al. Panic disorder: coronary spasm as a basis for cardiac risk? *Medical Journal of Australia*, Apr. 20, 1998; 168 (8): 390-392.
27. Bashour T, et al. Coronary spastic angina in middle-aged women: a psychosomatic disorder? *American Heart Journal*, 1983; 106: 609-613.
28. Tsutsumi A, et al. Association between job characteristics and plasma fibrinogen in a normal working population: a cross sectional analysis in referents of the SHEEP Study. Stockholm Heart Epidemiology Program. *Journal of Epidemiology and Community Health*, Jun, 1999; 53 (6): 348-354.
29. Vrijkotte TGM, et al. Effects of work stress on ambulatory blood pressure, heart rate, and heart rate variability. *Hypertension*, 2000; 35: 880-886.
30. Peter R, et al. High effort, low reward, and cardiovascular risk factors in employed Swedish men and women: baseline results from the WOLF study. *Journal of Epidemiology and Community Health*, 1998; 52: 540-547.
31. Bishop GD, et al. Job demands, decisional control, and cardiovascular responses. *Journal of Occupational Health Psychology*, Apr, 2003; 8 (2): 146-156.
32. Peter R, et al. Does a stressful psychosocial work environment mediate the effects of shift work on cardiovascular risk factors? *Scandinavian Journal of Work, Environment & Health*, Aug, 1999; 25 (4): 376-381.
33. Ross C, et al. Impact of the family on health: Decade in review. *Journal of Marriage and the Family*, Nov, 1990; 52: 1059-1078.
34. Glenn N, Weaver C. The contribution of marital happiness to global happiness. *Journal of Marriage and the Family*, 1981; 43: 161-168.
35. Tucker JS, et al. Marital history at midlife as a predictor of longevity alternative explanations to the protective effect of marriage. *Health Psychology*, 1996; 15: 94–101.
36. Burman B, Margolin G. Analysis of the association between marital relationships and health problems: an interactional perspective. *Psychological Bulletin*, Jul, 1992; 112 (1): 39-63.
37. Kiecolt Glaser JK, et al. Marriage and health: His and hers. *Psychological Bulletin*, Jul, 2001; 127 (4): 472-503.
38. Matthews KA, Gump BB. Chronic Work Stress and Marital Dissolution Increase Risk of Posttrial Mortality in Men From the Multiple Risk Factor Intervention Trial. *Archives of Internal Medicine*, Feb 11, 2002; 162 (3): 309-315.
39. Orth-Gomer K, et al. Marital Stress Worsens Prognosis in Women With Coronary Heart Disease: The Stockholm Female Coronary Risk Study. *Journal of the American Medical Association*, Dec 20, 2000; 284 (23): 3008-3014.
40. Gallo LC, et al. Marital Status, Marital Quality, and Atherosclerotic Burden in Postmenopausal Women. *Psychosomatic Medicine*, 2003; 65: 952-962.
41. Ewart CK, et al. High blood pressure and marital discord: not being nasty matters more than being nice. *Health Psychology*, 1991; 10: 155–63.
42. Kiecolt-Glaser JK, et al. Negative behavior during marital conflict is associated with immunological down-regulation. *Psychosomatic Medicine*, 1993; 55: 395-409.

43. Kiecolt-Glaser JK, et al. Marital Stress: Immunologic, Neuroendocrine, and Autonomic Correlates. *Annals of the New York Academy Of Sciences,* May 1, 1998; 840 (1): 656-663.

44. Smith TW, Brown PC. Cynical hostility, attempts to exert social control, and cardiovascular reactivity in married couples. *Journal of Behavioral Medicine,* 1991; 14: 581–92.

45. Smith TW, Gallo LC. Hostility and Cardiovascular Reactivity During Marital Interaction. *Psychosomatic Medicine,* 1999; 61: 436-445.

46. Fuller RG. What happens to mental patients after discharge from the hospital? *Psychiatric Quarterly,* 1935; 9: 95-104.

47. Malzberg B. Mortality among patients with involution melancholia. *American Journal of Psychiatry,* 1937; 93: 1231-1238.

48. Carney RM, Freedland KE. Depression, mortality, and medical morbidity in patients with coronary heart disease. *Biological Psychiatry,* 2003; 54: 241-247.

49. Wulsin LR, Singal BM. Do depressive symptoms increase the risk for the onset of coronary disease? A systematic quantitative review. *Psychosomatic Medicine,* 2003; 65: 201-210.

50. Rugulies R. Depression as a predictor for coronary heart disease. *American Journal of Preventive Medicine,* Jul, 2002; 23: 51-61.

51. Surgeon General. *The Health Consequences of Smoking: Cardiovascular Disease.* Department of Health & Human Services, MD, 1983. Available online: http://sgreports.nlm.nih.gov/NN/B/B/T/D/ (accessed September 8, 2005)

52. Jonas BS, Mussolino ME. Symptoms of depression as a prospective risk factor for stroke. *Psychosomatic Medicine,* Jul-Aug, 2000; 62 (4): 463-471.

53. Larson SL, et al. Depressive disorder, dysthymia, and risk of stroke: thirteen-year follow-up from the Baltimore epidemiologic catchment area study. *Stroke,* Sep, 2001; 32 (9): 1979-1983.

54. Frasure-Smith N, et al. Depression following myocardial infarction. Impact on 6-month survival. *Journal of the American Medical Association,* Oct, 1993; 270: 1819-1825.

55. Rudisch B, Nemeroff CB. Epidemiology of comorbid coronary artery disease and depression. *Biological Psychiatry,* 2003; 54: 227-240.

56. Suarez EC, Williams RB. Situational determinants of cardiovascular and emotional reactivity in high and low hostile men. *Psychosomatic Medicine,* 1989; 51: 404–18.

57. Smith TW, Allred KD. Blood pressure responses during social interaction in high- and low-cynically hostile males. *Journal of Behavioral Medicine,* 1989; 12: 125–143.

58. Everson SA, et al. Effect of trait hostility on cardiovascular responses to harassment in young men. *International Journal of Behavioral Medicine,* 1995; 2: 172-191.

59. Williams JE, et al. Effects of an angry temperament on coronary heart disease risk: The Atherosclerosis Risk in Communities Study. *American Journal of Epidemiology,* Aug 1, 2001; 154 (3): 230-235.

60. Matthews KA, et al. Hostile Behaviors Predict Cardiovascular Mortality Among Men Enrolled in the Multiple Risk Factor Intervention Trial. *Circulation,* Jan 6, 2004; 109 (1): 66-70.

61. Gallacher JE, et al. Anger and Incident Heart Disease in the Caerphilly Study. *Psychosomatic Medicine,* 1999; 61: 446-453.

62. Stroebe W, Stroebe MS. *Bereavement and Health: The Psychological and Physical Consequences of Partner Loss.* Cambridge University Press, New York, 1987: 151-167.

63. Bachen EA, et al. Effects of hemoconcentration and sympathetic activation on serum lipid responses to brief mental stress. *Psychosomatic Medicine,* Jul-Aug, 2002; 64 (4): 587-594.

356

64. Patterson SM, et al. Stress-induced hemoconcentration of blood cells and lipids in healthy women during acute psychological stress. *Health Psychology*, Jul, 1995; 14 (4): 319-324.
65. Muldoon MF, et al. Effects of acute psychological stress on serum lipid levels, hemoconcentration, and blood viscosity. *Archives of Internal Medicine*, Mar 27, 1995; 155 (6): 615-620.
66. Kendrick M. Does insulin resistance cause atherosclerosis in the post-prandial period? *Medical Hypotheses*, Jan, 2003; 60 (1): 6-11.
67. Morrow LA, et al. Effects of epinephrine on insulin secretion and action in humans. Interaction with aging. *Diabetes*, 1993; 42: 307-315.
68. Heise T, et al. Simulated postaggression metabolism in healthy subjects: Metabolic changes and insulin resistance. *Metabolism*, Oct, 1998; 47 (10): 1263-1268.
69. Hsueh WA, et al. Insulin Signaling in the Arterial Wall. *American Journal of Cardiology*, Jul 8, 1999; 84 (1A): 21J-24J.
70. Ceolotto G, et al. Insulin generates free radicals by an NAD(P)H, phosphatidylinositol 3'-kinase-dependent mechanism in human skin fibroblasts ex vivo. *Diabetes*, May, 2004; 53 (5): 1344-1351.
71. Charles MA, et al. Non-insulin-dependent diabetes in populations at risk: the Pima Indians. *Diabetes & Metabolism*, Nov, 1997; 23 (Suppl 4): 6-9.
72. Nelson RG, et al. Low incidence of fatal coronary heart disease in Pima Indians despite high prevalence of non-insulin-dependent diabetes. *Circulation*, Mar, 1990; 81: 987-995.
73. Tataranni PA, Hypothalamic-pituitary-adrenal axis and sympathetic nervous system activities in Pima Indians and Caucasians. *Metabolism*, Mar, 1999; 48 (3): 395-399.
74. Legrain M, Lecomte T. Psychotropic drug consumption in France and several European countries. *Bulletin De l'Academie Nationale De Medecine*, Jun-Jul, 1997; 181 (6): 1073-1084.
75. Young CM. Migration and mortality: the experience of birthplace groups in Australia. *International Migration Review*, Fall, 1987; 21 (3): 531-554.
76. Armstrong BK, et al. Coronary risk factors in Italian migrants to Australia. *American Journal of Epidemiology*, Nov, 1983; 118 (5): 651-658.
77. Kouris-Blazos A. Morbidity mortality paradox of 1st generation Greek Australians. *Asia Pacific Journal of Clinical Nutrition*, 2002; 11 Suppl 3: S569-S575.
78. Hodge AM, et al. Increased Diabetes Incidence in Greek and Italian Migrants to Australia: How much can be explained by known risk factors? *Diabetes Care*, Oct, 2004; 27 (10): 2330-2234.
79. Hayashi K, et al. Laughter lowered the increase in postprandial blood glucose. *Diabetes Care*, May, 2003; 26 (5): 1651.
80. The DECODE study group/European Diabetes Epidemiology Group: Glucose tolerance and mortality: comparison of WHO and American Diabetes Association diagnostic criteria. *Lancet*, 1999; 354: 617-621.
81. Rodriguez BL, et al. Glucose intolerance and 23-year risk of coronary heart disease and total mortality: the Honolulu Heart Program. *Diabetes Care*, 1999; 22: 1262-1265.
82. Hanefeld M,et al. Risk factors for myocardial infarction and death in newly detected NIDDM: the Diabetes Intervention Study, 11-year follow-up. *Diabetologia*, 1996; 39: 1577-1583.
83. Kaufmann PG. Depression in cardiovascular disease: Can the risk be reduced? *Biological Psychiatry*, 2003; 54: 187-190.

Chapter 15

1. Abrams HL Jr. The relevance of Paleolithic diet in determining contemporary nutritional needs. *Journal of Applied Nutrition*, 1979; 31 (1 & 2): 43-59.

2. Harlan JR. *The Living Fields: Our Agricultural Heritage.* Cambridge University Press, 1998.
3. Tudge C. *Neanderthals, Bandits, and Farmers: How Agriculture Really Began.* Yale University Press, 1999.
4. Stephen AM. Whole grains--impact of consuming whole grains on physiological effects of dietary fiber and starch. *Critical Reviews in Food Science and Nutrition*, 1994; 34 (5-6): 499-511.
5. Gahlawat P, Sehgal S. Protein and starch digestibilities and mineral availability of products developed from potato, soy and corn flour. *Plant Foods in Human Nutrition*, 1998; 52 (2): 151-160.
6. Bradbury JH, et al. Digestibility of proteins of the histological components of cooked and raw rice. *British Journal of Nutrition*, Nov, 1984; 52 (3): 507-513.
7. Aikens CM. First in the world: The Jomon pottery of Japan. In: *Emergence of Pottery: Technology and Innovation In Ancient Societies.* Eds: Barnett WK, Hoopes JW, McAdams R. Smithsonian Institution Press, Nov, 1995: 11-21.
8. *Paleopathology at the Origins of Agriculture.* Eds: Cohen MN, Armelagos GJ. Academic Press, New York, 1984.
9. Food and Agriculture Organization Food Balance Sheet for United States of America, 2002. Available online at: http://faostat.fao.org (accessed September 8, 2005).
10. Bohn T, et al. Phytic acid added to white-wheat bread inhibits fractional apparent magnesium absorption in humans. *American Journal of Clinical Nutrition*, March 2004; (79) 3: 418-423.
11. Torre M, et al. Effects of dietary fiber and phytic acid on mineral availability. *Critical Reviews in Food Science and Nutrition*, 1991; 30 (1): 1-22.
12. Reinhold JG, et al. Effects of purified phytate and phytate-rich bread upon metabolism of zinc, calcium, phosphorous, and nitrogen in man. *Lancet*, Feb. 10, 1973; 1 (7798): 283-288.
13. Ervin RB, et al. Dietary intakes of selected minerals for the United States population: 1999-2000. *Advance Data*, Apr 27, 2004; 341: 1-5.
14. Ford ES, Mokdad, AH. Dietary Magnesium Intake in a National Sample of U.S. Adults. *Journal of Nutrition*, 2003; 133: 2879-2882.
15. Hambidge M. Human zinc deficiency. *Journal of Nutrition*, May, 2000; 130 (Suppl. 5): 1344S-1349S.
16. Reinhold JG, et al. Effects of purified phytate and phytate-rich bread upon metabolism of zinc, calcium, phosphorous, and nitrogen in man. *Lancet*, Feb. 10, 1973; 1 (7798): 283-288.
17. Campbell BJ, et al. The effects of prolonged consumption of wholemeal bread upon metabolism of calcium, magnesium, zinc and phosphorus of two young American adults. *Pahlavi Medical Journal*, Jan, 1976; 7 (1): 1-17.
18. Reinhold JG, et al. Decreased absorption of calcium, magnesium, zinc and phosphorus by humans due to increased fiber and phosphorus consumption as wheat bread. *Journal of Nutrition*, Apr, 1976; 106 (4): 493-503.
19. Cummings JH, et al. Changes in fecal composition and colonic function due to cereal fiber. *American Journal of Clinical Nutrition*, 1976; 29, 1468-1473.
20. Walker ARP, et al. Studies in human mineral metabolism. I. The effect of bread rich in phytate phosphorous on the metabolism of certain mineral salts with special reference to calcium. *Biochemical Journal*, 1948; 42: 452.
21. Reynolds RD. Bioavailability of vitamin B6 from plant foods. *American Journal of Clinical Nutrition*, 1988; 48: 863-867.
22. Kabir H, et al. Comparative vitamin B-6 bioavailability from tuna, whole wheat bread and peanut butter. *Journal of Nutrition*, 1983; 113: 2412-2420.

23. Gregory JF. Bioavailability of vitamin B6 in nonfat dry milk and a fortified rice breakfast cereal product. *Journal of Food Science,* 1980; 45: 84-86.
24. Leklem JE, et al. Bioavailability of vitamin B6 from wheat bread in humans. *Journal of Nutrition,* 1980; 110: 1819-1828.
25. Lindberg AS, et al. The effect of wheat bran on the bioavailability of vitamin B6 in young men. *Journal of Nutrition,* 1983; 113: 2578-2586.
26. Dollahite J, et al. Problems encountered in meeting the Recommended Dietary Allowances for menus designed according to the Dietary Guidelines for Americans. *Journal of the American Dietetic Association,* Mar, 1995; 95 (3): 341-344.
27. Hansen CM, et al. Assessment of vitamin B-6 status in young women consuming a controlled diet containing four levels of vitamin B-6 provides an estimated average requirement and recommended dietary allowance. *Journal of Nutrition,* Jun, 2001; 131 (6): 1777-1786.
28. Ewer TK: Rachitogenicity of green oats. *Nature,* 1950; 166: 732-733.
29. Hidiroglou M, et al. Effect of a single intramuscular dose of vitamin D on concentrations of liposoluble vitamins in the plasma of heifers winter-fed oat silage, grass silage or hay. *Canadian Journal of Animal Science,* 1980; 60: 311-318.
30. Batchelor AJ, Compston JE: Reduced plasma half-life of radio-labelled 25-hydroxyvitamin D3 in subjects receiving a high fiber diet. *British Journal of Nutrition,* 1983; 49 (2): 213-216.
31. Hollick MF. Vitamin D: importance in the prevention of cancers, type 1 diabetes, heart disease, and osteoporosis. *American Journal of Clinical Nutrition,* 2004; 79 (3): 362-371.
32. Bischoff-Ferrari HA, et al. Effect of Vitamin D on Falls: A Meta-analysis. *Journal of the American Medical Association,* Apr, 2004; 291: 1999-2006.
33. Papadimitropoulos E, et al. VIII: Meta-Analysis of the Efficacy of Vitamin D Treatment in Preventing Osteoporosis in Postmenopausal Women. *Endocrine Reviews,* Aug 1, 2002; 23 (4): 560-569.
34. Hypponen E, Laara E, Reunanen A, Intake of vitamin D and risk of type 1 diabetes: a birth-cohort study. *Lancet,* Nov 3, 2001; 358 (9292): 1500-1503.
35. McAlindon TE, et al. Relation of dietary intake and serum levels of vitamin D to progression of osteoarthritis of the knee among participants in the Framingham Study. *Annals of Internal Medicine,* 1996; 125: 353-359.
36. Lane NE, et al. Serum levels of vitamin D and hip osteoarthritis in elderly women: a longitudinal study. *Arthritis and Rheumatism,* 1997; 40 (suppl): S238.
37. Thys-Jacobs S. Micronutrients and the premenstrual syndrome: the case for calcium. *Journal of the American College of Nutrition,* 2000; 19: 220-227.
38. Vieth R, et al. Randomized comparison of the Effects of the Vitamin D3 Adequate Intake Versus 100 mcg (4000 IU) Per Day on Biochemical Responses and the Wellbeing of Patients. *Nutrition Journal,* Jul 1, 2004; 3 (1): 8.
39. Gloth FM III, et al. Vitamin D vs broad spectrum phototherapy in the treatment of seasonal affective disorder. *Journal of Nutrition, Health & Aging,* 1999; 3 (1): 5-7.
40. Hayes CE. Vitamin D: a natural inhibitor of multiple sclerosis. *Proceedings of the Nutrition Society,* Nov, 2000; 59 (4): 531-535.
41. McMichael AJ, Hall AJ. Multiple sclerosis and ultraviolet radiation: time to shed more light. *Neuroepidemiology,* Aug, 2001; 20 (3): 165-167.
42. Al Faraj S, Al Mutairi K. Vitamin D deficiency and chronic low back pain in Saudi Arabia. *Spine,* Jan 15, 2003; 28 (2): 177-179.
43. Ortlepp JR, et al. The vitamin D receptor gene variant is associated with the prevalence of type 2 diabetes mellitus and coronary artery disease. *Diabetic Medicine,* Oct. 2001; 18 (10): 842-845.
44. Segall JJ. Latitude and ischaemic heart disease. *Lancet,* 1989; 1: 1146.
45. Williams FL, Lloyd OL. Latitude and heart disease. *Lancet,* 1989; 1: 1072-1073.

46. Burr ML, et al. Effects of changes in fat, fish, and fibre intakes on death and myocardial reinfarction: diet and reinfarction trial (DART). *Lancet*, 1989; 2: 757-761.
47. Jenkins DJ, et al. Effect of wheat bran on glycemic control and risk factors for cardiovascular disease in type 2 diabetes. *Diabetes Care*, Sep, 2002; 25 (9): 1522-1528.
48. Hu FB, et al. Dietary protein and risk of ischemic heart disease in women. *American Journal of Clinical Nutrition*, Aug, 1999; 70 (2): 221-227.
49. Acosta PB. Availability of essential amino acids and nitrogen in vegan diets. *American Journal of Clinical Nutrition*, 1988; 48: 868-874.
50. Antony AC. Vegetarianism and vitamin B-12 (cobalamin) deficiency. *American Journal of Clinical Nutrition,* 2003; 78: 3-6.
51. Chan KM, Decker EA. Endogenous skeletal muscle antioxidants. *Critical Reviews in Food Science and Nutrition*, 1994; 34 (4): 403-26.
52. Hipkiss AR. Carnosine. a protective, anti-ageing peptide? *International Journal of Biochemistry & Cell Biology*, 1998; 30: S63-868.
53. Price DL, et al. Chelating Activity of Advanced Glycation End-product Inhibitors. *Journal of Biological Chemistry*, 2001; 276 (52): 48967-48972.
54. Davini P, et al. Controlled study on L-carnitine therapeutic efficacy in post-infarction. *Drugs Under Experimental and Clinical Research,* 1992; 18: 355-365.
55. Sebekova K, et al. Plasma levels of advanced glycation end products in healthy, long-term vegetarians and subjects on a western mixed diet. *European Journal of Nutrition,* Dec, 2001; 40 (6): 275-281.
56. Rizos I. Three-year survival of patients with heart failure caused by dilated cardiomyopathy and L-carnitine administration. *American Heart Journal,* Feb, 2000; 139 (2, Pt 3): S120-123.
57. Iliceto S, et al. Effects of L-carnitine administration on left ventricular remodeling after acute anterior myocardial infarction: the L-Carnitine Ecocardiografia Digitalizzata Infarto Miocardico (CEDIM) Trial. *Journal of the American College Of Cardiology*, Aug, 1995; 26 (2): 380-387.
58. Kreider RB. Effects of creatine supplementation on performance and training adaptations. *Molecular and Cellular Biochemistry*, Feb, 2003; 244 (1-2): 89-94.
59. Andrews R, et al. The effect of dietary creatine supplementation on skeletal muscle metabolism in congestive heart failure. *European Heart Journal*, Apr, 1998; 19 (4): 617-622.
60. Gordon A, et al. Creatine supplementation in chronic heart failure increases skeletal muscle creatine phosphate and muscle performance. *Cardiovascular Research,* Sep, 1995; 30 (3): 413-418.
61. Lukaszuk JM, et al. Effect of creatine supplementation and a lacto-ovo-vegetarian diet on muscle creatine concentration. *International Journal of Sport Nutrition & Exercise Metabolism,* Sept, 2002; 12 (3): 336-348.
62. Harris RC, et al. Absorption of creatine supplied as a drink, in meat or in solid form. *Journal of Sports Sciences*, Feb, 2002; 20 (2): 147-151.
63. Laidlow SA, et al. The taurine content of common foodstuffs. *Journal of Parenteral Enteral Nutrition*, Mar-Apr, 1990; 14 (2): 183-188.
64. Pasantes-Morales H, et al. Taurine content in foods. *Nutrition Reports International*, 1989; 40: 793-801.
65. Schaffer SW, et al. Interaction between the actions of taurine and angiotensin II. *Amino Acids*, 2000; 18 (4): 305-318.
66. Azuma J, et al. Therapeutic effect of taurine in congestive heart failure: a double-blind crossover trial. *Clinical Cardiology*, May, 1985; 8 (5): 276-282.
67. Azuma J, et al. Double-blind randomized crossover trial of taurine in congestive heart failure. *Current Therapeutic Research, Clinical and Experimental*, 1983; 34 (4): 543-57.

68. Laidlaw SA, et al. Plasma and urine taurine levels in vegans. *American Journal of Clinical Nutrition*, 1988; 47: 660-663.
69. Pasantes-Morales H, et al. Taurine content in breast milk of Mexican women from urban and rural areas. *Archives of Medical Research*, Spring, 1995; 26 (1): 47-52.
70. Rice-Evans CA, et al. The relative antioxidant activities of plant-derived polyphenolic flavonoids. *Free Radical Research,* Apr, 1995; 22 (4): 375-83.
71. Wang SY, Jiao H. Scavenging capacity of berry crops on superoxide radicals, hydrogen peroxide, hydroxyl radicals, and singlet oxygen. *Journal of Agricultural and Food Chemistry,* Nov, 2000; 48 (11): 5677-5684.
72. Elliott AJ, et al. Inhibition of glutathione reductase by flavonoids. A structure-activity study. *Biochemical Pharmacology*, Oct 20, 1992; 44 (8): 1603-8.
73. Andriambeloson E, et al. Natural dietary polyphenolic compounds cause endothelium-dependent vasorelaxation in rat thoracic aorta. *Journal of Nutrition*, Dec, 1998; 128 (12): 2324-2333.
74. Bertuglia S, et al. Effect of Vaccinium myrtillus anthocyanosides on ischaemia reperfusion injury in hamster cheek pouch microcirculation. *Pharmacological Research*, Mar-Apr, 1995; 31(3-4): 183-187.
75. Cohen-Boulakia F. In vivo sequential study of skeletal muscle capillary permeability in diabetic rats: effect of anthocyanosides. *Metabolism,* Jul, 2000; 49 (7): 880-885.
76. Tsuda T, et al. Dietary Cyanidin 3-O-ß-d-Glucoside Increases ex vivo Oxidation Resistance of Serum in Rats. *Lipids*, Jun, 1998; 33: 583-588.
77. Preuss HG, et al. Effects of niacin-bound chromium and grape seed proanthocyanidin extract on the lipid profile of hypercholesterolemic subjects: a pilot study. *Journal of Medicine*, 2000; 31 (5-6): 227-246.
78. Pawlowicz P, et al. Administration of natural anthocyanins derived from chokeberry retardation of idiopathic and preeclamptic origin. Influence on metabolism of plasma oxidized lipoproteins: the role of autoantibodies to oxidized low density lipoproteins. *Ginekologia Polska*, Aug, 2000; 71 (8): 848-53.
79. Rissanen TH, et al. Low intake of fruits, berries and vegetables is associated with excess mortality in men: the Kuopio Ischaemic Heart Disease Risk Factor (KIHD) Study. *Journal of Nutrition*, Jan, 2003; 133 (1): 199-204.
80. Ramirez-Tortosa C, et al. Anthocyanin-rich extract decreases indices of lipid peroxidation and DNA damage in vitamin E-depleted rats. *Free Radical Biology & Medicine*, Nov 1, 2001; 31 (9): 1033-1037.
81. Hagiwara A, et al. Pronounced inhibition by a natural anthocyanin, purple corn color, of 2-amino-1-methyl-6-phenylimidazo[4,5-b]pyridine (PhIP)-associated colorectal carcinogenesis in male F344 rats pretreated with 1,2-dimethylhydrazine. *Cancer Letters*, Sep 28, 2001; 171 (1): 17-25.
82. Briviba K, et al. Neurotensin-and EGF-induced metabolic activation of colon carcinoma cells is diminished by dietary flavonoid cyanidin but not by its glycosides. *Nutrition and Cancer*, 2001; 41 (1-2): 172-179.
83. Meiers S, et al. The anthocyanidins cyanidin and delphinidin are potent inhibitors of the epidermal growth-factor receptor. *Journal of Agricultural and Food Chemistry,* Feb, 2001; 49 (2): 958-962.
84. Magistretti MJ, et al. Antiulcer activity of an anthocyanidin from Vaccinium myrtillus. *Arzneimittelforschung*, 1988; 38: 686-90.
85. Cristoni A, Magistretti MJ. Antiulcer and healing activity of Vaccinium myrtillus anthocyanosides. *Farmaco*, 1987; 42: 29-43.
86. Bravetti GO, et al. Preventive Medical Treatment of Senile Cataract with Vitamin E and Vaccinium myrtillus Anthocianosides: Clinical Evaluation, *Annali di Ottalmologia e Clinica Oculistica*, 1987; 115: 109-116.

87. Boniface R. Effect of anthocyanins on human connective tissue metabolism in the human. *Klinische Monatsblatter fur Augenheilkunde*, Dec, 1996; 209 (6): 368-377.
88. Perossini M, et al. Diabetic and Hypertensive Retinopathy Therapy with Vaccinium Myrtillus Anthocianosides (Tegens) Double Blind Placebo-Controlled Clinical Trial, *Annali di Ottalmologia e Clinica Oculistica*, 1987; 12: 1173-1190.
89. Borissova P, et al. Antiinflammatory effect of flavonoids in the natural juice from Aronia melanocarpa, rutin and rutin-magnesium complex on an experimental model of inflammation induced by histamine and serotonin. *Acta Physiologica et Pharmacologica Bulgarica*, 1994; 20 (1): 25-30.
90. Borrud L, et al. What we eat in America: USDA surveys food consumption changes. *Food Review*, Sept-Dec. 1996: 14-19. Available online: http://ers.usda.gov/publications/foodreview/sep1996/sept96d.pdf (accessed September 8, 2005).
91. No listed author. Americans Don't Eat Healthy. *CBSNews.com*, Aug 23, 2004.
92. Johnston CS, et al. More Americans Are Eating "5 A Day" but Intakes of Dark Green and Cruciferous Vegetables Remain Low. *Journal of Nutrition*, 2000; 130: 3063-3067.
93. Halvorsen BL, et al. A systematic screening of total antioxidants in dietary plants. *Journal of Nutrition*, Mar, 2002; 132 (3): 461-471.
94. Wu X, et al. Lipophilic and hydrophilic antioxidant capacities of common foods in the United States. *Journal of Agricultural and Food Chemistry*, Jun 16, 2004; 52 (12): 4026-4037.
95. Liu RH. Health benefits of fruit and vegetables are from additive and synergistic combinations of phytochemicals. *American Journal of Clinical Nutrition*, Sep, 2003; 78 (Suppl 3): 517S-520S.

Chapter 16

1. USDA National Nutrient Database for Standard Reference. Available at USDA web site: http://www.nal.usda.gov/fnic/foodcomp/search/
2. Foster-Powell K, et al. International table of glycemic index and glycemic load values: 2002. *American Journal of Clinical Nutrition*, Jul, 2002; 76 (1): 5-56.
3. Vincent JB. Recent advances in the nutritional biochemistry of trivalent chromium. *Proceedings of the Nutrition Society*, Feb, 2004; 63 (1): 41-47.
4. Kozlovsky AS, et al. Effects of diets high in simple sugars on urinary chromium losses. *Metabolism*, Jun, 1986; 35 (6): 515-518.
5. Mahoney AW, et al. Effects of level and source of dietary fat on the bioavailability of iron from turkey meat for the anemic rat. *Journal of Nutrition*, 1980: 110 (8): 1703-1708.
6. Johnson PE, et al. The effects of stearic acid and beef tallow on iron utilization by the rat. *Proceedings of the Society for Experimental Biology and Medicine*, 1992; 200 (4): 480-486.
7. Koo SI, Ramlet JS. Effect of dietary linoleic acid on the tissue levels of zinc and copper, and serum high-density lipoprotein cholesterol. *Atherosclerosis*, 1984; 50 (2): 123-132.
8. Van Dokkum W, et al. Effect of variations in fat and linoleic acid intake on the calcium, magnesium and iron balance of young men. *Annals of Nutrition & Metabolism*, 1983; 27 (5): 361-369.
9. Lukaski HC, et al. Interactions among dietary fat, mineral status, and performance of endurance athletes: a case study. *International Journal Of Sport Nutrition And Exercise Metabolism*, Jun, 2001; 11 (2): 186-198.
10. Puupponen-Pimiä R, et al. Blanching and long-term freezing affect various bioactive compounds of vegetables in different ways. *Journal of the Science of Food and Agriculture*, 2003; 83 (14): 1389-1402.

11. Vallejo F, et al. Phenolic compound contents in edible parts of broccoli inflorescences after domestic cooking. *Journal of the Science of Food and Agriculture*, Oct, 2003; 83 (14): 1511-1516.

12. Kimura M, Itokawa Y. Cooking losses of minerals in foods and its nutritional significance. *Journal of Nutritional Science and Vitaminology*, 1990; 36, S25-S31.

13. Schroeder H. Losses of vitamins and trace minerals resulting from processing and preservation of foods. *American Journal of Clinical Nutrition*, 1971; 24: 562-573.

14. Maeda N, et al. Aortic wall damage in mice unable to synthesize ascorbic acid. *Proceedings of the National Academy of Sciences USA*, Jan 18, 2000; 97 (2): 841-846.

15. Nakata Y, Maeda N. Vulnerable atherosclerotic plaque morphology in apolipoprotein E-deficient mice unable to make ascorbic Acid. *Circulation*, Mar 26, 2002; 105 (12): 1485-1490.

16. Gey KF, et al. Poor plasma status of carotene and vitamin C is associated with higher mortality from ischemic heart disease and stroke: Basel Prospective Study. *Clinical Investigation*, Jan, 1993; 71 (1): 3-6.

17. Osganian SK, et al. Vitamin C and risk of coronary heart disease in women. *Journal of the American College of Cardiology*, Jul 16, 2003; 42 (2): 246-252.

18. Kurl S, et al. Plasma vitamin C modifies the association between hypertension and risk of stroke. *Stroke*, Jun, 2002; 33 (6): 1568-1573.

19. Yokoyama T, et al. Serum vitamin C concentration was inversely associated with subsequent 20-year incidence of stroke in a Japanese rural community. The Shibata study. *Stroke*, Oct, 2000; 31 (10): 2287-2294.

20. Daviglus ML, et al. Dietary vitamin C, beta-carotene and 30-year risk of stroke: results from the Western Electric Study. *Neuroepidemiology*, 1997; 16 (2): 69-77.

21. Eaton SB, et al. An evolutionary perspective enhances understanding of human nutritional requirements. *Journal of Nutrition*, 1996; 126: 1732-1740. Note: Eaton et al calculated that the average daily vitamin C intake during the late Paleolithic era was 440 milligrams, based on an estimated ratio of animal/plant food intake among Paleolithic hunter-gatherers of 35:65. The authors later performed a re-analysis and revised this estimated ratio to 65:35 (Cordain L, et al. Plant-animal subsistence ratios and macronutrient energy estimations in worldwide hunter-gatherer diets. *American Journal of Clinical Nutrition*, Mar, 2000; 71 (3): 682-692). Assuming average calorie intakes among hunter-gatherers of between 1,800-3,500 per day, such a ratio would still deliver far higher amounts of vitamin C than that consumed by most modern populations.

22. *Vitamin C in Health and Disease*. Eds: Packer L, Fuchs J. Marcel Dekker Inc., New York, 1997.

23. Hampl JS, et al. Vitamin C Deficiency and Depletion in the United States: The Third National Health and Nutrition Examination Survey, 1988-1994. *American Journal of Public Health,* May, 2004; 94, 5; 870-875.

24. Heart Protection Study Collaborative Group. MRC/BHF Heart Protection Study of antioxidant vitamin supplementation in 20,536 high-risk individuals: a randomised placebo-controlled trial. *Lancet*, Jul 6, 2002; 360 (9326): 23-33.

25. Age-Related Eye Disease Study Research Group. A Randomized, Placebo-Controlled, Clinical Trial of High-Dose Supplementation With Vitamins C and E and Beta Carotene for Age-Related Cataract and Vision Loss: AREDS Report No. 9. *Archives of Ophthalmology*, Oct, 2001; 119: 1439-1452.

26. Blot WJ, et al. Nutrition intervention trials in Linxian, China: supplementation with specific vitamin/mineral combinations, cancer incidence, and disease-specific mortality in the general population. *Journal of the National Cancer Institute*, Sep 15, 1993; 85 (18): 1483-1492.

27. Samman S, et al. A mixed fruit and vegetable concentrate increases plasma antioxidant vitamins and folate and lowers plasma homocysteine in men. *Journal of Nutrition*, Jul, 2003; 133 (7): 2188-2193.
28. Freese R, et al. High intakes of vegetables, berries, and apples combined with a high intake of linoleic or oleic acid only slightly affect markers of lipid peroxidation and lipoprotein metabolism in healthy subjects. *American Journal of Clinical Nutrition*, Nov, 2002; 76 (5): 950-960.
29. Record IR, et al. Changes in plasma antioxidant status following consumption of diets high or low in fruit and vegetables or following dietary supplementation with an antioxidant mixture. *British Journal of Nutrition*, Apr, 2001; 85 (4): 459-464.
30. Broekmans WM, et al. Fruits and vegetables increase plasma carotenoids and vitamins and decrease homocysteine in humans. *Journal of Nutrition*, Jun, 2000; 130 (6): 1578-1583.
31. Huxley RR, Neil HA. The relation between dietary flavonol intake and coronary heart disease mortality: a meta-analysis of prospective cohort studies. *European Journal of Clinical Nutrition*, Aug, 2003; 57 (8): 904-908.
32. Knekt P, et al. Flavonoid intake and risk of chronic diseases. *American Journal of Clinical Nutrition*, Sep, 2002; 76 (3): 560-568.
33. Ohtsuki K, et al. Effects of long-term administration of hesperidin and glucosyl hesperidin to spontaneously hypertensive rats. *Journal of Nutritional Science and Vitaminology*, Oct, 2002; 48 (5): 420-422.
34. Havsteen B. Flavonoids, a class of natural products of high pharmacological potency. *Biochemical Pharmacology*, Apr 1, 1983; 32 (7): 1141-1148.
35. Tixier JM, et al. Evidence by in vivo and in vitro studies that binding of pycnogenols to elastin affects its rate of degradation by elastases. *Biochemical Pharmacology*, Dec 15, 1984; 33 (24): 3933-3939.
36. Duarte J, et al. Antihypertensive effects of the flavonoid quercetin in spontaneously hypertensive rats. *British Journal of Pharmacology*, May, 2001; 133 (1): 117-124.
37. Mokrzycki K. Anti-atherosclerotic efficacy of quercetin and sodium phenylbutyrate in rabbits. *Annales Academiae Medicae Stetinensis,* 2000; 46: 189-200.
38. Yamakoshi J, et al. Proanthocyanidin-rich extract from grape seeds attenuates the development of aortic atherosclerosis in cholesterol-fed rabbits. *Atherosclerosis,* Jan, 1999; 142 (1): 139-149.
39. Aviram M, et al. Pomegranate juice consumption reduces oxidative stress, atherogenic modifications to LDL, and platelet aggregation: studies in humans and in atherosclerotic apolipoprotein E-deficient mice. *American Journal of Clinical Nutrition*, May, 2000; 71 (5): 1062-1076.
40. Vinson JA, Bose P. Comparative bioavailability to humans of ascorbic acid alone or in a citrus extract. *American Journal of Clinical Nutrition*, Sep, 1988; 48 (3): 601-604.
41. Milde J, et al. Synergistic inhibition of low-density lipoprotein oxidation by rutin, gamma-terpinene, and ascorbic acid. *Phytomedicine*, Feb, 2004; 11 (2-3): 105-113.
42. Tesoriere L, et al. Supplementation with cactus pear (Opuntia ficus-indica) fruit decreases oxidative stress in healthy humans: a comparative study with vitamin C. *American Journal of Clinical Nutrition*, 2004; 80: 391-395.

Chapter 17

1. Miller RA, Britigan BE. Role of oxidants in microbial pathophysiology. *Clinical Microbiology Reviews*, Jan, 1997; 10 (1): 1-18.
2. Gordillo GM, Sen CK. Revisiting the essential role of oxygen in wound healing. *American Journal of Surgery,* Sep, 2003; 186 (3): 259-263.

3. Ridker PM, et al. Comparison of C-reactive protein and low density lipoprotein cholesterol levels in the prediction of first cardiovascular events. *New England Journal of Medicine*, 2002; 347 (20): 1557-1565.

4. Steinberg D. Lewis A. Conner Memorial Lecture: Oxidative Modification of LDL and Atherogenesis. *Circulation*, Feb, 1997; 95: 1062-1071.

5. Goldstein JL, et al. Binding site on macrophages that mediates uptake and degradation of acetylated low density lipoprotein, producing massive cholesterol deposition. *Proceedings of the National Academy of Sciences USA*, 1979; 76: 333-337.

6. Weinstein DB, et al. Uptake and degradation of low density lipoprotein by swine arterial smooth muscle cells with inhibition of cholesterol biosynthesis. *Biochimica et Biophysica Acta*, 1976; 424: 404-421.

7. Sasahara M, et al. Inhibition of hypercholesterolemia-induced atherosclerosis in the nonhuman primate by probucol, I: is the extent of atherosclerosis related to resistance of LDL to oxidation? *Journal of Clinical Investigation*, 1994; 94: 155-164

8. Tangirala RK, et al. Effect of the antioxidant N,N'-diphenyl 1,4-phenylenediamine (DPPD) on atherosclerosis in apo E–deficient mice. *Arteriosclerosis, Thrombosis, and Vascular Biology,* 1995;15:1625-1630

9. Carew TE, et al. Antiatherogenic effect of probucol unrelated to its hypocholesterolemic effect: evidence that antioxidants in vivo can selectively inhibit low density lipoprotein degradation in macrophage-rich fatty streaks and slow the progression of atherosclerosis in the Watanabe heritable hyperlipidemic rabbit. *Proceedings of the National Academy of Sciences USA*, 1987; 84: 7725-7729.

10. Daugherty A, et al. Probucol attenuates the development of aortic atherosclerosis in cholesterol-fed rabbits. *British Journal of Pharmacology*, 1989; 98: 612-618.

11. Bjorkhem I, et al. The antioxidant butylated hydroxytoluene protects against atherosclerosis. *Arteriosclerosis and Thrombosis*, 1991;11:15-22.

12. Holvoet P, et al. The Metabolic Syndrome, Circulating Oxidized LDL, and Risk of Myocardial Infarction in Well-Functioning Elderly People in the Health, Aging, and Body Composition Cohort. *Diabetes*, Apr 1, 2004; 53(4): 1068-1073.

13. Holvoet P, et al. Association of High Coronary Heart Disease Risk Status With Circulating Oxidized LDL in the Well-Functioning Elderly: Findings From the Health, Aging, and Body Composition Study. *Arteriosclerosis, Thrombosis, and Vascular Biology,* Aug 1, 2003; 23(8): 1444 - 1448.

14. Nishi K, et al. Oxidized LDL in Carotid Plaques and Plasma Associates With Plaque Instability. *Arteriosclerosis, Thrombosis, and Vascular Biology*, Oct 1, 2002; 22 (10): 1649-1654.

15. Kristenson M, et al. Antioxidant state and mortality from coronary heart disease in lithuanian and swedish men: concomitant cross sectional study of men aged 50. *British Medical Journal*, Mar, 1997; 314: 629.

16. Hecht HS, Harman SM. Relation of aggressiveness of lipid-lowering treatment to changes in calcified plaque burden by electron beam tomography. *American Journal of Cardiology,* Aug 1, 2003; 92 (3): 334-336.

17. Ammouche A, et al. Effect of ingestion of thermally oxidized sunflower oil on the fatty acid composition and antioxidant enzymes of rat liver and brain in development. *Annals of Nutrition and Metabolism*, 2001; 46: 268-275.

18. Giani E, et al. Heated fat, vitamin E and vascular eicosanoids. *Lipids*, Jul, 1985; 20 (7): 439-448.

19. Hageman G, et al. Biological effects of short-term feeding to rats of repeatedly used deep-frying fats in relation to fat mutagen content. *Food and Chemical Toxicology*, Oct, 1991; 29 (10): 689-698.

20. Liu JF, Lee YW. Vitamin C supplementation restores the impaired vitamin E status of guinea pigs fed oxidized frying oil. *Journal of Nutrition*, Jan, 1998; 128 (1): 116-122.

21. Eder K. The effects of a dietary oxidized oil on lipid metabolism in rats. *Lipids*, Jul, 1999; 34 (7): 717-725.
22. Sutherland WHF. Effect of meals rich in heated olive and safflower oils on oxidation of postprandial serum in healthy men. *Atherosclerosis*, 2002 ; 160 (1) : 195-203.
23. Jenkinson A, et al. Dietary intakes of polyunsaturated fatty acids and indices of oxidative stress in human volunteers. *European Journal of Clinical Nutrition*, Jul, 1999; 53 (7): 523-528.
24. Turpeinen AM, et al. A high linoleic acid diet increases oxidative stress in vivo and affects nitric oxide metabolism in humans. *Prostaglandins, Leukotrienes and Essential Fatty Acids*, 1998; 59 (3): 229-233.
25. Reaven P, et al. Feasibility of using an oleate-rich diet to reduce the susceptibility of low-density lipoprotein to oxidative modification in humans. *American Journal of Clinical Nutrition*, Oct, 1991; 54: 701-706.
26. Nenseter MS, Drevon CA. Dietary polyunsaturates and peroxidation of low density lipoprotein. *Current Opinion in Lipidology*, Feb, 1996; 7 (1): 8-13.
27. Rose GA, et al. Corn oil in treatment of ischaemic heart disease. *British Medical Journal*, 1965; 1: 1531-1533.
28. Kristenson M, et al. Antioxidant state and mortality from coronary heart disease in Lithuanian and Swedish men: concomitant cross sectional study of men aged 50. *British Medical Journal*, Mar 1, 1997; 314: 629.
29. Kristenson M, et al. Lower serum levels of beta-carotene in Lithuanian men are accompanied by higher urinary excretion of the oxidative DNA adduct, 8-hydroxydeoxyguanosine. The LiVicordia study. *Nutrition*, Jan, 2003; 19 (1): 11-15.
30. Phelps S, Harris WS. Garlic supplementation and lipoprotein oxidation susceptibility. *Lipids*, May, 1993; 28 (5): 475-477.
31. Staprans I, et al. Oxidized cholesterol in the diet is a source of oxidized lipoproteins in human serum. *Journal of Lipid Research*, Apr 1, 2003; 44 (4): 705 - 715.
32. Chopra M, et al. Influence of increased fruit and vegetable intake on plasma and lipoprotein carotenoids and LDL oxidation in smokers and nonsmokers. *Clinical Chemistry*, Nov, 2000; 46 (11): 1818-1829.
33. Harats D, et al. Citrus fruit supplementation reduces lipoprotein oxidation in young men ingesting a diet high in saturated fat: presumptive evidence for an interaction between vitamins C and E in vivo. *American Journal of Clinical Nutrition*, Feb, 1998; 67 (2): 240-245.
34. Folts JD. Potential health benefits from the flavonoids in grape products on vascular disease. *Advances in Experimental Medicine and Biology*, 2002; 505: 95-111.
35. Bub A, et al. Moderate intervention with carotenoid-rich vegetable products reduces lipid peroxidation in men. *Journal of Nutrition*, Sep, 2000; 130 (9): 2200-2206.
36. Samman S, et al. A mixed fruit and vegetable concentrate increases plasma antioxidant vitamins and folate and lowers plasma homocysteine in men. *Journal of Nutrition*, Jul, 2003; 133 (7): 2188-2193.
37. Takyi EE. Children's consumption of dark green, leafy vegetables with added fat enhances serum retinol. *Journal of Nutrition*, 1999; 129 (8): 1549-1554.
38. Jalal F, et al. Serum retinol concentrations are affected by food sources of ß-carotene, fat intake, and anthehelmintic drug treatment. *American Journal of Clinical Nutrition*, 1998; 68: 623-629.
39. Drammeh BS, et al. A Randomized, 4-Month Mango and Fat Supplementation Trial Improved Vitamin A Status among Young Gambian Children. *Journal of Nutrition*, 2002; 132 (12): 3693 - 3699.
40. Brown MJ, et al. Carotenoid bioavailabilty is higher from salads ingested with full-fat than with fat-reduced salad dressings as measured with electrochemical detection. *American Journal of Clinical Nutrition*, Aug, 2004; 80: 396-403.

41. Dwyer JH, et al. Progression of Carotid Intima-Media Thickness and Plasma Antioxidants: The Los Angeles Atherosclerosis Study. *Arteriosclerosis, Thrombosis, and Vascular Biology*, Feb 1, 2004; 24 (2): 313-319.
42. Mares-Perlman JA, et al. The Body of Evidence to Support a Protective Role for Lutein and Zeaxanthin in Delaying Chronic Disease. Overview. *Journal of Nutrition*, Mar 1, 2002; 132 (3): 518S-524.
43. Roodenburg JA, et al. Amount of fat in the diet affects bioavailability of lutein esters but not of {alpha}-carotene, {beta}-carotene, and vitamin E in humans. *American Journal of Clinical Nutrition*, 2000; 71 (5): 1187-1193.
44. Capps O, et al. Dietary behaviors associated with total fat and saturated fat intake. *Journal of the American Dietetic Association*, 2002; 102: 490-502.
45. Iuliano L, et al. Bioavailability of Vitamin E as Function of Food Intake in Healthy Subjects: Effects on Plasma Peroxide–Scavenging Activity and Cholesterol-Oxidation Products. *Arteriosclerosis, Thrombosis, and Vascular Biology*, 2001; 21: e34.
46. Kaushik S, et al. Removal of fat from cow's milk decreases the vitamin E contents of the resulting dairy products. *Lipids,* Jan, 2001; 36 (1): 73-78.
47. Elosua R, et al. Response of oxidative stress biomarkers to a 16-week aerobic physical activity program, and to acute physical activity, in healthy young men and women. *Atherosclerosis*, Apr, 2003; 167 (2): 327-334.
48. Powers SK, et al. Exercise training-induced alterations in skeletal muscle antioxidant capacity: a brief review. *Medicine and Science in Sports and Exercise*, Jul, 1999; 31 (7): 987-997.
49. Bergholm R, et al. Intense physical training decreases circulating antioxidants and endothelium-dependent vasodilatation in vivo. *Atherosclerosis*, Aug, 1999; 145(2):341-349.
50. Watson TA, et al. Antioxidant restricted diet increases oxidative stress during acute exhaustive exercise. *Asia Pacific Journal of Clinical Nutrition*, 2003; 12 (Suppl): S9.

Chapter 18

1. Narayan KM, et al. Lifetime risk for diabetes mellitus in the United States. *Journal of the American Medical Association*, Oct 8, 2003; 290 (14): 1884-1890.
2. Tominaga M, et al. Impaired glucose tolerance is a risk factor for cardiovascular disease, but not impaired fasting glucose: the Funagata Diabetes Study. *Diabetes Care*, 1999; 22: 920-924.
3. Barzilay JI, et al. Cardiovascular disease in older adults with glucose disorders: comparison of American Diabetes Association criteria for diabetes mellitus with WHO criteria. *Lancet*, 1999; 354: 622–625.
4. Barrett-Connor E, Ferrara A. Isolated postchallenge hyperglycemia and the risk of fatal cardiovascular disease in older women and men: The Rancho Bernardo Study. *Diabetes Care*, 1998; 21: 1236–1239.
5. Shaw JE, et al. Isolated post-challenge hyperglycaemia confirmed as a risk factor for mortality. *Diabetologia*, 1999; 42: 1050–1054.
6. Saydah SH, et al. Postchallenge Hyperglycemia and Mortality in a National Sample of U.S. Adults. *Diabetes Care*, 2001; 24: 1397-1402.
7. Meigs JB, et al. Fasting and Postchallenge Glycemia and Cardiovascular Disease Risk. The Framingham Offspring Study. *Diabetes Care*, 2002; 25: 1845-1850.
8. Glucose tolerance and mortality: comparison of WHO and American Diabetes Association diagnostic criteria: the DECODE study group: European Diabetes Epidemiology Group. Diabetes epidemiology: collaborative analysis of diagnostic criteria in Europe. *Lancet*, 1999; 354: 617-621.
9. Tuomilehto J, et al. The effect of diabetes and impaired glucose tolerance on mortality in Malta. *Diabetic Medicine,* 1994; 11: 170-176.

10. Tominaga M, et al. Impaired glucose tolerance is a risk factor for cardiovascular disease, but not impaired fasting glucose: the Funagata Diabetes Study. *Diabetes Care*, 1999; 22: 920-924.
11. Stengard JH, et al. Diabetes mellitus, impaired glucose tolerance and mortality among elderly men: the Finnish cohorts of the Seven Countries Study. *Diabetologia*, 1992; 35: 760-765.
12. Shaw JE, et al. Isolated post-challenge hyperglycaemia confirmed as a risk factor for mortality. *Diabetologia*, 1999; 42: 1050-1054.
13. Barrett-Connor E, Ferrara A. Isolated postchallenge hyperglycemia and the risk of fatal cardiovascular disease in older women and men: the Rancho Bernardo Study. *Diabetes Care*, 1998; 21: 1236-1239.
14. Knowler W, et al. Glucose tolerance and mortality including a sub-study of tolbutamide treatment. *Diabetologia*, 1997; 40:680-686.
15. Burchfiel C, et al. Cardiovascular risk factors and impaired glucose tolerance: the San Luis Valley Diabetes Study. *American Journal of Epidemiology*, 1990; 131: 57-70.
16. Wei M, et al. Effects of diabetes and level of glycemia on all-cause and cardiovascular mortality: the San Antonio Heart Study. *Diabetes Care*, 1998; 21: 1167-1172.
17. Saydah SH, et al. Postchallenge Hyperglycemia and Mortality in a National Sample of U.S. Adults. *Diabetes Care*, 2001; 24: 1397-1402.
18. Lowe LP, et al. Diabetes, asymptomatic hyperglycemia, and 22-year mortality in black and white men: the Chicago Heart Association Detection Project in Industry Study. *Diabetes Care*, 1997; 20: 163-169.
19. Yano K, et al. Glucose intolerance and nine-year mortality in Japanese men in Hawaii. *American Journal of Medicine*, 1982; 72: 71-80.
20. Sala J, et al. Short-term mortality of myocardial infarction patients with diabetes or hyperglycaemia during admission. *Journal of Epidemiology and Community Health*, 2002; 56: 707-712.
21. Coutinho M, et al. The relationship between glucose and incident cardiovascular events. A metaregression analysis of published data from 20 studies of 95,783 individuals followed for 12.4 years. *Diabetes Care*, 1999; 22: 233-240.
22. Centers for Disease Control and Prevention (CDC). Prevalence of diabetes and impaired fasting glucose in adults--United States, 1999-2000. *MMR Weekly*, Sep 5, 2003; 52 (35): 833-837.
23. Bjornholt JV, et al. Fasting blood glucose: an underestimated risk factor for cardiovascular death. Results from a 22-year follow-up of healthy nondiabetic men. *Diabetes Care*, 1999; 22: 45-49.
24. Wei M, et al. Low Fasting Plasma Glucose Level as a Predictor of Cardiovascular Disease and All-Cause Mortality. *Circulation*, May, 2000; 101: 2047-2052.
25. The DECODE Study Group. Is the Current Definition for Diabetes Relevant to Mortality Risk From All Causes and Cardiovascular and Noncardiovascular Diseases? *Diabetes Care*, 2003; 26: 688-696.
26. Smith NL, et al. Fasting and 2-hour postchallenge serum glucose measures and risk of incident cardiovascular events in the elderly. *Archives of Internal Medicine*, Jan 28, 2002; 162: 209-216.
27. Reid DD, et al. Cardiorespitory disease and diabetes among middle-aged civil servants: a study of screening and intervention. *Lancet*, 1974; i: 469-473.
28. Ducimetiere P, et al. Relationship of plasma insulin levels to the incidence of myocardial infarction and coronary heart disease mortality in a middle-aged population. *Diabetiologia*, 1980; 19: 205-210.
29. Pyorala K, et al. Glucose intolerance and coronary heart disease: Helsinki Policeman Study. *Journal of Chronic Diseases*, 1979; 32: 729-745.

30. Lyons TJ. Glycation and oxidation: A role in the pathogenesis of atherosclerosis. *American Journal of Cardiology*, Feb 25, 1993; 71: 26B-31B.
31. Marfella R, et al. Glutathione reverses systemic hemodynamic changes induced by acute hyperglycemia in healthy subjects. *American Journal of Physiology*, Jun, 1995; 268 (6 Pt 1): E1167-1173.
32. Williams SB, et al. Acute hyperglycemia attenuates endothelium-dependent vasodilation in humans in vivo. *Circulation*, 1998; 97: 1695-1701.
33. Ceriello A, et al. Hyperglycemia-induced thrombin formation in diabetes. The possible role of oxidative stress. *Diabetes*, 1995; 44: 924-928.
34. Ceriello A, et al. Meal-generated oxidative stress in type 2 diabetic patients. *Diabetes Care*, 1998; 21: 1529-1533.
35. Ceriello A, et al. Antioxidant defenses are reduced during oral glucose tolerance test in normal and non-insulin-dependant subjects. *European Journal of Clinical Investigation*, 1998; 28: 329-333.
36. Mohanty P, et al. Glucose Challenge Stimulates Reactive Oxygen Species (ROS) Generation by Leucocytes. *Journal of Clinical Endocrinology & Metabolism*, 2000; 85: 2970-2973.
37. Sanchez A, et al. Role of sugars in human neutrophilic phagocytosis. *American Journal of Clinical Nutrition,* 1973; 26: 1180-1184.
38. Price KD, et al. Hyperglycemia-induced ascorbic acid deficiency promotes endothelial dysfunction and the development of atherosclerosis. *Atherosclerosis*, Sep, 2001; 158 (1): 1-12.
39. Will JC, Byers T. Does diabetes mellitus increase the requirement for vitamin C? *Nutrition Reviews*, Jul, 1996; 54 (7): 193-202.
40. Tessier D, et al. Effects of an oral glucose challenge on free radicals/antioxidants balance in an older population with type II diabetes. *Journals of Gerontology. Series A, Biological Sciences and Medical Sciences,* Nov, 1999; 54 (11): M541-M545.
41. O'Riordan M. Early and intensive glucose control significantly reduces the risk of future cardiovascular events. *TheHeart.org HeartWire*, Jun 14, 2005. Available online: http://www.theheart.org/viewArticle.do?primaryKey=505423 (accessed Jun 15, 2005).
42. Benjamin SM, et al. Estimated number of adults with prediabetes in the US in 2000: opportunities for prevention. *Diabetes Care*, Mar, 2003; 26 (3): 645-649.
43. Yudkin J. Diet and coronary thrombosis. Hypothesis and fact. *Lancet,* Jul 27, 1957; ii: 155-162.
44. Liu S, et al. A prospective study of dietary glycemic load, carbohydrate intake, and risk of coronary heart disease in US women. *American Journal of Clinical Nutrition,* 2000; 71: 1455–1461.
45. USDA US Food Supply database. Available online at: http://www.nal.usda.gov/fnic/foodcomp/search/
46. Olshansky SJ, et al. A Potential Decline in Life Expectancy in the United States in the 21st Century. *New England Journal of Medicine*, Mar 17, 2005; 352 (11): 1138-1145.
47. Obesity Threatens to Cut U.S. Life Expectancy, New Analysis Suggests. National Institute on Aging (NIA) Press Release, Wed, Mar 16, 2005. Available online: http://www.nih.gov/news/pr/mar2005/nia-16.htm (accessed September 8, 2005).
48. Baba NH, et al. High Protein vs High Carbohydrate Hypoenergetic Diet for the Treatment of Obese Hyperinsulinemic Subjects. *International Journal of Obesity*, 1999; 11: 1202-1206.
49. Volek JS, et al. Comparison of a Very Low-Carbohydrate and Low-Fat Diet on Fasting Lipids, LDL Subclasses, Insulin Resistance, and Postprandial Lipemic Responses in Overweight Women. *Journal of the American College of Nutrition*, 2004; 23 (2): 177-184.

50. Brehm BJ, et al., A Randomized Trial Comparing a Very Low Carbohydrate Diet and a Calorie-Restricted Low Fat Diet on Body Weight and Cardiovascular Risk Factors in Healthy Women. *Journal of Clinical Endocrinology and Metabolism*, 2003; 88 (4): 1617-1623.

51. Lewis SB, et al. Effect of Diet Composition on Metabolic Adaptations to Hypocaloric Nutrition: Comparison of High Carbohydrate and High Fat Isocaloric Diets. *American Journal of Clinical Nutrition*, 1977; 30 (2): 160-170.

52. Volek JS, et al. Body Composition and Hormonal responses to a Carbohydrate Restricted Diet. *Metabolism*, 51(7), 2002, pages 864-870.

53. Layman DK, et al. Increased Dietary Protein Modifies Glucose and Insulin Homeostasis in Adult Women during Weight Loss. *Journal of Nutrition*, 2003; 133 (2): 405-410.

54. Farnsworth E, et al. Effect of a high-protein, energy-restricted diet on body composition, glycemic control, and lipid concentrations in overweight and obese hyperinsulinemic men and women. *American Journal of Clinical Nutrition*, Jul, 2003; 78: 31-39.

55. Heilbronn LK, et al. Effect of Energy Restriction, Weight Loss, and Diet Composition on Plasma Lipids and Glucose in Patients With Type 2 Diabetes. *Diabetes Care*, 1999; 22 (6): 889-895.

56. Gumbiner B, et al. Effects of diet composition and ketosis on glycemia during very-low-energy-diet therapy in obese patients with non-insulin-dependent diabetes mellitus. *American Journal of Clinical Nutrition*, 1996; 63: 110-115.

57. Piatti PM, et al. Hypocaloric high protein diet improves glucose oxidation and spares lean body mass. Comparison to hypocaloric high-CHO diet. *Metabolism*, Dec, 1994; 43 (12): 1481-1487.

58. Rabast U, et al. Dietetic treatment of obesity with low and high carbohydrate diets: Comparitive studies and clinical results. *International Journal of Obesity*, 1979; 3 (3): 201-211.

59. Fujita Y, et al. Basal and postprotein insulin and glucagon levels during a high and low carbohydrate intake and their relationships to plasma triglycerides. *Diabetes*, 1975; 24 (6): 552-558.

60. Brehm B, et al. A randomized trial comparing a very low carbohydrate diet and a calorie-restricted low fat diet on body weight and cardiovascular risk factors in healthy women. *Journal of Clinical Endocrinology and Metabolism*, 2003; 88 (4): 1617-1623.

61. Foster GD, et al. A randomized trial of a low-carbohydrate diet for obesity. *New England Journal of Medicine*, May 22, 2003; 348: 2082-2090.

62. Samaha FF, et al. A low-carbohydrate diet as compared with a low fat diet in severe obesity. *New England Journal of Medicine*, May 22, 2003; 348: 2074-2081.

63. Yudkin J, Carey M. The treatment of obesity by the "high fat" diet: the inevitability of calories. *Lancet*, Oct 29, 1960; 2: 939-941.

64. Yancy WS, et al. A Low-Carbohydrate, Ketogenic Diet versus a Low-Fat Diet To Treat Obesity and Hyperlipidemia: A Randomized, Controlled Trial. *Annals of Internal Medicine*, 2004; 140: 769-777.

65. Hays JH, et al. Effect of a high saturated fat diet and no-starch diet on serum lipid subfractions in patients with documented atherosclerotic cardiovascular disease. *Mayo Clinic Proceedings*, 2003; 78: 1331-1336.

66. Dashti HM, et al. Ketogenic diet modifies the risk factors of heart disease in obese patients. *Nutrition*, 2003; 19: 901-902.

67. Golay A, et al. Similar weight loss with low- or high-carbohydrate diets. *American Journal of Clinical Nutrition*, Feb, 1996; 63: 174-178.

68. Torbay N, et al. High protein vs high carbohydrate hypoenergetic diet in treatment of obese normoinsulinemic and hyperinsulinemic subjects. *Nutrition Research*, May, 2002; 22 (5): 587-598.

69. Samaha FF, et al. A low-carbohydrate diet as compared with a low fat diet in severe obesity. *New England Journal of Medicine*, May 22, 2003; 348: 2074-2081.
70. Coulston AM, et al. Deleterious metabolic effects of high-carbohydrate, sucrose-containing diets in patients with non-insulin-dependent diabetes mellitus. *American Journal of Medicine*, Feb, 1987; 82 (2): 213-220.
71. Garg A, et al. Effects of varying carbohydrate content of diet in patients with non-insulin-dependent diabetes mellitus. *Journal of the American Medical Association*, 1994; 271: 1421-1428.
72. Sestoft L, et al. High-carbohydrate, low-fat diet: effect on lipid and carbohydrate metabolism, GIP and insulin secretion in diabetics. *Danish Medical Bulletin*, 1985 Mar; 32 (1): 64-69.
73. Gannon MC, et al. An increase in dietary protein improves the blood glucose response in persons with type 2 diabetes. *American Journal of Clinical Nutrition*, 2003; 78: 734-741.
74. Bisschop PH, et al. Dietary fat content alters insulin-mediated glucose metabolism in healthy men. *American Journal of Clinical Nutrition*, 2001; 73: 554-559.
75. McLaughlin T, et al. Carbohydrate-Induced Hypertriglyceridemia: An Insight into the Link between Plasma Insulin and Triglyceride Concentrations. *Journal of Clinical Endocrinology & Metabolism*, Sep, 2000; 85: 3085-3088.
76. Gutierrez M, et al. Utility of a Short-Term 25% Carbohydrate Diet on Improving Glycemic Control in Type 2 Diabetes Mellitus. *Journal of the American College of Nutrition*, 1998; 17 (6): 595-600.

Chapter 19
1. Gerster H. Can adults adequately convert alpha-linolenic acid (18:3n-3) to eicosapentaenoic acid (20:5n-3) and docosahexaenoic acid (22:6n-3)? *International Journal for Vitamin and Nutrition Research*, 1998; 68 (3): 159-173.
2. Pawlosky RJ, et al. Physiological compartmental analysis of alpha-linolenic acid metabolism in adult humans. *Journal of Lipid Research*, 2001; 42: 1257–1265.
3. Simopoulos AP. The importance of the ratio of omega-6/omega-3 essential fatty acids. *Biomedicine & Pharmacotherapy*, Oct, 2002; 56 (8): 365-379.
4. Simopoulos AP. Essential fatty acids in health and chronic disease. *American Journal of Clinical Nutrition*, Sep, 1999; 70 (3 Suppl): 560S-569S.
5. Lands WE. Eicosanoids and health. *Annals of the New York Academy of Sciences*, 1993; 676: 46-59.
6. Lands WE. Biosynthesis of prostaglandins. *Annual Review of Nutrition*, 1991; 11: 41-60.
7. Carpenter KL, et al. Lipids and oxidised lipids in human atheroma and normal aorta. *Biochimica et Biophysica Acta*, Apr 7, 1993 ; 1167 (2): 121-130.
8. Felton CV, et al. Dietary polyunsaturated fatty acids and composition of human aortic plaques. *Lancet*, 1994; 344: 1195-1196.
9. Felton CV, et al. Relation of Plaque Lipid Composition and Morphology to the Stability of Human Aortic Plaques. *Arteriosclerosis, Thrombosis, and Vascular Biology*, 1997; 17: 1337-1345.
10. Thies F, et al. Association of n-3 polyunsaturated fatty acids with stability of atherosclerotic plaques: a randomised controlled trial. *Lancet*, 2003; 361: 477-485.
11. Lands WE, et al. Changing dietary patterns. *American Journal of Clinical Nutrition*, Jun, 1990; 51 (6): 991-993.
12. Burr ML, et al. Effects of changes in fat, fish, and fibre intakes on death and myocardial reinfarction: diet and reinfarction trial (DART). *Lancet*, 1989; 2: 757–761.
13. Marchioli R, et al. Early protection against sudden death by n-3 polyunsaturated fatty acids after myocardial infarction: time-course analysis of the results of the Gruppo Italiano per lo Studio della Sopravvivenza nell'Infarto Miocardico (GISSI)-Prevenzione. *Circulation*, 2002; 105: 1897–1903.

14. Oomen CM, et al. Association between trans fatty acid intake and 10-year risk of coronary heart disease in the Zutphen Elderly Study: a prospective population-based study. *Lancet*, Mar 10, 2001; 357 (9258): 746-751.
15. Rozenn N, et al, Cell Membrane Trans-Fatty Acids and the Risk of Primary Cardiac Arrest, *Circulation*, 2002; 105: 697.
16. Pedersen JI, et al, Adipose tissue fatty acids and risk of myocardial infarction--a case-control study. *European Journal of Clinical Nutrition*, Aug, 2000; 54 (8): 618-625.
17. Han SN, et al, Effect of hydrogenated and saturated, relative to polyunsaturated, fat on immune and inflammatory responses of adults with moderate hypercholesterolemia. *Journal of Lipid Research*, Mar, 2002; 43 (3): 445-52.
18. Muller H, et al, Partially hydrogenated soybean oil reduces postprandial t-PA activity compared with palm oil. *Atherosclerosis*, Apr, 2001; 155 (2): 467-476.
19. Kummerow FA, et al. Effect of trans fatty acids on calcium influx into human arterial endothelial cells. *American Journal of Clinical Nutrition*, Nov, 1999; 70 (5): 832-838.
20. Kummerow FA, et al. Trans fatty acids in hydrogenated fat inhibited the synthesis of the polyunsaturated fatty acids in the phospholipid of arterial cells. *Life Sciences*, Apr 16, 2004; 74 (22): 2707-2723.
21. Ascherio A, et al. Trans fatty acids and coronary heart disease. *New England Journal of Medicine*, 1999; 340: 1994-1998.
22. de Roos, et al, Consumption of a solid fat rich in lauric acid results in a more favorable serum lipid profile in healthy men and women than consumption of a solid fat rich in trans-fatty acids. *Journal of Nutrition*, 2001; 131: 242-245.
23. Hamazaki T, Okuyama H. The Japan Society for Lipid Nutrition recommends to reduce the intake of linoleic acid: a review and critique of the scientific evidence. *World Review of Nutrition and Dietetics*, 2003; 92: 109-132.
24. International Society for the Study of Fatty Acids and Lipids (ISSFAL). *Workshop on the essentiality of and recommended dietary intakes for omega-6 and omega-3 fatty acids*. Available online: http://www.issfal.org.uk/adequateintakes.htm (accessed September 8, 2005).

Chapter 20

1. Moncada S, Higgs A. The L-arginine-nitric oxide pathway. *New England Journal of Medicine*, 1993; 329: 2002-2012.
2. Freedman JE, et al. Impaired Platelet Production of Nitric Oxide Predicts Presence of Acute Coronary Syndromes. *Circulation*, Oct 13, 1998; 98 (15): 1481-1486.
3. Ludmer P, et al. Paradoxical vasoconstriction induced by acetylcholine in atherosclerotic coronary arteries. *New England Journal of Medicine*, 1986; 315: 1046-1051.
4. Haight JS, Djupesland PG. Nitric oxide (NO) and obstructive sleep apnea (OSA). *Sleep & Breathing*, Jun, 2003; 7 (2): 53-62.
5. Gazzaruso C, et al. Relationship Between Erectile Dysfunction and Silent Myocardial Ischemia in Apparently Uncomplicated Type 2 Diabetic Patients. *Circulation*, Jun, 2004; 110: 22-26.
6. Greenstein A, et al. Does severity of ischemic coronary disease correlate with erectile function? *International Journal of Impotence Research*, Sep, 1997; 9 (3): 123-126.
7. Lauer T, et al. Indexes of NO Bioavailability in Human Blood. *News in Physiological Sciences*, Dec 1, 2002; 17 (6): 251-255.
8. Cooke JP. Does ADMA Cause Endothelial Dysfunction? *Arteriosclerosis, Thrombosis, and Vascular Biology*, Sep 1, 2000; 20 (9): 2032-2037.
9. Lu TM, et al. Asymmetrical dimethylarginine: a novel risk factor for coronary artery disease. *Clinical Cardiology*, Oct, 2003; 26 (10): 458-464.

10. Boger RH, et al. Asymmetric dimethylarginine (ADMA): a novel risk factor for endothelial dysfunction: its role in hypercholesterolemia. *Circulation,* 1998; 98: 1842–1847.
11. Miyazaki H, et al. Endogenous nitric oxide synthase inhibitor. A novel marker of atherosclerosis. *Circulation,* 1999; 99: 1141-1146.
12. Zoccali C, et al. Plasma concentration of asymmetrical dimethylarginine and mortality in patients with end-stage renal disease: a prospective study. *Lancet,* 2001; 358: 2113-2117.
13. Loscalzo J. Oxidative stress in endothelial cell dysfunction and thrombosis. *Pathophysiology of Haemostasis and Thrombosis,* 2002; 32: 359-360.
14. Gielen S, et al. Exercise training in coronary artery disease and coronary vasomotion. *Circulation,* 2001; 103: e1-e6.
15. Higashi Y, et al. Regular Aerobic Exercise Augments Endothelium-Dependent Vascular Relaxation in Normotensive As Well As Hypertensive Subjects: Role of Endothelium-Derived Nitric Oxide. *Circulation,* Sep, 1999; 100: 1194-1202.
16. Edwards DG, Effect of exercise training on endothelial function in men with coronary artery disease. *American Journal of Cardiology,* Mar 1, 2004; 93 (5): 617-620.
17. Higashi Y, et al. Daily Aerobic Exercise Improves Reactive Hyperemia in Patients With Essential Hypertension. *Hypertension,* Jan, 1999; 33: 591-597.
18. Niebauer J, et al. NOS inhibition accelerates atherogenesis: reversal by exercise. *American Journal of Physiology. Heart and Circulatory Physiology,* Jul 11, 2003; 285(2): H535-540.
19. Ziccardi P, et al. Reduction of inflammatory cytokine concentrations and improvement of endothelial functions in obese women after weight loss over one year. *Circulation,* Feb 19, 2002; 105 (7): 804-809.
20. Esposito K, et al. Effect of lifestyle changes on erectile dysfunction in obese men: a randomized controlled trial. *Journal of the American Medical Association,* Jun 23, 2004; 291 (24): 2978-2984.
21. Freedman JE, et al. Select Flavonoids and Whole Juice From Purple Grapes Inhibit Platelet Function and Enhance Nitric Oxide Release. *Circulation,* Jun 12, 2001; 103(23): 2792-2798.
22. Liu M, et al. Mixed tocopherols inhibit platelet aggregation in humans: potential mechanisms. *American Journal of Clinical Nutrition,* Mar 1, 2003; 77 (3): 700-706.
23. Neil A, Silagy C. Garlic: its cardio-protective properties. *Current Opinion in Lipidology,* 1994; 5: 6-10.
24. Heinle H, Betz E. Effects of garlic supplementation in a rat model of atherosclerosis. *Arzneimittelforschung,* 1994; 44: 614-617.
25. Orekhov AN, et al. Direct antiatherosclerosis-related effects of garlic. *Annals of Medicine,* 1995; 27: 63-65.
26. Breithaupt-Grögler K, et al. Protective Effect of Chronic Garlic Intake on Elastic Properties of Aorta in the Elderly. *Circulation,* Oct, 1997; 96: 2649-2655.
27. Das I, et al. Potent activation of nitric oxide synthase by garlic: a basis for its therapeutic applications. *Current Medical Research and Opinion,* 1995; 13: 257-263.
28. Brodsky SV, et al. Glucose scavenging of nitric oxide. *American Journal of Physiology. Renal Physiology,* Mar 1, 2001; 280 (3): F480-486.
29. James PE, et al. Vasorelaxation by red blood cells and impairment in diabetes: reduced nitric oxide and oxygen delivery by glycated hemoglobin. *Circulation Research,* Apr 16, 2004; 94 (7): 976-983.
30. Giugliano D, et al. Reversed by L-Arginine: Evidence for Reduced Availability of Nitric Oxide During Hyperglycemia. *Circulation,* Apr 1, 1997; 95(7): 1783-1790.
31. Tsuchiya M, et al. Smoking a single cigarette rapidly reduces combined concentrations of nitrate and nitrite and concentrations of antioxidants in plasma. *Circulation,* Mar 12, 2002; 105 (10): 1155-1157.

32. Node K, et al. Reversible reduction in plasma concentration of nitric oxide induced by cigarette smoking in young adults. *American Journal of Cardiology*, 1997; 79: 1538–1541.
33. Tentolouris C, et al. Effects of smoking on nitric oxide synthesis in epicardial normal and atheromatous coronary arteries. *International Journal of Cardiology*, May, 2004; 95 (1): 69-73.
34. Barua RS, et al. Heavy and light cigarette smokers have similar dysfunction of endothelial vasoregulatory activity: an in vivo and in vitro correlation. *Journal of the American College of Cardiology*, Jun 5, 2002; 39 (11): 1758-1563.
35. Barua RS, et al. Dysfunctional endothelial nitric oxide biosynthesis in healthy smokers with impaired endothelium-dependent vasodilatation. *Circulation*, Oct 16, 2001; 104 (16): 1905-1910.
36. Barua RS, et al. Smoking is associated with altered endothelial-derived fibrinolytic and antithrombotic factors: an in vitro demonstration. *Circulation*, Aug 20, 2002; 106 (8): 905-908.
37. Takajo Y, et al. Augmented oxidative stress of platelets in chronic smokers. Mechanisms of impaired platelet-derived nitric oxide bioactivity and augmented platelet aggregability. *Journal of the American College of Cardiology*, Nov 1, 2001; 38 (5): 1320-1327.
38. Adams MR, et al. Cigarette smoking is associated with increased human monocyte adhesion to endothelial cells: reversibility with oral L-arginine but not vitamin C. *Journal of the American College of Cardiology*, Mar 1, 1997; 29 (3): 491-497.
39. Surgeon General. *The Health Consequences of Smoking: Cardiovascular Disease*. Department of Health & Human Services, MD, 1983. Available online: http://sgreports.nlm.nih.gov/NN/B/B/T/D/ (accessed September 8, 2005)
40. He J, et al. Passive Smoking and the Risk of Coronary Heart Disease -- A Meta-Analysis of Epidemiologic Studies. *New England Journal of Medicine*, Mar 25, 1999; 340 (12): 920-926.
41. Pitsavos C, et al. Association between exposure to environmental tobacco smoke and the development of acute coronary syndromes: the CARDIO2000 case-control study. *Tobbacco Control*, Sep 1, 2002; 11(3): 220 - 225.
42. Thun MJ. More misleading science from the tobacco industry. *British Medical Journal*, Oct 6, 2003; 327 (7418): E237-238.
43. Whincup PH, et al. Passive smoking and risk of coronary heart disease and stroke: prospective study with cotinine measurement. *British Medical Journal*, Jul 24, 2004; 329 (7459): 200-205.
44. Celermayer D, Adams M, Clarkson P, Robinson J, McCredie R, Donald A, Deanfield JE. Passive smoking is associated with impaired endothelium-dependent dilation in healthy young adults. *New England Journal of Medicine*, 1996; 334: 150–154.
45. Valkonen M, Kuusi T. Passive Smoking Induces Atherogenic Changes in Low-Density Lipoprotein. *Circulation*, May 26, 1998; 97 (20): 2012-2016.
46. Penn A, et al. Inhalation of steady-state sidestream smoke from one cigarette promotes arteriosclerotic plaque development. *Circulation*, 1994; 90: 1363-1367.
47. Morita H, et al. Only two-week smoking cessation improves platelet aggregability and intraplatelet redox imbalance of long-term smokers. *Journal of the American College of Cardiology*, 2005; 45:589-594.
48. Zhou JF, et al. Effects of cigarette smoking and smoking cessation on plasma constituents and enzyme activities related to oxidative stress. *Biomedical and Environmental Sciences*, Mar, 2000; 13 (1): 44-55.
49. Wilson K, et al. Effect of smoking cessation on mortality after myocardial infarction: meta-analysis of cohort studies. *Archives of Internal Medicine*, 2000; 160: 939-944.

Chapter 21

1. Saikku P. Epidemiology of Chlamydia pneumoniae in atherosclerosis. *American Heart Journal*, 1999; 138 (5 Pt 2): S500-503.
2. Saikku P, et al. Serological evidence of an association of a novel Chlamydia, TWAR, with chronic coronary heart disease and acute myocardial infarction. *Lancet*, Oct 29, 1988; 2 (8618): 983-986.
3. Saikku P, et al. Chronic Chlamydia pneumoniae infection as a risk factor for coronary heart disease in the Helsinki Heart Study. *Annals of Internal Medicine*, Feb 15, 1992; 116 (4): 273-278.
4. Belland RJ, et al. Chlamydia pneumoniae and atherosclerosis. *Cellular Microbiology*, Feb, 2004; 6 (2): 117-127.
5. Danesh J, et al. Chronic infections and coronary heart disease: is there a link? *Lancet*, Aug 9, 1997; 350 (9075): 430-436.
6. Joshipura KJ, et al. Poor oral health and coronary heart disease. *Journal of Dental Research*, Sep, 1996; 75 (9): 1631-1636.
7. Scannapieco FA. Position paper of The American Academy of Periodontology: periodontal disease as a potential risk factor for systemic diseases. *Journal of Periodontology*, Jul, 1998; 69 (7): 841-850.
8. Mattila KJ, et al. Association between dental health and acute myocardial infarction. *British Medical Journal*, Mar 25, 1989; 298 (6676): 779-781.
9. Hung HC, et al. Oral health and peripheral arterial disease. *Circulation*, Mar 4, 2003; 107 (8): 1152-1157.
10. Haraszthy VI, et al. Identification of periodontal pathogens in atheromatous plaques. *Journal of Periodontology*, 2000; 71: 1554-1560.
11. Chiu B. Multiple infections in carotid atherosclerotic plaques. *American Heart Journal*, 1999; 138 (5 Pt 2): 534-536.
12. Muhlestein JB, Anderson JL. Chronic infection and coronary artery disease. *Cardiology Clinics*, Aug, 2003; 21(3): 333-362.
13. Huittinen T, et al. Synergistic effect of persistent Chlamydia pneumoniae infection, autoimmunity, and inflammation on coronary risk. *Circulation*, May 27, 2003; 107 (20): 2566-2570.
14. Muhlestein JB. Antibiotic treatment of atherosclerosis. *Current Opinions in Lipidology*, Dec, 2003; 14 (6): 605-614.
15. Jeffrey S. PROVE IT-TIMI 22, ACES: New trial results a blow to the infection hypothesis in CVD. *TheHeart.org HeartWire*, Sep 1, 2004. Available online www.theheart.org.
16. O'Connor CM, et al. Azithromycin for the secondary prevention of coronary heart disease events: the WIZARD study: a randomized controlled trial. *Journal of the American Medical Association*, 2003; 290: 1459-1466.
17. Arcavi L, Benowitz NL. Cigarette smoking and infection. *Archives of Internal Medicine*, Nov 8, 2004; 164 (20): 2206-2216.
18. Shah BR, Hux JE. Quantifying the Risk of Infectious Diseases for People With Diabetes. *Diabetes Care*, 2003; 26: 510-513.
19. Gillum RF. Infection with Helicobacter pylori, coronary heart disease, cardiovascular risk factors, and systemic inflammation: the Third National Health and Nutrition Examination Survey. *Journal of the National Medical Association*, Nov, 2004; 96 (11): 1470-1476.
20. Elizalde JI, et al. Effects of Helicobacter pylori eradication on platelet activation and disease recurrence in patients with acute coronary syndromes. *Helicobacter*, Dec, 2004; 9 (6): 681-689.
21. Zhu J, et al. Effects of total pathogen burden on coronary artery disease risk and C-reactive protein levels. *American Journal of Cardiology*, 2000; 85: 140–146.

22. Jespersen CM, et al. Randomised placebo controlled multicentre trial to assess short term clarithromycin for patients with stable coronary heart disease: CLARICOR trial. *British Medical Journal*, 2006; 332: 22-27.

23. Sinisalo J, et al. Effect of 3 months of antimicrobial treatment with clarithromycin in acute non-Q-wave coronary syndrome. *Circulation*, 2002; 105: 1555-1560.

24. Berg HF, et al. Treatment with clarithromycin prior to coronary artery bypass graft surgery does not prevent subsequent cardiac events. *Clinical Infectious Diseases*, 2005; 40: 358-65.

25. Reichert TA, et al. Influenza and the Winter Increase in Mortality in the United States, 1959–1999. *American Journal of Epidemiology*, 2004; 160 (5): 492-502.

26. Woodhouse PR, et al. Seasonal variations of plasma fibrinogen and factor VII activity in the elderly: winter infections and death from cardiovascular disease. *Lancet*, 1994; 343 (8895): 435–439.

27. Tillet HE, et al. Excess death attributable to influenza in England and Wales: age at death and certified cause. *International Journal of Epidemiology*, 1983; 12 (3): 344–352.

28. The Eurowinter Group. Cold exposure and winter mortality from ischaemic heart disease, cerebrovascular disease, respiratory disease, and all causes in warm and cold regions of Europe. *Lancet*, 1997; 349: 1341–1343.

29. Hak E, et al. Clinical Effectiveness of Influenza Vaccination in Persons Younger Than 65 Years With High-Risk Medical Conditions: The PRISMA Study. *Archives of Internal Medicine*, 2005; 165: 274-280.

30. Siscovick DS, et al. Influenza vaccination and the risk of primary cardiac arrest. *American Journal of Epidemiology*, 2000; 152: 674–677.

31. Naghavi M, et al. Association of influenza vaccination and reduced risk of recurrent myocardial infarction. *Circulation*, 2000; 102: 3039–3045.

32. Lavallee P, et al. Association between influenza vaccination and reduced risk of brain infarction. *Stroke*, 2002; 33: 513–518.

33. Nichol KL, et al. Influenza vaccination and reduction in hospitalisations for cardiac disease and stroke among the elderly. *New England Journal of Medicine*, 2003; 348: 1322–1332.

34. Gurfinkel EP, et al. Flu vaccination in acute coronary syndromes and planned percutaneous coronary interventions (FLUVACS) Study: One-year follow-up. *European Heart Journal*, Jan, 2004; 25 (1): 25-31.

35. Cavaillon JM, et al. Cytokine response by monocytes and macrophages to free and lipoprotein-bound lipopolysaccharide. *Infection and Immunity*, 1990; 58: 2375-2382.

36. Weinstock C, et al. Low density lipoproteins inhibit endotoxin activation of monocytes. *Arteriosclerosis Thrombosis and Vascular Biology*, 1992; 12: 341-347.

37. Flegel WA, et al. Prevention of endotoxin-induced monokine release by human low- and high-density lipoproteins and by apolipoprotein A-I. *Infection and Immunity*, 1993; 61: 5140-5146.

38. Grunfel C. Lipoproteins inhibit macrophage activation by lipoteichoic acid. *Journal of Lipid Research*, Feb, 1999; 40: 245-252.

39. Bhakdi S, et al. Binding and partial inactivation of Staphylococcus aureus a-toxin by human plasma low density lipoprotein. *Journal of Biological Chemistry*, 1983; 258: 5899–5904.

40. Netera MG, et al. Low-density lipoprotein receptor-deficient mice are protected against lethal endotoxemia and severe Gram-negative infections. *Journal of Clinical Investigation*, 1996; 97: 1366–1372.

41. Feingold KR, et al. Role for circulating lipoproteins in protection from endotoxin toxicity. *Infection and Immunity*, 1995; 63: 2041–2046.

42. Pajkrt D, et al. Antiinflammatory effects of reconstituted high-density lipoprotein during human endotoxemia. *Journal of Experimental Medicine*, Nov 1, 1996; 184 (5): 1601-1608.
43. Muldoon MF, et al. Immune system differences in men with hypo- or hypercholesterolemia. *Clinical Immunology and Immunopathology*, 1997; 84: 145–149.
44. Losche W, et al. Functional behavior of mononuclear blood cells from patients with hypercholesterolemia. *Thrombosis Research*, 1992; 65: 337–342.
45. Fiser RH, et al. Effects of acute infection on cholesterogenesis in the rhesus monkey. *Proceedings of the Society for Experimental Biology and Medicine*, Nov, 1971; 138 (2): 605-609.
46. Gallin JI, et al. Serum lipids in infection. *New England Journal of Medicine*, 1969; 281: 1081–1086.
47. Jacobs D, et al. Report of the conference on low blood cholesterol: Mortality associations. *Circulation,* 1992; 86: 1046–1060.
48. Iribarren C, et al. Cohort study of serum total cholesterol and in-hospital incidence of infectious diseases. *Epidemiology and Infection*, 1998; 121: 335–347.
49. Claxton AJ, et al. Association between serum total cholesterol and HIV infection in a high-risk cohort of young men. *Journal of Acquired Immune Deficiency Syndromes and Human Retrovirology*, 1998; 17: 51–57.
50. Neaton JD, Wentworth DN. Low serum cholesterol and risk of death from AIDS. *AIDS,* 1997; 11: 929–930.
51. Pacelli F, et al. Prognosis in intra-abdominal infections. Multivariate analysis on 604 patients. *Archives of Surgery*, 1996; 131: 641–645.
52. Fraunberger P, et al. Serum cholesterol levels in neutropenic patients with fever. *Clinical Chemistry and Laboratory Medicine*, 2002; 40: 304–307.
53. Rauchhaus M, et al. The endotoxin-lipoprotein hypothesis. *Lancet*, 2000; 356: 930–933.
54. Scientific steering committee on behalf of the Simon Broome Register group. Risk of fatal coronary heart disease in familial hypercholesterolaemia. *British Medical Journal,* 1991; 303: 893–896.
55. Anderson KM, et al. Cholesterol and mortality. 30 years of follow-up from the Framingham study. *Journal of the American Medical Association*, 1987; 257: 2176–2180.
56. Forette F, et al. The prognostic significance of isolated systolic hypertension in the elderly. Results of a ten year longitudinal survey. *Clinical and Experimental Hypertension. Part A, Theory and Practice,* 1982; 4: 1177–1191.
57. Siegel D, et al. Predictors of cardiovascular events and mortality in the Systolic Hypertension in the Elderly Program pilot project. *American Journal of Epidemiology*, 1987; 126: 385–389.
58. Nissinen A, et al. Risk factors for cardiovascular disease among 55 to 74 year-old Finnish men: a 10-year follow-up. *Annals of Medicine,* 1989; 21: 239–240.
59. Krumholz HM, et al. Lack of association between cholesterol and coronary heart disease mortality and morbidity and all-cause mortality in persons older than 70 years. *Journal of the American Medical Association*, 1994; 272: 1335–1340.
60. Weijenberg MP, et al. Serum total cholesterol and systolic blood pressure as risk factors for mortality from ischemic heart disease among elderly men and women. *Journal of Clinical Epidemiology*, 1994; 47: 197–205.
61. Simons LA, et al. Diabetes, mortality and coronary heart disease in the prospective Dubbo study of Australian elderly. *Australian and New Zealand Journal of Medicine,* 1996; 26:66–74.
62. Weijenberg MP, et al. Total and high density lipoprotein cholesterol as risk factors for coronary heart disease in elderly men during 5 years of follow-up. The Zutphen Elderly Study. *American Journal of Epidemiology*, 1996; 143: 151–158.

63. Simons LA, et al. Cholesterol and other lipids predict coronary heart disease and ischaemic stroke in the elderly, but only in those below 70 years. *Atherosclerosis*, 2001; 159: 201–208.

64. Abbott RD, et al. Age-related changes in risk factor effects on the incidence of coronary heart disease. *Annals of Epidemiology*, 2002; 12: 173–181.

65. Zimetbaum P, et al. Plasma lipids and lipoproteins and the incidence of cardiovascular disease in the very elderly. The Bronx aging study. *Arteriosclerosis Thrombosis and Vascular Biology*, 1992; 12: 416–423.

66. Fried LP, et al. Risk factors for 5-year mortality in older adults: the Cardiovascular Health Study. *Journal of the American Medical Association*, 1998; 279: 585–592.

67. Chyou PH, Eaker ED. Serum cholesterol concentrations and all-cause mortality in older people. *Age and Ageing*, 2000; 29: 69–74.

68. Menotti A, et al. Cardiovascular risk factors and 10-year all-cause mortality in elderly European male populations; the FINE study. *European Heart Journal*, 2001; 22: 573–579.

69. Räihä I, et al. Effect of serum lipids, lipoproteins, and apolipoproteins on vascular and nonvascular mortality in the elderly. *Arteriosclerosis Thrombosis and Vascular Biology*, 1997; 17: 1224–1232.

70. Brescianini S, et al. Low total cholesterol and increased risk of dying: are low levels clinical warning signs in the elderly? Results from the Italian Longitudinal Study on Aging. *Journal of the American Geriatrics Society*, Jul, 2003; 51 (7): 991-996.

71. Forette B, et al. Cholesterol as risk factor for mortality in elderly women. *Lancet*, 1989; 1: 868–870.

72. Schatz IJ, et al. Cholesterol and all-cause mortality in elderly people from the Honolulu Heart Program: a cohort study. *Lancet*, 2001; 358: 351–355.

73. Jonsson A, et al. Total cholesterol and mortality after age 80 years. *Lancet*, 1997; 350: 1778–1779.

74. Weverling-Rijnsburger AW, et al. Total cholesterol and risk of mortality in the oldest old. *Lancet*, 1997; 350: 1119–1123.

75. Psaty BM, et al. The association between lipid levels and the risks of incident myocardial infarction, stroke, and total mortality: The Cardiovascular Health Study. *Journal of the American Geriatrics Society*, 2004; 52: 1639–1647.

76. Marsland AL, et al. Stress, immune reactivity and susceptibility to infectious disease. *Physiology & Behavior*, Dec, 2002; 77 (4-5): 711-716.

77. Welsh CJ, et al. The effects of restraint stress on the neuropathogenesis of Theiler's virus infection II: NK cell function and cytokine levels in acute disease. *Brain, Behavior, and Immunity*, Mar, 2004; 18 (2): 166-174.

78. Yu WK, et al. Influence of acute hyperglycemia in human sepsis on inflammatory cytokine and counterregulatory hormone concentrations. *World Journal of Gastroenterology*, Aug, 2003; 9 (8): 1824-1827.

79. Sanchez A, et al. Role of sugars in human neutrophilic phagocytosis. *American Journal of Clinical Nutrition*, 1973; 26: 1180-1184.

80. Bernstein J, et al. Depression of lymphocyte transformation following oral glucose ingestion. *American Journal of Clinical Nutrition*, 1977, 30: 613.

81. Sammon AM. Dietary linoleic acid, immune inhibition and disease. *Postgraduate Medical Journal*, Mar, 1999; 75 (881): 129-132.

82. Boulay M, et al. Dietary protein and zinc restrictions independently modify a Heligmosomoides polygyrus (Nematoda) infection in mice. *Parasitology*, May, 1998; 116 (Pt 5): 449-462.

83. McGee DW, McMurray DN. Protein malnutrition reduces the IgA immune response to oral antigen by altering B-cell and suppressor T-cell functions. *Immunology*, Aug, 1988; 64 (4): 697-702.

84. Slater AF, Keymer AE. The influence of protein deficiency on immunity to Heligmosomoides polygyrus (Nematoda) in mice. *Parasite Immunology*, Sep, 1988; 10 (5): 507-522.
85. Pena-Cruz V, et al. Sendai virus infection of mice with protein malnutrition. *Journal of Virology*, Aug, 1989; 63 (8): 3541-3544.
86. Price P, et al. Modulation of immunocompetence by cyclosporin A, cyclophosphamide or protein malnutrition potentiates murine cytomegalovirus pneumonitis. *Pathology, Research and Practice*, Dec, 1991; 187 (8): 993-1000.
87. Deitch EA, et al. Protein malnutrition alone and in combination with endotoxin impairs systemic and gut-associated immunity. *JPEN: Journal of Parenteral and Enteral Nutrition*, Jan-Feb, 1992; 16 (1): 25-31.
88. Nimmanwudipong T, et al. Effect of protein malnutrition and immunomodulation on immune cell populations. *Journal of Surgical Research*, Mar, 1992; 52 (3): 233-238.
89. Sullivan DA, et al. Influence of severe protein malnutrition on rat lacrimal, salivary and gastrointestinal immune expression during development, adulthood and ageing. *Immunology*, Feb, 1993; 78 (2): 308-317.
90. Szabo G. Consequences of alcohol consumption on host defence. *Alcohol and Alcoholism*, 1999; 34 (6): 830-841.
91. Zeidel A, et al. Immune response in asymptomatic smokers. *Acta Anaesthesiologica Scandinavica*, Sep, 2002; 46 (8): 959-964.
92. Friedman H, et al. Microbial infections, immunomodulation, and drugs of abuse. *Clinical Microbiology Reviews*, Apr, 2003; 16 (2): 209-219.
93. Irwin M, et al. Partial night sleep deprivation reduces natural killer and cellular immune responses in humans. *FASEB Journal*, Apr, 1996; 10 (5): 643-653.
94. Irwin M, et al. Partial sleep deprivation reduces natural killer cell activity in humans. *Psychosomatic Medicine*, Nov-Dec, 1994; 56 (6): 493-498.
95. Spiegel K, et al. Effect of sleep deprivation on response to immunization. *Journal of the American Medical Association*, Sep 25, 2002; 288 (12): 1471-1472.

Chapter 22
1. Writing Group for the Women's Health Initiative. Risks and Benefits of Estrogen Plus Progestin in Healthy Postmenopausal Women: Principal Results From the Women's Health Initiative Randomized Controlled Trial. *Journal of the American Medical Association*, Jul 17, 2002; 288 (3): 321-333.
2. Grady D, et al. Cardiovascular Disease Outcomes During 6.8 Years of Hormone Therapy: Heart and Estrogen/Progestin Replacement Study Follow-up (HERS II). *Journal of the American Medical Association*, Jul 3, 2002; 288 (1): 49-57.
3. The Women's Health Initiative Steering Committee. Effects of conjugated equine estrogen in postmenopausal women with hysterectomy: the Women's Health Initiative randomized controlled trial. *Journal of the American Medical Association*, 2004; 291: 1701-1712.
4. Cook JD, et al. Evaluation of the iron status in a population. *Blood*, 1976; 48: 449-455.
5. Jehn M, et al. Serum Ferritin and Risk of the Metabolic Syndrome in U.S. Adults. *Diabetes Care,* 2004; 27: 2422-2428.
6. Stoltzfus RJ, et al. Hookworm Control as a Strategy to Prevent Iron Deficiency. *Nutrition Reviews*, 1997; 55: 223-232.
7. Hopkins RM, et al. The prevalence of hookworm infection, iron deficiency and anaemia in an aboriginal community in north-west Australia. *Medical Journal of Australia*, Mar 3, 1997; 166 (5): 241-244.
8. Sullivan JL. Iron and the sex difference in heart disease risk. *Lancet*, 1981;1:1293-1294.
9. Salonen JT, et al. High stored iron levels are associated with excess risk of myocardial infarction in eastern Finnish men. *Circulation*, Sep 1992; 86: 803-811.

10. Danesh J, Appleby P. Coronary Heart Disease and Iron Status: Meta-Analyses of Prospective Studies. *Circulation*, Feb, 1999; 99: 852-854.
11. Smith C, et al. Stimulation of lipid peroxidation and hydroxyl-radical generation by the contents of human atherosclerotic lesions. *Biochemical Journal*, 1992; 286: 901-905.
12. Lee TS, et al. Iron-deficient diet reduces atherosclerotic lesions in apoE-deficient mice. *Circulation*, 1999; 99: 1222-1229.
13. Lee HT, et al. Dietary iron restriction increases plaque stability in apolipoprotein-e-deficient mice. *Journal of Biomedical Science*, Sep-Oct, 2003; 10 (5): 510-517.
14. Pool GF, van Jaarsveld H. Dietary iron elevates LDL-cholesterol and decreases plasma antioxidant levels: influence of antioxidants. *Research Communications in Molecular Pathology and Pharmacology*, May, 1998; 100 (2):139-150.
15. Duffy SJ, et al. Iron Chelation Improves Endothelial Function in Patients With Coronary Artery Disease. *Circulation*, Jun 12, 2001; 103 (23): 2799-2804.
16. Nitenberg A, et al. Coronary artery responses to physiological stimuli are improved by deferoxamine but not by L-arginine in non–insulin-dependent diabetic patients with angiographically normal coronary arteries and no other risk factors. *Circulation*, 1998; 97: 736-743.
17. Fernandez-Real JM, et al. Blood Letting in High-Ferritin Type 2 Diabetes: Effects on vascular reactivity. *Diabetes Care*, Dec 1, 2002; 25 (12): 2249-2255.
18. Fernandez-Real JM, et al. Blood Letting in High-Ferritin Type 2 Diabetes : Effects on Insulin Sensitivity and {beta}-Cell Function. *Diabetes*, Apr 1, 2002; 51 (4): 1000-1004.
19. Facchini FS, Saylor KL. Effect of iron depletion on cardiovascular risk factors: Studies in carbohydrate-intolerant patients. *Annals of the New York Academy of Sciences*, 2002; 967: 342-351.
20. Facchini FS, et al. Effect of iron depletion in carbohydrate-intolerant patients with clinical evidence of nonalcoholic fatty liver disease. *Gastroenterology*, 2002 Apr; 122 (4): 931-939.
21. Zacharski LR, et al. The iron (Fe) and atherosclerosis study (FeAST): a pilot study of reduction of body iron stores in atherosclerotic peripheral vascular disease. *American Heart Journal*, 2000; 139: 337-345.
22. Hua N, et al. Low iron status and enhanced insulin sensitivity in lacto-ovo vegetarians. *British Journal of Nutrition*, 2001; 86: 515-519.
23. Ascherio A, et al. Blood donations and risk of coronary heart disease in men. *Circulation*, Jan 2, 2001; 103 (1): 52-57.
24. Meyers DG, et al. Possible association of a reduction in cardiovascular events with blood donation. *Heart*, 1997; 78: 188-193.
25. Salonen JT, et al. Donation of blood is associated with reduced risk of myocardial infarction: the Kuopio Ischaemic Heart Disease Risk Factor Study. *American Journal of Epidemiology*, 1998; 148: 445-451.
26. Tuomainen TP, et al. Cohort study of relation between donating blood and risk of myocardial infarction in 2682 men in eastern Finland. *British Medical Journal*, Mar 15, 1997; 314 (7083): 793-794.
27. Jiang R, et al. Dietary iron intake and blood donations in relation to risk of type 2 diabetes in men: a prospective cohort study. *American Journal of Clinical Nutrition*, Jan 1, 2004; 79 (1): 70-75.
28. Sullivan JL, et al. Blood Donation Without Adequate Iron Depletion: An Invalid Test of the Iron Hypothesis. *Circulation*, Dec 11, 2001; 104 (24): e149-149.
29. Hawkins PT, et al. Inhibition of iron-catalysed hydroxyl radical formation by inositol polyphosphates: a possible physiological function for *myo*-inositol hexakisphosphate. *Biochemical Journal*, 1993; 294: 929-934.
30. Fox CH, Eberl M. Phytic acid (IP6), novel broad spectrum anti-neoplastic agent: a systematic review. *Complementary Therapies in Medicine*, 2002; 10: 229–234.

31. Shamsuddin AM, Vucenik I. Mammary tumor inhibition by IP6: a review. *Anticancer Research*, 1999; 19 (5A): 3671–3674.
32. Jenab M, Thompson LU. Phytic acid in wheat bran affects colon morphology, cell differentiation and apoptosis. *Carcinogenesis*, 2000; 21 (8): 1547–1552.
33. Asano T, McLeod RS. Dietary fibre for the prevention of colorectal adenomas and carcinomas (Cochrane Review). In: *The Cochrane Library*, Issue 2, 2002. Oxford.
34. Facchini FS, Saylor KL. A Low-Iron-Available, Polyphenol-Enriched, Carbohydrate-Restricted Diet to Slow Progression of Diabetic Nephropathy. *Diabetes*, 52 (5), 2003: 1204-1209.
35. Lakka T, et al. Higher levels of conditioning leisure time physical activity are associated with reduced levels of stored iron in Finnish men. *American Journal of Epidemiology*, 1994; 140 (2): 148-160.
36. Dallongeville J, et al. Iron deficiency among active men. *Journal of the American College of Nutrition*, 1989; 8 (3): 195-202.
37. Lauffer RB. Exercise as prevention: do the health benefits derive in part from lower iron levels? *Medical Hypotheses*, Jun, 1991; 35 (2): 103-107.
38. Verdon F, et al. Iron supplementation for unexplained fatigue in non-anaemic women: double-blind randomised placebo controlled trial. *British Medical Journal*, May 24, 2003; 326: 1124-1128.
39. Patterson AJ, et al. Dietary and Supplement Treatment of Iron Deficiency Results in Improvements in General Health and Fatigue in Australian Women of Childbearing Age. *Journal of the American College of Nutrition*, 2001; 20 (4): 337-342.
40. Hinton PS, et al. Iron supplementation improves endurance after training in iron-depleted, nonanemic women. *Journal of Applied Physiology*, Mar 1, 2000; 88 (3): 1103 - 1111.
41. Lyle RM, et al. Iron status in exercising women: the effect of oral iron therapy vs increased consumption of muscle foods. *American Journal of Clinical Nutrition*, Dec, 1992; 56: 1049-1055.
42. Donovan UM, Gibson RS. Iron and zinc status of young women aged 14 to 19 years consuming vegetarian and omnivorous diets. *Journal of the American College of Nutrition*, Oct, 1995; 14 (5): 463-472.
43. Alexander D, et al. Nutrient intake and haematological status of vegetarians and age-sex matched omnivores. *European Journal of Clinical Nutrition*, Aug, 1994; 48 (8): 538-46.
44. Hunt JR, Roughead ZK. Adaptation of iron absorption in men consuming diets with high or low iron bioavailability. *American Journal of Clinical Nutrition*, Jan, 2000; 71: 94 - 102.
45. The Vegetarian Resource Group. How Many Vegetarians Are There? Available online: http://www.vrg.org/nutshell/poll2000.htm (accessed September 8, 2005).

Chapter 23

1. Bradford RH et al. Expanded Clinical Evaluation of Lovastatin (EXCEL) study results. I. Efficacy in modifying plasma lipoproteins and adverse event profile in 8245 patients with moderate hypercholesterolemia. *Archives of Internal Medicine*, Jan, 1991; 151 (1): 43-49.
2. Downs JR, et al. Primary prevention of acute coronary events with lovastatin in men and women with average cholesterol levels. *Journal of the American Medical Association*, 1998; 279: 1615-1622.
3. Scandinavian Simvastatin Survival Study Group. Randomised trial of cholesterol lowering in 4444 patients with coronary heart disease: the Scandinavian Simvastatin Survival Study (4S). *Lancet*, 1994. 344; 1383-1389.

4. Shepherd J, et al. Prevention of Coronary Heart Disease with Pravastatin in Men with Hypercholesterolemia. *New England Journal of Medicine*, Nov 16, 1995; 333 (20): 1301-1308.
5. Sacks FM, et al. The Effect of Pravastatin on Coronary Events after Myocardial Infarction in Patients with Average Cholesterol Levels. *New England Journal of Medicine*, Oct 3, 1996; 335 (14): 1001-1009.
6. The Long-Term Intervention with Pravastatin In ischaemic Disease (LIPID) Study Group. Prevention of cardiovascular events and death with pravastatin in patients with coronary heart disease and a broad range of initial cholesterol levels. *New England Journal of Medicine,* 1998; 339: 1349-1357.
7. Heart Protection Study Collaborative Group. MRC/BHF Heart Protection Study of cholesterol lowering with simvastatin in 20,536 high risk individuals: a randomised placebo-controlled trial. *Lancet*, 2002; 360: 7-22M.
8. Serruys PW, et al. Fluvastatin for prevention of cardiac events following successful first percutaneous coronary intervention: a randomized controlled trial. *Journal of the American Medical Association*, Jun 26, 2002; 287 (24): 3215-3222.
9. Shepherd J, et al. Pravastatin in elderly individuals at risk of vascular disease (PROSPER): a randomised controlled trial. *Lancet*, 2002; 360: 1623-1630.
10. The ALLHAT Officers and Coordinators for the ALLHAT Collaborative Research Group. Major Outcomes in Moderately Hypercholesterolemic, Hypertensive Patients Randomized to Pravastatin vs Usual Care: The Antihypertensive and Lipid-Lowering Treatment to Prevent Heart Attack Trial (ALLHAT-LLT). *Journal of the American Medical Association,* 2002; 288: 2998-3007.
11. Sever PS, et al. Prevention of coronary and stroke events with atorvastatin in hypertensive patients who have average or lower-than-average cholesterol concentrations, in the Anglo-Scandinavian Cardiac Outcomes Trial-Lipid Lowering Arm (ASCOT-LLA): a multi-centre randomised controlled trial. *Lancet*, Apr 5, 2003; 361: 1149-1158.
12. Colhoun HM, et al. Primary prevention of cardiovascular disease with atorvastatin in type 2 diabetes in the Collaborative Atorvastatin Diabetes Study (CARDS): multicentre randomised placebo-controlled trial. *Lancet*, 2004; 364: 685-696.
13. Amarenco P, et al. High-dose atorvastatin after stroke or transient ischemic attack. *New England Journal of Medicine*, Aug 10, 2006; 355 (6): 549-559.
14. Nakamura H, et al. Primary prevention of cardiovascular disease with pravastatin in Japan (MEGA study): a prospective randomised controlled trial. *Lancet*, 2006; 368: 1155-1163.
15. Walsh JE, Pignone M. Drug Treatment of Hyperlipidemia in Women. *Journal of the American Medical Association*, May, 2004; 291: 2243-2252.
16. Antithrombotic Trialists' Collaboration. Collaborative meta-analysis of randomised trials of antiplatelet therapy for prevention of death, myocardial infarction, and stroke in high risk patients. *British Medical Journal*, Jan 12, 2002; 324: 71-86.
17. Hennekens CH. Update on aspirin in the treatment and prevention of cardiovascular disease. *American Journal of Managed Care*, Dec, 2002; 8 (22 Suppl): S691-700.
18. Hennekens CH, et al. Additive Benefits of Pravastatin and Aspirin to Decrease Risks of Cardiovascular Disease: Randomized and Observational Comparisons of Secondary Prevention Trials and Their Meta-analyses. *Archives of Internal Medicine*, Jan 12, 2004; 164 (1): 40-44.
19. ETDRS Investigators. Aspirin effects on mortality and morbidity in patients with diabetes mellitus. Early treatment diabetic retinopathy study report 14. *Journal of the American Medical Association*, 1992; 268: 1292-1300.

20. Sacco M, et al. Collaborative Group: Primary prevention of cardiovascular events with low-dose aspirin and vitamin E in type 2 diabetic patients: results of the Primary Prevention Project (PPP) trial. *Diabetes Care*, 2003; 26: 3264–3272.
21. Cleland JG, et al. The Warfarin/Aspirin Study in Heart failure (WASH): a randomized trial comparing antithrombotic strategies for patients with heart failure. *American Heart Journal*, Jul, 2004; 148 (1): 157-164.
22. Peto R, et al. Randomised trial of prophylactic daily aspirin in British male doctors. *British Medical Journal,* 1988; 296: 313-316.
23. The Steering Committee of the Physicians' Health Study Research Group. Final report on the aspirin component of the ongoing Physicians' Health Study. *New England Journal of Medicine*, 1989; 321: 129-135.
24. The Medical Research Council's General Practice Research Framework. Thrombosis prevention trial: randomised trial of low intensity oral anticoagulation with warfarin and low-dose aspirin in the primary prevention of ischaemic heart disease in men at increased risk. *Lancet,* 1998; 351: 233-241.
25. Hansson L, et al. Effects of intensive blood-pressure lowering and low dose aspirin in patients with hypertension: principal results of the Hypertension Optimal Treatment (HOT) randomised trial. *Lancet*, 1998; 351: 1755-1762.
26. Ridker PM, et al. A randomized trial of low-dose aspirin in the primary prevention of cardiovascular disease in women. *New England Journal of Medicine*, 2005; 352 (13): 1293-1304.
27. Fischer LM, et al. Discontinuation of nonsteroidal anti-inflammatory drug therapy and risk of acute myocardial infarction. *Archives of Internal Medicine*, Dec 13-27, 2004; 164 (22): 2472-2476.

Chapter 24

1. Watts GF, et al. Effects on coronary artery disease of lipid-lowering diet, or diet plus cholestyramine, in the St Thomas' atherosclerosis regression study (STARS). *Lancet*, 1992; 339: 563-569.
2. De Lorgeril M, et al. Mediterranean alpha-linolenic acid-rich diet in secondary prevention of coronary heart disease. *Lancet*, 1994; 343: 1454-1459.
3. Burr ML, et al. Effects of changes in fat, fish, and fibre intakes on death and myocardial reinfarction: diet and reinfarction trial (DART). *Lancet*, 1989; 2: 757–761.
4. Marchioli R, et al. Early protection against sudden death by n-3 polyunsaturated fatty acids after myocardial infarction: time-course analysis of the results of the Gruppo Italiano per lo Studio della Sopravvivenza nell'Infarto Miocardico (GISSI)-Prevenzione. *Circulation*, 2002; 105: 1897–1903.
5. Kuklinski B, et al. Coenzyme Q10 and antioxidants in acute myocardial infarction. *Molecular Aspects of Medicine*, 1994; 15 (Suppl): S143-147.
6. Korpela H, et al. Effect of selenium supplementation after acute myocardial infarction. *Research Communications in Chemical Pathology and Pharmacology*, Aug, 1989; 65 (2): 249-252.
7. Davini P, et al. Controlled study on L-carnitine therapeutic efficacy in post-infarction. *Drugs Under Experimental And Clinical Research,* 1992; 18: 355-365.
8. Jolliffe JA, et al. Exercise-based rehabilitation for coronary heart disease (Cochrane Review). In: The Cochrane Library, Issue 2, 2004. Chichester, UK: John Wiley & Sons, Ltd.
9. Ip, et al. Requirement of essential fatty acid for mammary tumorigenesis in the rat. *Cancer Research,* 1985; 45 (5): 1997-2001.
10. Rose DP. Effects of dietary fatty acids on breast and prostate cancers: evidence from in vitro experiments and animal studies. *American Journal of Clinical Nutrition,* Dec, 1997; 66 (6 Suppl): 1513S-1522S.

11. Fernandez E, et al. Fish consumption and cancer risk. *American Journal of Clinical Nutrition,* Jul 1, 1999; 70(1): 85-90.
12. Terry P, et al. Fatty fish consumption and risk of prostate cancer. *Lancet,* Jun 2, 2001; 357 (9270): 1764-1766.
13. Terry P, et al. Fatty fish consumption lowers the risk of endometrial cancer: a nationwide case-control study in Sweden. *Cancer Epidemiology, Biomarkers & Prevention,* Jan, 2002; 11 (1): 143-145.
14. Maillard V, et al. N-3 and N-6 fatty acids in breast adipose tissue and relative risk of breast cancer in a case-control study in Tours, France. *International Journal of Cancer,* Mar 1, 2002; 98 (1): 78-83.
15. Kato I, et al. Prospective study of diet and female colorectal cancer: the New York University Women's Health Study. *Nutrition and Cancer,* 1997; 28: 276–281.
16. Hakim IA, et al. Fat intake and risk of squamous cell carcinoma of the skin. *Nutrition and Cancer,* 2000; 36 (2): 155-162.
17. Tanskanen A, et al. Fish Consumption and Depressive Symptoms in the General Population in Finland. *Psychiatric Services,* Apr, 2001; 52: 529-531.
18. Adams PB, et al. Arachidonic acid to eicosapentaenoic acid ratio in blood correlates positively with clinical symptoms of depression. *Lipids,* Mar, 1996; 31 (Suppl): S157-161.
19. Mamalakis G, et al. Depression and adipose essential polyunsaturated fatty acids. *Prostaglandins, Leukotrienes, and Essential Fatty Acids,* Nov, 2002; 67 (5): 311-318.
20. Laugharne JD, et al. Fatty acids and schizophrenia. *Lipids,* Mar, 1996; 31 (Suppl): S163-165.
21. Olsen SF, Secher NJ. Low consumption of seafood in early pregnancy as a risk factor for preterm delivery: prospective cohort study. *British Medical Journal,* Feb 23, 2002; 324: 447.
22. Williams MA, et al. Omega-3 fatty acids in maternal erythrocytes and risk of preeclampsia. *Epidemiology,* May, 1995; 6 (3): 232-237.
23. Hibbeln JR. Seafood consumption, the DHA content of mothers' milk and prevalence rates of postpartum depression: a cross-national, ecological analysis. *Journal of Affective Disorders,* May, 2002; 69(1-3): 15-29.
24. Turek JJ, et al. Dietary polyunsaturated fatty acids modulate responses of pigs to Mycoplasma hyopneumoniae infection. *Journal of Nutrition,* Jun, 1996; 126 (6): 1541-1548.
25. Tully AM, et al. Low serum cholesteryl ester-docosahexaenoic acid levels in Alzheimer's disease: a case-control study. *British Journal of Nutrition,* Apr, 2003; 89 (4): 483-489.
26. Requirand P, et al. Serum fatty acid imbalance in bone loss: example with periodontal disease. *Clinical Nutrition,* Aug, 2000; 19 (4): 271-276.
27. Watkins BA, et al. Nutraceutical Fatty Acids as Biochemical and Molecular Modulators of Skeletal Biology. *Journal of the American College of Nutrition,* 2001; 20 (90005): 410S-416S.
28. Reinwald S, et al. Repletion with (n-3) Fatty Acids Reverses Bone Structural Deficits in (n-3)–Deficient Rats. *Journal of Nutrition,* Feb 2004; 134: 388-394.
29. Schwartz J. Role of polyunsaturated fatty acids in lung disease. *American Journal of Clinical Nutrition,* Jan 2000; 71 (suppl): 393S-96S.
30. Shahar E, et al. Dietary n-3 polyunsaturated fatty acids and smoking-related chronic obstructive pulmonary disease. *New England Journal of Medicine,* Jul 28, 1994: 331 (4): 228-233.
31. Deutch B. Menstrual pain in Danish women correlated with low n-3 polyunsaturated fatty acid intake. *European Journal of Clinical Nutrition,* 1995; 49: 508-516.
32. Kalmijn, S., et al. Polyunsaturated fatty acids, antioxidants, and cognitive function in very old men. *American Journal of Epidemiology,* Jan 1, 1997: 145: 33-41.

384

33. Seddon JM, et al. Dietary Fat and Risk for Advanced Age-Related Macular Degeneration. *Archives of Ophthalmology*, 2001; 119 (8): 1191-1199.
34. Hodge L, et al. Consumption of oily fish and childhood asthma risk. *Medical Journal of Australia*, 1996; 164: 137-140.
35. Burgess JR, et al. Long-chain polyunsaturated fatty acids in children with attention-deficit hyperactivity disorder. *American Journal of Clinical Nutrition*, 2000; 71: 327-330.
36. Dry J, Vincent D. Effect of a fish oil diet on asthma: results of a 1-year double-blind study. *International Archives of Allergy and Applied Immunology*, 1991; 95 (2/3): 156-157.
37. Yehuda S, et al. Essential fatty acids preparation (SR-3) improves Alzheimer's patients quality of life. *International Journal of Neuroscience*, Nov, 1996; 87 (3-4): 141-149.
38. Geusens P et al. Long-term effect of omega-3 fatty acid supplementation in active rheumatoid arthritis, a 12-month, double-blind, controlled study. *Arthritis & Rheumatism*, Jun, 1994; 37 (6): 824-829.
39. Schiz Peet M, Horrobin DF. A dose-ranging study of the effects of ethyl-eicosapentaenoate in patients with ongoing depression despite apparently adequate treatment with standard drugs. *Archives of General Psychiatry*, Oct, 2002; 59 (10): 913-919.
40. Stoll AL, et al. Omega 3 fatty acids in bipolar disorder: a preliminary double-blind, placebo-controlled trial. *Archives of General Psychiatry*, May, 1999; 56 (5): 407-412.
41. Peet M, et al. Two double-blind placebo-controlled pilot studies of eicosapentaenoic acid in the treatment of schizophrenia. *Schizophrenia Research*, Apr 30, 2001; 49 (3): 243-251.
42. Peet M, Horrobin DF. A dose-ranging exploratory study of the effects of ethyl-eicosapentaenoate in patients with persistent schizophrenic symptoms. *Journal of Psychiatric Research,* Jan-Feb, 2002; 36 (1): 7-18.
43. Hamazaki T, et al. The Effect of Docosahexaenoic Acid on Aggression in Young Adults. A Placebo-controlled Double-blind Study. *Journal of Clinical Investigation,* Feb, 1996; 97 (4): 1129-1134.
44. Jorgensen MH, et al. Effect of formula supplemented with docosahexaenoic acid and gamma-linolenic acid on fatty acid status and visual acuity in term infants. *Journal of Pediatric Gastroenterology and Nutrition*, 1998; 26: 412–421.
45. Carlson SE, et al. Visual acuity and fatty acid status of term infants fed human milk and formulas with and without docosahexaenoate and arachidonate from egg yolk lecithin. *Pediatric Research*, 1996; 39: 882–888.
46. O'Connor DL, et al. Growth and Development in Preterm Infants Fed Long-Chain Polyunsaturated Fatty Acids: A Prospective, Randomized Controlled Trial. *Pediatrics*, Aug 1, 2001; 108 (2): 359-371.
47. Helland IB, et al. Maternal Supplementation With Very-Long-Chain n-3 Fatty Acids During Pregnancy and Lactation Augments Children's IQ at 4 Years of Age. *Pediatrics*, Jan, 2003; 111 (1): e39-e44.
48. Dunstan JA, et al. Fish oil supplementation in pregnancy modifies neonatal allergen-specific immune responses and clinical outcomes in infants at high risk of atopy: a randomized, controlled trial. *Journal of Allergy and Clinical Immunology*, Dec, 2003; 112 (6): 1178-1184.
49. Olsen SF, et al. Randomised controlled trial of effect of fish-oil supplementation on pregnancy duration. *Lancet*, Apr 25, 1992; 339 (8800): 1003-1007.
50. Olsen SF, Secher NJ. A possible preventive effect of low-dose fish oil on early delivery and pre-eclampsia: indications from a 50-year-old controlled trial. *British Journal of Nutrition*, Nov, 1990; 64 (3): 599-609.

51. De Caterina R et al. n-3 fatty acids and renal diseases. *American Journal of Kidney Diseases*, Sept, 1994; 24 (3): 397-415.
52. Harel Z et al. Supplementation with omega-3 polyunsaturated fatty acids in the management of dysmenorrhea in adolescents. *American Journal of Obstetrics & Gynecology*, Apr, 1996; 174 (4): 1335-1338.
53. Aslan A, Triadafilopoulos G. Fish oil fatty acid supplementation in active ulcerative colitis: A double-blind, placebo-controlled, crossover study. *American Journal of Gastroenterology*, Apr, 1992; 87: 432-37.
54. Salomon, P., et al. Treatment of ulcerative colitis with fish oil n-3 omega fatty acid: an open trial. *Journal of Clinical Gastroenterology,* Apr, 1990; (12): 157-1161.
55. Belluzzi A et al. Effect of an enteric-coated fish-oil preparation on relapses in Crohn's disease. *New England Journal of Medicine*, Jun 13, 1996; 334 (24): 1557-1560.
56. Lawrence R, Sorrell T. Eicosapentaenoic acid in cystic fibrosis: evidence of a pathogenetic role for leukotriene B4. *Lancet*, Aug 21, 1993; 342: 465-469.
57. US Food and Drug Administration, Center for Food Safety and Applied Nutrition, Office of Seafood. Mercury Levels in Seafood Species. May, 2001. Available online: http://www.cfsan.fda.gov/~frf/sea-mehg.html (accessed September 8, 2005).
58. Hites RA, et al. Global assessment of organic contaminants in farmed salmon. *Science*, Jan 9, 2004; 303 (5655): 226-229.
59. Foran SE, et al. Measurement of mercury levels in concentrated over-the-counter fish oil preparations: is fish oil healthier than fish? *Archives of Pathology and Laboratory Medicine,* 2003; 127 (12): 1603-1605.
60. Schaller JL. Mercury and Fish Oil Supplements. *Medscape General Medicine,* April 13, 2001; 3 (2). Available online: http://www.medscape.com/viewarticle/408125 (accessed September 8, 2005).
61. ConsumerLab.com Product Review: Omega-3 Fatty Acids (EPA and DHA) from Fish/Marine Oils. Available online: http://www.consumerlab.com/results/omega3.asp (accessed September 8, 2005).
62. Eritsland J, et al. Long-term effects of n-3 polyunsaturated fatty acids on haemostatic variables and bleeding episodes in patients with coronary artery disease. *Blood Coagulation & Fibrinolysis,* Feb, 1995; 6 (1): 17-22.
63. Saynor R, et al. The long-term effect of dietary supplementation with fish lipid concentrate on serum lipids, bleeding time, platelets and angina. *Atherosclerosis*, Jan, 1984; 50 (1): 3-10.
64. Eritsland J, et al. Effects of highly concentrated omega-3 polyunsaturated fatty acids and acetylsalicylic acid, alone and combined, on bleeding time and serum lipid profile. *Journal of the Oslo City Hospitals*, Aug-Sep, 1989; 39 (8-9): 97-101.
65. Buckley MS, et al. Fish oil interaction with warfarin. *Annals of Pharmacotherapy*, Jan, 2004; 38 (1): 50-52.
66. Montori VM, et al. Fish oil supplementation in type 2 diabetes: a quantitative systematic review. *Diabetes Care*, 2000; 23: 1407-1415.
67. Friedberg CE, et al. Fish oil and glycemic control in diabetes. A meta-analysis. *Diabetes Care*, Apr, 1998; 21: 494-500.
68. Burr ML, et al. Lack of benefit of dietary advice to men with angina: results of a controlled trial. *European Journal of Clinical Nutrition*, 2003; 57 (2): 193-200.
69. Mori TA, Woodman RJ. The independent effects of eicosapentaenoic acid and docosahexaenoic acid on cardiovascular risk factors in humans. Current Opinion in Clinical Nutrition and Metabolic Care, Mar, 2006; 9 (2): 95-104.
70. 70. Food and Agriculture Organization database. Available online: http://faostat.fao.org/faostat/form?collection=FBS&Domain=FBS&servlet=1&hasbulk=&version=ext&language=EN (accessed March 31, 2006).

71. Raitt MH, et al. Fish oil supplementation and risk of ventricular tachycardia and ventricular fibrillation in patients with implantable defibrillators: a randomized controlled trial. *Journal of the American Medical Association*, 2005; 293: 2884–2891.

72. Burr ML, Dunstan FD, George CH. Is fish oil good or bad for heart disease? Two trials with apparently conflicting results. *Journal of Membrane Biology*, Jul, 2005; 206 (2): 155-163.

73. Ross R, et al. Reduction in Obesity and Related Comorbid Conditions after Diet-Induced Weight Loss or Exercise-Induced Weight Loss in Men: A Randomized, Controlled Trial. *Annals of Internal Medicine*, Jul, 2000; 133: 92-103.

74. Fenicchia LM, et al. Influence of resistance exercise training on glucose control in women with type 2 diabetes. *Metabolism*, Mar, 2004; 53 (3): 284-289.

75. Carlson JE, et al. Disability in Older Adults 2: Physical Activity as Prevention. *Behavioral Medicine, Disability in Older Adults*, Winter, 1999; 24 (4): 157-168.

76. Kelley GA, et al. Resistance training and bone mineral density in women: a meta-analysis of controlled trials. *American Journal of Physical Medicine & Rehabilitation*, Jan, 2001; 80 (1): 65-77.

77. Batty D, Thune I. Does physical activity prevent cancer? *British Medical Journal*, Dec 2000; 321: 1424-1425.

78. Cuff DJ, et al. Effective exercise modality to reduce insulin resistance in women with type 2 diabetes. *Diabetes Care*, Nov, 2003; 26 (11): 2977-2982.

79. Hertog MG, et al. Fruit and vegetable consumption and cancer mortality in the Caerphilly Study. *Cancer Epidemiology, Biomarkers & Prevention*, Sep 1996; 5 (9): 673-677.

80. Sauvaget C, et al. Vegetables and fruit intake and cancer mortality in the Hiroshima/Nagasaki Life Span Study. *British Journal of Cancer*, Mar 10, 2003; 88 (5): 689-694.

81. Terry P, et al. Protective effect of fruits and vegetables on stomach cancer in a cohort of Swedish twins. *International Journal of Cancer*, Mar 30, 1998; 76 (1): 35-37.

82. Smith-Warner SA, et al. Fruits, vegetables and lung cancer: A pooled analysis of cohort studies. *International Journal of Cancer*, Dec 20, 2003; 107 (6): 1001-1011.

83. Smith-Warner SA, et al. Intake of fruits and vegetables and risk of breast cancer: a pooled analysis of cohort studies. *Journal of the American Medical Association*, Feb 14, 2001; 285 (6): 769-776.

84. Michels KB, et al. Prospective study of fruit and vegetable consumption and incidence of colon and rectal cancers. *Journal of the National Cancer Institute*, Nov 1, 2000; 92 (21): 1740-1752.

85. Engelhart MJ, et al. Dietary Intake of Antioxidants and Risk of Alzheimer Disease. *Journal of the American Medical Association*, 2002; 287: 3223-3229.

86. New SA, et al. Nutritional influences on bone mineral density: a cross-sectional study in premenopausal women. *American Journal of Clinical Nutrition,* 1997; 65: 1831-1839.

87. New SA, et al. Dietary influences on bone mass and bone metabolism: further evidence of a positive link between fruit and vegetable consumption and bone health? *American Journal of Clinical Nutrition,* Jan, 2000; 71 (1): 142-151.

88. Tucker KL, et al. Bone mineral density and dietary patterns in older adults: the Framingham Osteoporosis Study. *American Journal of Clinical Nutrition,* Jul, 2002; 76 (1): 245-252.

89. Tylavsky FA, et al. Fruit and vegetable intakes are an independent predictor of bone size in early pubertal children. *American Journal of Clinical Nutrition*, Feb, 2004; 79 (2): 311-317.

90. Muhlbauer RC, et al. Various selected vegetables, fruits, mushrooms and red wine residue inhibit bone resorption in rats. *Journal of Nutrition,* Nov, 2003; 133 (11): 3592-3597.

91. Muhlbauer RC, et al. Onion and a mixture of vegetables, salads, and herbs affect bone resorption in the rat by a mechanism independent of their base excess. *Journal of Bone and Mineral Research*, Jul, 2002; 17 (7): 1230-1236.

92. Rissanen TH, et al. Low intake of fruits, berries and vegetables is associated with excess mortality in men: the Kuopio Ischaemic Heart Disease Risk Factor (KIHD) Study. *Journal of Nutrition*, Jan, 2003; 133 (1): 199-204.

93. Sahyoun NR, et al. Carotenoids, vitamins C and E, and mortality in an elderly population. *American Journal of Epidemiology*, 1996; 144: 501-511.

94. Huijbregts P, et al. Dietary pattern and 20 year mortality in elderly men in Finland, Italy, and the Netherlands: longitudinal cohort study. *British Medical Journal*, 1997; 315: 13-17.

95. Kalen A, et al. Age-related changes in the lipid compositions of rat and human tissues. *Lipids*, 1989; 24: 579-584.

96. Rosenfeldt F, et al. Systematic review of effect of coenzyme Q10 in physical exercise, hypertension and heart failure. *Biofactors*, 2003; 18 (1-4): 91-100.

97. Weber C, et al. Coenzyme Q10 in the diet--daily intake and relative bioavailability. *Molecular Aspects of Medicine*, 1997; 18 Suppl: S251-254.

98. Weis M, et al. Bioavailability of four oral coenzyme Q10 formulations in healthy volunteers. *Molecular Aspects of Medicine*, 1994; 15 Suppl: S273-280.

99. Lu WL, et al. Total coenzyme Q10 concentrations in Asian men following multiple oral 50-mg doses administered as coenzyme Q10 sustained release tablets or regular tablets. *Biological & Pharmaceutical Bulletin*, Jan, 2003; 26 (1): 52-55.

100. Engelsen J, et al. Effect of coenzyme Q10 and Ginkgo biloba on warfarin dosage in stable, long-term warfarin treated outpatients. A randomised, double blind, placebo-crossover trial. *Thrombosis and Haemostasis*, Jun, 2002; 87 (6): 1075-1076.

101. Henriksen JE, et al. Impact of ubiquinone (coenzyme Q10) treatment on glycaemic control, insulin requirement and well-being in patients with Type 1 diabetes mellitus. *Diabetic Medicine*, 1999 Apr; 16 (4): 312-318.

102. Eriksson JG, et al. The effect of coenzyme Q10 administration on metabolic control in patients with type 2 diabetes mellitus. *Biofactors*, 1999; 9 (2-4): 315-318.

103. Playford DA, et al. Combined effect of coenzyme Q10 and fenofibrate on forearm microcirculatory function in type 2 diabetes. *Atherosclerosis*, 2003 May; 168 (1): 169-179.

104. Hodgson JM, et al. Coenzyme Q10 improves blood pressure and glycaemic control: a controlled trial in subjects with type 2 diabetes. *European Journal of Clinical Nutrition*, Nov, 2002; 56 (11): 1137-1142.

105. Watts GF, et al. Coenzyme Q(10) improves endothelial dysfunction of the brachial artery in Type II diabetes mellitus. *Diabetologia*, Mar, 2002; 45 (3): 420-426.

106. Bargossi AM, et al. Exogenous CoQ10 supplementation prevents plasma ubiquinone reduction induced by HMG-CoA reductase inhibitors. *Molecular Aspects of Medicine*, 1994; 15 (Suppl): S187-193.

107. Langsjoen P, et al. Treatment of statin adverse effects with supplemental Coenzyme Q10 and statin drug discontinuation. *BioFactors*, 2005; 25: 147-152.

108. Folkers K, et al. The activities of coenzyme Q10 and vitamin B6 for immune responses. *Biochemical and Biophysical Research Communications*, May 28, 1993; 193(1): 88-92.

109. Barbieri B, et al. Coenzyme Q10 administration increases antibody titer in hepatitis B vaccinated volunteers--a single blind placebo-controlled and randomized clinical study. *Biofactors*, 1999; 9 (2-4): 351-357.

110. Hodges S, et al. CoQ10: could it have a role in cancer management? *Biofactors*, 1999; 9 (2-4): 365-370.

388

111.	Lockwood K, et al. Partial and complete regression of breast cancer in patients in relation to dosage of coenzyme Q10. *Biochemical and Biophysical Research Communications*, Mar 30, 1994; 199 (3): 1504-1508.
112.	Rosenfeldt F, et al. Systematic review of effect of coenzyme Q10 in physical exercise, hypertension and heart failure. *Biofactors*, 2003; 18 (1-4): 91-100.
113.	Hanioka T, et al. Effect of topical application of coenzyme Q10 on adult periodontitis. *Molecular Aspects of Medicine*, 1994; 15 (Suppl): S241-248.
114.	Shults CW, et al. Effects of coenzyme Q10 in early Parkinson disease: evidence of slowing of the functional decline. *Archives of Neurology*, Oct, 2002; 59 (10): 1541-1550.
115.	Chan A, et al. Metabolic changes in patients with mitochondrial myopathies and effects of coenzyme Q10 therapy. *Journal of Neurology*, Oct, 1998; 245 (10): 681-685.
116.	Chen RS, et al. Coenzyme Q10 treatment in mitochondrial encephalomyopathies. Short-term double-blind, crossover study. *European Neurology*, 1997; 37 (4): 212-218.
117.	Brigelius-Flohe R, et al. Selenium-dependent enzymes in endothelial cell function. *Antioxidants and Redox Signaling*, Apr, 2003; 5 (2): 205-215.
118.	Clark LC, et al. Effects of selenium supplementation for cancer prevention in patients with carcinoma of the skin. A randomized controlled trial. Nutritional Prevention of Cancer Study Group. *Journal of the American Medical Association*, Dec 25, 1996; 276 (24): 1957-1963.
119.	Yu SY, et al. Protective role of selenium against hepatitis B virus and primary liver cancer in Qidong. *Biological Trace Element Research*, 1997; 56 (1): 117-124.
120.	Blot WJ, et al. Nutrition intervention trials in Linxian, China: supplementation with specific vitamin/mineral combinations, cancer incidence, and disease-specific mortality in the general population. *Journal of the National Cancer Institute*, Sep 15, 1993; 85 (18): 1483-1492.
121.	Hercberg S, et al. The SU.VI.MAX Study: A Randomized, Placebo-Controlled Trial of the Health Effects of Antioxidant Vitamins and Minerals. *Archives of Internal Medicine*, Nov 2004; 164: 2335-2342. Note: The lack of protection against cancer in women may have been due to their superior antioxidant status at the start of the study; blood tests revealed lower baseline blood sugar levels and higher baseline blood levels of vitamin C and beta-carotene than the male subjects. As for the null effect on cardiovascular disease risk, this may have been an artifact of the already low risk of cardiovascular ailments enjoyed by the French population.
122.	Becker DJ, et al. Oral selenate improves glucose homeostasis and partly reverses abnormal expression of liver glycolytic and gluconeogenic enzymes in diabetic rats. *Diabetologia*, Jan, 1996; 39 (1): 3-11.
123.	Ghosh R, et al. A novel effect of selenium on streptozotocin-induced diabetic mice. *Diabetes Research*, 1994; 25 (4): 165-171.
124.	Stapleton SR. Selenium: an insulin-mimetic. *Cellular and Molecular Life Sciences*, Dec, 2000; 57 (13-14): 1874-1879.
125.	Foster HD. AIDS: The seleno-enzyme solution. *Nexus Magazine*, December-January 2004; 11 (1). Available online: http://www.nexusmagazine.com/AIDS.Selenium.html#44. (accessed February 1, 2004).
126.	Cowgill UM. The distribution of selenium and mortality owing to acquired immune deficiency syndrome in the continental United States. *Biological Trace Element Research*, Jan 1997; 56 (1): 43-61.
127.	Rubin RN, et al. Relationship of serum antioxidants to asthma prevalence in youth. *American Journal of Respiratory and Critical Care Medicine*, Feb 1, 2004; 169 (3): 393-398.
128.	Omland O, et al. Selenium serum and urine is associated to mild asthma and atopy. The SUS study. *Journal of Trace Elements in Medicine and Biology*, 2002; 16 (2): 123-127.

129. Shaheen SO, et al. Dietary antioxidants and asthma in adults: population-based case-control study. *American Journal of Respiratory and Critical Care Medicine*, Nov 15, 2001; 164 (10 Pt 1): 1823-1828.

130. Lyons G, et al. High-selenium wheat: biofortification for better health. *Nutrition Research Reviews,* 2003; 16: 45-60.

131. Hasselmark L, et al. Selenium supplementation in intrinsic asthma. *Allergy*, Jan, 1993; 48 (1): 30-36.

132. Benton D, Cook R. The impact of selenium supplementation on mood. *Biological Psychiatry*, 1991; 29: 1092-1098.

133. Tolonen M, et al. Vitamin E and selenium supplementation in geriatric patients A double-blind preliminary clinical trial. *Biological Trace Element Research*, 1985; 7: 161-168.

134. Girodon F, et al. Effect of micronutrient supplementation on infection in institutionalized elderly subjects: a controlled trial. *Annals of Nutrition and Metabolism*, 1997; 41 (2): 98-107.

135. Broome CS, et al. An increase in selenium intake improves immune function and poliovirus handling in adults with marginal selenium status. *American Journal of Clinical Nutrition*, Jul, 2004; 80 (1): 154-162.

136. Girodon F, et al. Impact of trace elements and vitamin supplementation on immunity and infections in institutionalized elderly patients: a randomized controlled trial. MIN. VIT. AOX. geriatric network. *Archives of Internal Medicine*, Apr 12 1999; 159 (7): 748-754.

137. The American Cancer Society, *Cancer Facts and Figures 2003*: 30.

138. Combs GF Jr. Selenium in global food systems. *British Journal of Nutrition,* May, 2001; 85 (5): 517-47.

139. Kelly GS. L-Carnitine: Therapeutic Applications of a Conditionally-Essential Amino Acid. *Alternative Medicine Review*, 1998; 3 (5): 345-360.

140. Cavallini G, et al. Carnitine versus androgen administration in the treatment of sexual dysfunction, depressed mood, and fatigue associated with male aging. *Urology*, Apr, 2004; 63 (4): 641-646.

141. Cederblad G. Effect of diet on plasma carnitine levels and urinary carnitine excretion in humans. *American Journal of Clinical Nutrition*, 1987; 45: 725-729.

Chapter 25

1. Jacobs DR, et al. Whole-grain intake may reduce the risk of ischemic heart disease death in postmenopausal women: the Iowa Women's Health Study. *American Journal of Clinical Nutrition,* 1998; 68: 248-257.

2. Burr ML, et al. Effects of changes in fat, fish, and fibre intakes on death and myocardial reinfarction: diet and reinfarction trial (DART). *Lancet*, 1989; 2: 757-761.

3. Challen AD, et al. The effect of pectin and wheat bran on platelet function and haemostatis in man. *Human Nutrition: Clinical Nutrition*, May, 1983; 37 (3): 209-217.

4. Jenkins DJ, et al. Effect of wheat bran on glycemic control and risk factors for cardiovascular disease in type 2 diabetes. *Diabetes Care*, Sep, 2002; 25 (9): 1522-1528.

5. Asano T, McLeod RS. Dietary fibre for the prevention of colorectal adenomas and carcinomas (Cochrane Review). In: *The Cochrane Library*, Issue 2, 2002. Oxford.

6. Food and Drug Administration, HHS. Food Labeling: Health Claims; Soy Protein and Coronary Heart Disease. *Federal Register*, Oct 26, 1999; 64 (206): 57699-57733. Available online: http://vm.cfsan.fda.gov/~lrd/fr991026.html (accessed September 8, 2005).

7. Anderson JW, et al. Meta-analysis of the effects of soy protein intake on serum lipids. *New England Journal of Medicine,* 1995; 333 (5): 276-282.

8. Jenkins DJ, et al. Effects of high- and low-isoflavone soyfoods on blood lipids, oxidized LDL, homocysteine, and blood pressure in hyperlipidemic men and women. *American Journal of Clinical Nutrition*, Aug, 2002; 76 (2): 365-372.

9. Hwang J, et al. Synergistic inhibition of LDL oxidation by phytoestrogens and ascorbic acid. *Free Radical Biology & Medicine*, Jul 1, 2000; 29 (1): 79-89.

10. Ashton EL, et al. Effect of meat replacement by tofu on CHD risk factors including copper induced LDL oxidation. *Journal of the American College of Nutrition*, Nov-Dec, 2000; 19 (6): 761-767.

11. Cuevas AM, et al. Isolated soy protein improves endothelial function in postmenopausal hypercholesterolemic women. *European Journal of Clinical Nutrition*, Aug, 2003; 57 (8): 889-894.

12. Hale G, et al. Isoflavone supplementation and endothelial function in menopausal women. *Clinical Endocrinology*, Jun, 2002; 56 (6): 693-701.

13. Yamashita T, et al. Arterial compliance, blood pressure, plasma leptin, and plasma lipids in women are improved with weight reduction equally with a meat-based diet and a plant-based diet. *Metabolism*, Nov, 1998; 47 (11): 1308-1314.

14. Teede HJ, et al. Dietary soy has both beneficial and potentially adverse cardiovascular effects: a placebo-controlled study in men and postmenopausal women. *Journal of Clinical Endocrinology and Metabolism*, Jul, 2001; 86 (7): 3053-3060.

15. Kreijkamp-Kaspers S, et al. Randomized controlled trial of the effects of soy protein containing isoflavones on vascular function in postmenopausal women. *American Journal of Clinical Nutrition*, Jan, 2005; 81: 189-195.

16. Gooderham MH, et al. A soy protein isolate rich in genistein and daidzein and its effects on plasma isoflavone concentrations, platelet aggregation, blood lipids and fatty acid composition of plasma phospholipid in normal men. *Journal of Nutrition,* Aug, 1996; 126 (8): 2000-2006.

17. Nilausen K, Meinertz H. Lipoprotein(a) and dietary proteins: casein lowers lipoprotein(a) concentrations as compared with soy protein. *American Journal of Clinical Nutrition,* Mar, 1999; 69 (3): 419-425.

18. Stauffer BL, et al. Soy diet worsens heart disease in mice. *Journal of Clinical Investigation*, 2006; 116: 209-216.

19. Martin PM, et al. Phytoestrogen interaction with estrogen receptors in human breast cancer cells. *Endocrinology*, 1978; 103: 1860-1867.

20. Hsieh CY, et al. Estrogenic effects of genistein on the growth of estrogen receptor-positive human breast cancer (MCF-7) cells in vitro and in vivo. *Cancer Research*, 1998; 58: 3833-3838.

21. Allred CD, et al. Dietary genistin stimulates growth of estrogen-dependent breast cancer tumors similar to that observed with genistein. *Carcinogenesis*, Oct 1, 2001; 22(10): 1667 - 1673.

22. Ju YH, et al. Physiological Concentrations of Dietary Genistein Dose-Dependently Stimulate Growth of Estrogen-Dependent Human Breast Cancer (MCF-7) Tumors Implanted in Athymic Nude Mice. *Journal of Nutrition*, 2001; 131 (11): 2957-2962.

23. Ju YH, et al. Dietary Genistein Negates the Inhibitory Effect of Tamoxifen on Growth of Estrogen-dependent Human Breast Cancer (MCF-7) Cells Implanted in Athymic Mice. *Cancer Research*, 2002; 62 (9): 2474-2477.

24. Petrakis NL, et al. Stimulatory influence of soy protein isolate on breast fluid secretion in pre- and postmenopausal women. *Cancer Epidemiology, Biomarkers & Prevention*, 1996; 5: 785-794.

25. Hargreaves DF, et al. Two-week dietary soy supplementation has an estrogenic effect on normal premenopausal breast. *Journal of Clinical Endocrinology and Metabolism*, 1999; 84: 4017-4024.

26. Kimura S et al. Development of malignant goiter by defatted soybean with iodine-free diet in rats. *Gann*, 1976; 67: 763-765.
27. Rao CV, et al. Enhancement of experimental colon cancer by genistein. *Cancer Research*, 1997; 57: 3717-3722.
28. Sun CL, et al. Dietary Soy and Increased Risk of Bladder Cancer: the Singapore Chinese Health Study. *Cancer Epidemiology, Biomarkers & Prevention,* 2002; 11 (12): 1674-1677.
29. Yellayi S, et al. The phytoestrogen genistein induces thymic and immune changes: a human health concern? *Proceedings of the National Academy of Sciences*, 2002; 99 (11): 7616-7621.
30. Zoppi G, et al. Immunocompetence and dietary protein intake in early infancy. *Journal of Pediatric Gastroenterology and Nutrition*, 1982; 1 (2): 175-182.
31. Zoppi G, et al. Diet and antibody response to vaccinations in healthy infants. *Lancet*, Jul 2, 1983; 2 (8340): 11-14.
32. Van Wyk JJ, et al. The effects of a soybean product on thyroid function in humans. *Pediatrics*, Nov, 1959; 24: 752-760.
33. Shepard TH, et al. Soybean goiter: Report of three cases. *New England Journal of Medicine*, 1960; 262: 1099–1103.
34. Hydovitz JD. Occurrence of goiter in an infant on a soy diet. *New England Journal of Medicine,* 1960; 26: 351-353.
35. Ripp J. Soybean-induced goiter. *American Journal of Diseases of Children,* Jul, 1961; 102: 106-109.
36. Pinchera A, et al. Thyroid refractoriness in an athyreotic cretin fed soybean formula. *New England Journal of Medicine,* 1965; 265, 83-87.
37. Chorazy PA, et al. Persistent hypothyroidism in an infant receiving a soy formula: Case report and review of the literature. *Pediatrics,* 148-150, 1995.
38. Jabbar MA et al. Abnormal thyroid function tests in infants with congenital hypothyroidism: the influence of soy-based formula. *Journal of the American College of Nutrition,* 1997; 16: 280-282.
39. Labib M, et al. Dietary maladvice as a cause of hypothyroidism and short stature. *British Medical Journal*, 1989; 298: 232-233.
40. Bell DS, Ovalle F. Use of soy protein supplement and resultant need for increased dose of levothyroxine. *Endocrine Practice,* May-Jun, 2001; 7 (3): 193-194.
41. Ishizuki Y, et al. The effects on the thyroid gland of soybeans administered experimentally in healthy subjects. *Nippon Naibunpi Gakkai Zasshi*, 1991; 67: 622-629.
42. Duncan AM, et al. Soy isoflavones exert modest hormonal effects in premenopausal women. *Journal of Clinical Endocrinology and Metabolism*, 1999; 84:192–197.
43. Watanabe S, et al. Effects of isoflavone supplement on healthy women. *Biofactors*, 2000; 12 (1-4): 233-241.
44. Ham JO, et al. Endocrinological response to soy protein and fiber in mildly hypercholesterolemic men. *Nutrition Research*, 1993; 13: 873–884.
45. Persky VW, et al. Effect of soy protein on endogenous hormones in postmenopausal women. *American Journal of Clinical Nutrition*, 2002; 75 (1): 145-153.
46. Huszno B, et al. Influence of iodine deficiency and iodine prophylaxis on thyroid cancer histotypes and incidence in endemic goiter area. *Journal of Endocrinological Investigation*, 2003; 26 (2 Suppl): 71-76.
47. Fort P et al. Breast and soy-formula feedings in early infancy and the prevalence of autoimmune thyroid disease in children. *Journal of the American College of Nutrition*, 1990; 9 (2): 164-167.
48. Fort P et al. Breast feeding and insulin-dependent diabetes mellitus in children. *Journal of the American College of Nutrition*, 1986; 5 (5): 439-441.

49. Nagata C, et al. Inverse association of soy product intake with serum androgen and estrogen concentrations in Japanese men. *Nutrition and Cancer*, 2000; 36 (1): 14-18.
50. Habito RC, et al. Effects of replacing meat with soyabean in the diet on sex hormone concentrations in healthy adult males. *British Journal of Nutrition*, 2000; 84: 557-563.
51. Raben A, et al. Serum sex hormones and endurance performance after a lacto-ovo vegetarian and a mixed diet. *Medicine and Science in Sports and Exercise*, 1992; 24: 1290-1297.
52. Gardner-Thorpe D, et al. Dietary supplements of soya flour lower serum testosterone concentrations and improve markers of oxidative stress in men. *European Journal of Clinical Nutrition*, Jan, 2003; 57 (1): 100-106.
53. Zhong, et al. Effects of dietary supplement of soy protein isolate and low fat diet on prostate cancer. *FASEB Journal*, 2000; 14 (4): A531.11.
54. North K, Golding J. A maternal vegetarian diet in pregnancy is associated with hypospadias. *British Journal of Urology International*, Jan, 2000 85:107-113.
55. Hurrell RF, et al. Soy protein, phytate, and iron absorption in humans. *American Journal of Clinical Nutrition*, Sep, 1992; 56 (3): 573-578.
56. Koo WWK, Kaplan LA, Krug-Wispe SK. Aluminum contamination of infant formulas. *JPEN: Journal of Parenteral and Enteral Nutrition*, 1988; 12: 170-173.
57. Massey LK, et al. Oxalate content of soybean seeds (Glycine max: Leguminosae), soyfoods, and other edible legumes. *Journal of Agricultural and Food Chemistry*, Sep, 2001; 49 (9): 4262-4266.
58. Shu XO, et al. Soyfood intake during adolescence and subsequent risk of breast cancer among Chinese women. *Cancer Epidemiology, Biomarkers & Prevention,* May, 2001; 10: 483-488.
59. Nagata C, et al. Decreased serum total cholesterol concentration is associated with high intake of soy products in Japanese men and women. *Journal of Nutrition*, 1998; 128: 209-213.
60. Rose GA, et al. Corn oil in treatment of ischaemic heart disease. *British Medical Journal*, 1965; 1: 1531-1533.
61. Mutanen M., et al. Rapeseed oil and sunflower oil diets enhance platelet in vitro aggregation and thromboxane production in healthy men when compared with milk fat or habitual diets. *Thrombosis and Haemostasis*, 1992; 67: 352-356.
62. Turpeinen AM, et al. Replacement of dietary saturated by unsaturated fatty acids: effects of platelet protein kinase C activity, urinary content of 2,3-dinor-TXB2 and in vitro platelet aggregation in healthy man. *Thrombosis and Haemostasis*, 1998; 80: 649-655.
63. Turpeinen AM, et al. A high linoleic acid diet increases oxidative stress in vivo and affects nitric oxide metabolism in humans. *Prostaglandins, Leukotrienes and Essential Fatty Acids*, 1998; 59 (3): 229-233.
64. Liu L, et al. Xuezhikang decreases serum lipoprotein(a) and C-reactive protein concentrations in patients with coronary heart disease. *Clinical Chemistry*, Aug, 2003; 49 (8): 1347-1352.
65. Zhao SP, et al. Effect of xuezhikang, a cholestin extract, on reflecting postprandial triglyceridemia after a high-fat meal in patients with coronary heart disease. *Atherosclerosis*, Jun, 2003; 168 (2): 375-380.
66. Yang HT, et al. Acute administration of red yeast rice (Monascus purpureus) depletes tissue coenzyme Q(10) levels in ICR mice. *British Journal of Nutrition*, Jan, 2005; 93 (1): 131-135.
67. Smith DJ, Olive KE. Chinese Red Rice-induced Myopathy. *Southern Medical Journal*, Dec, 2003; 96 (12): 1265.
68. Prasad GV, et al. Rhabdomyolysis due to red yeast rice (Monascus purpureus) in a renal transplant recipient. *Transplantation*, Oct 27, 2002; 74 (8): 1200-1201.

69. Rees K, et al. Psychological interventions for coronary heart disease (Cochrane Review). In: *The Cochrane Library*, Issue 2, 2004. Chichester, UK: John Wiley & Sons, Ltd.
70. Schneider RH, et al. A Randomized Controlled Trial of Stress Reduction for Hypertension in Older African Americans. *Hypertension*, 1995; 26: 820.
71. Castillo-Richmond A, et al. Effects of Stress Reduction on Carotid Atherosclerosis in Hypertensive African Americans. *Stroke*, Mar 1, 2000; 31 (3): 568-573.
72. Schneider RH, et al. Long-Term Effects of Stress Reduction on Mortality in Persons >55 Years of Age With Systemic Hypertension. *American Journal of Cardiology*, 2005; 95: 1060-1064.
73. Personal email communication with Robert H. Schneider, M.D., Director and Professor, Institute for Natural Medicine and Prevention, Maharishi University of Management, Iowa, USA.
74. Thayer RE, et al. Self-regulation of mood: strategies for changing a bad mood, raising energy, and reducing tension. *Journal of Personality and Social Psychology*, Nov, 1994; 67 (5): 910-925.
75. Jin P. Efficacy of Tai Chi, brisk walking, meditation, and reading in reducing mental and emotional stress. *Journal of Psychosomatic Medicine*, May, 1992; 36 (4): 361-370.
76. Roth DL, Holmes DS. Influence of aerobic exercise training and relaxation training on physical and psychologic health following stressful life events. *Psychosomatic Medicine*, Jul-Aug, 1987; 49 (4): 355-65.
77. Blumenthal JA, et al. Effects of Exercise Training on Older Patients With Major Depression. *Archives of Internal Medicine*, 1999; 159: 2349-2356.
78. Babyak M, et al. Exercise treatment for major depression: maintenance of therapeutic benefit at 10 months. *Psychosomatic Medicine*, Sep-Oct, 2000; 62: 633–638.

Chapter 26
1. Gutierrez M, et al. Utility of a Short-Term 25% Carbohydrate Diet on Improving Glycemic Control in Type 2 Diabetes Mellitus. *Journal of the American College of Nutrition,* 1998; 17 (6): 595-600.
2. Coulston AM, et al. Deleterious metabolic effects of high-carbohydrate, sucrose-containing diets in patients with non-insulin-dependent diabetes mellitus. *American Journal of Medicine*, Feb, 1987; 82 (2): 213-220.
3 Garg A, et al. Effects of varying carbohydrate content of diet in patients with non-insulin-dependent diabetes mellitus. *Journal of the American Medical Association*, 1994; 271: 1421-1428.
4. Sestoft L, et al. High-carbohydrate, low-fat diet: effect on lipid and carbohydrate metabolism, GIP and insulin secretion in diabetics. *Danish Medical Bulletin*, Mar, 1985; 32 (1): 64-69.
5. Gannon MC, et al. An increase in dietary protein improves the blood glucose response in persons with type 2 diabetes. *American Journal of Clinical Nutrition*, 2003; 78: 734-741.
6. The Diabetes Food Pyramid: Starches. American Diabetes Association web site. Available online: http://www.diabetes.org/nutrition-and-recipes/nutrition/starches.jsp (accessed September 8, 2005).
7. McKewen MW, et al. Glycemic control, muscle glycogen and exercise performance in IDDM athletes on diets of varying carbohydrate content. *International Journal of Sports Medicine,* 1999; 20: 349-353.
8. Wing RR, et al. Cognitive effects of weight-reducing diets. *International Journal of Obesity*, 1995; 19: 811-816.
9. Meckling KA, et al. Effects of a hypocaloric, low-carbohydrate diet on weight loss, blood lipids, blood pressure, glucose tolerance, and body composition in free-living overweight women. *Canadian Journal of Physiology and Pharmacology*, Nov, 2002; 80 (11): 1095-1105.

10. Allan CB, Lutz W. *Life Without Bread: How a Low-Carbohydrate Diet Can Save Your Life*. McGraw-Hill/Contemporary Books, July 2000.
11. Bisschop PH, et al. Dietary fat content alters insulin-mediated glucose metabolism in healthy men. *American Journal of Clinical Nutrition*, 2001; 73: 554-559.
12. Takyi EE. Children's consumption of dark green, leafy vegetables with added fat enhances serum retinol. *Journal of Nutrition*, 1999; 129 (8): 1549-1554.
13. Jalal F, et al. Serum retinol concentrations are affected by food sources of ß-carotene, fat intake, and anthehelmintic drug treatment. *American Journal of Clinical Nutrition*, 1998; 68: 623-629.
14. Roodenburg JA, et al. Amount of fat in the diet affects bioavailability of lutein esters but not of {alpha}-carotene, {beta}-carotene, and vitamin E in humans. *American Journal of Clinical Nutrition*, 2000; 71 (5): 1187-1193.
15. Drammeh BS, et al. A Randomized, 4-Month Mango and Fat Supplementation Trial Improved Vitamin A Status among Young Gambian Children. *Journal of Nutrition*, 2002; 132 (12): 3693-3699.
16. Chung H-Y, et al. Lutein Bioavailability Is Higher from Lutein-Enriched Eggs than from Supplements and Spinach in Men. *Journal of Nutrition*, 2004; 134: 1887-1893.
17. Brown MJ, et al. Carotenoid bioavailability is higher from salads ingested with full-fat than with fat-reduced salad dressings as measured with electrochemical detection. *American Journal of Clinical Nutrition*, Aug, 2004; 80: 396-403.
18. Unlu NZ, et al. Carotenoid Absorption from Salad and Salsa by Humans Is Enhanced by the Addition of Avocado or Avocado Oil. *Journal of Nutrition,* Mar, 2005; 135: 431-436.
19. USDA National Nutrient Database for Standard Reference. Available online: http://www.nal.usda.gov/fnic/foodcomp/search/
20. Giacobini E. Cholinergic function and Alzheimer's disease. *International Journal of Geriatric Psychiatry*, Sep, 2003; 18 (Suppl 1): S1-S5.
21. Adams CW, et al. Modification of aortic atheroma and fatty liver in cholesterol-fed rabbits by intravenous injection of saturated and polyunsaturated lecithins. *Journal of Pathology and Bacteriology*, Jul, 1967; 94 (1): 77-87.
22. Howard A, et al. Atherosclerosis induced in hypercholesterolaemic baboons by immunological injury, and the effects of intravenous polyunsaturated PPC. *Atherosclerosis*, 1971; 14 (1): 17-29.
23. Mahoney AW, et al. Effects of level and source of dietary fat on the bioavailability of iron from turkey meat for the anemic rat. *Journal of Nutrition,* 1980: 110 (8): 1703-1708.
24. Johnson PE, et al. The effects of stearic acid and beef tallow on iron utilization by the rat. *Proceedings of the Society for Experimental Biology and Medicine,* 1992; 200 (4): 480-486.
25. Koo SI, Ramlet JS. Effect of dietary linoleic acid on the tissue levels of zinc and copper, and serum high-density lipoprotein cholesterol. *Atherosclerosis*, 1984; 50 (2): 123-132.
26. Lukaski HC, et al. Interactions among dietary fat, mineral status, and performance of endurance athletes: a case study. *International Journal of Sport Nutrition and Exercise Metabolism,* Jun, 2001; 11 (2): 186-198.
27. Van Dokkum W, et al. Effect of variations in fat and linoleic acid intake on the calcium, magnesium and iron balance of young men. *Annals of Nutrition & Metabolism,* 1983; 27 (5): 361-369.
28. Emken EA, et al. Dietary linoleic acid influences desaturation and acylation of deuterium-labeled linoleic and linolenic acids in young adult males. *Biochimica et Biophysica Acta*, Aug 4, 1994; 1213 (3): 277-288.
29. Garg ML, et al. Dietary saturated fat level alters the competition between alpha-linolenic and linoleic acid. *Lipids*, Apr, 1989; 24 (4): 334-339.
30. Koopman JS, et al. Milk fat and gastrointestinal illness. *American Journal of Public Health*, 1984; 74: 1371-1373.

31. Puertollano MA, et al. Relevance of Dietary Lipids as Modulators of Immune Functions in Cells Infected with Listeria monocytogenes. *Clinical and Diagnostic Laboratory Immunology*, Mar, 2002; 9 (2): 352-357.
32. de Pablo MA, et al. Determination of natural resistance of mice fed dietary lipids to experimental infection induced by Listeria monocytogenes. *FEMS Immunology and Medical Microbiology*, Feb, 2000; 27 (2): 127-133.
33. Volek JS, et al. Testosterone and cortisol in relationship to dietary nutrients and resistance exercise. *Journal of Applied Physiology*, Jan, 1997; 82 (1): 49-54.
34. Hamalainen EK, et al. Decrease of serum total and free testosterone during a low-fat high-fibre diet. *Journal of Steroid Biochemistry*, Mar, 1983; 18 (3): 369-370.
35. Reed MJ, et al. Dietary lipids: an additional regulator of plasma levels of sex hormone binding globulin. *Journal of Clinical Endocrinology and Metabolism,* 1987; 64: 1083-1085.
36. Dorgan JF, et al. Effects of dietary fat and fiber on plasma and urine androgens and estrogens in men: a controlled feeding study. *American Journal of Clinical Nutrition*, Dec, 1996; 64 (6): 850-855.
37. Cha YS, Sachan DS. Opposite effects of dietary saturated and unsaturated fatty acids on ethanol-pharmacokinetics, triglycerides and carnitines. *Journal of the American College of Nutrition*, Aug, 1994; 13 (4): 338-343.
38. Polavarapu R, et al. Increased lipid peroxidation and impaired antioxidant enzyme function is associated with pathological liver injury in experimental alcoholic liver disease in rats fed diets high in corn oil and fish oil. *Hepatology*, May, 1998; 27 (5): 1317-1323
39. Nanji AA, et al. Dietary Saturated Fatty Acids Reverse Inflammatory and Fibrotic Changes in Rat Liver Despite Continued Ethanol Administration. *Journal of Pharmacology and Experimental Therapeutics*, Nov, 2001; 299 (2): 638-644.
40. Ronis MJ, et al. Dietary Saturated Fat Reduces Alcoholic Hepatotoxicity in Rats by Altering Fatty Acid Metabolism and Membrane Composition. *Journal of Nutrition,* Apr, 2004; 134: 904-912.
41. Nanji AA, French SW. Dietary factors and alcoholic cirrhosis. *Alcoholism, Clinical and Experimental Research*, Jun, 1986; 10 (3): 271-273.
42. Xu H, et al. Vitamin E stimulates trabecular bone formation and alters epiphyseal cartilage morphometry. *Calcified Tissue International*, Oct, 1995; 57 (4): 293-300.
43. Watkins BA, et al. Dietary Lipids Modulate Bone Prostaglandin E2 Production, Insulin-Like Growth Factor-I Concentration and Formation Rate in Chicks. *Journal of Nutrition*, Jun, 1997; 127 (6): 1084-1091.
44. Macdonald HM, et al. Nutritional associations with bone loss during the menopausal transition: evidence of a beneficial effect of calcium, alcohol, and fruit and vegetable nutrients and of a detrimental effect of fatty acids. *American Journal of Clinical Nutrition*, Jan, 2004; 79 (1): 155-165.
45. Chin SF, et al. Dietary sources of conjugated dienoic isomers of linoleic acid, a newly recognized class of anticarcinogens. *Journal of Food Composition and Analysis*, 1992; 5: 185-197.
46. Belury MA. Inhibition of Carcinogenesis by Conjugated Linoleic Acid: Potential Mechanisms of Action. *Journal of Nutrition*, 2002; 132: 2995-2998.
47. Albers R, et al. Effects of cis-9, trans-11 and trans-10, cis-12 conjugated linoleic acid (CLA) isomers on immune function in healthy men. *European Journal of Clinical Nutrition,* Apr, 2003; 57 (4): 595-603.
48. Belury MA, et al. The Conjugated Linoleic Acid (CLA) Isomer, t10c12-CLA, Is Inversely Associated with Changes in Body Weight and Serum Leptin in Subjects with Type 2 Diabetes Mellitus. *Journal of Nutrition,* 2003; 133: 257S-260S.

49. Gaullier JM, et al. Conjugated linoleic acid supplementation for 1 y reduces body fat mass in healthy overweight humans. *American Journal of Clinical Nutrition*, Jun, 2004; 79: 1118-1125.
50. Kamphuis MM, et al. The effect of conjugated linoleic acid supplementation after weight loss on body weight regain, body composition, and resting metabolic rate in overweight subjects. *International Journal Of Obesity & Related Metabolic Disorders,* Jul, 2003; 27 (7): 840-847.
51. Thom E, et al. Conjugated linoleic acid reduces body fat in healthy exercising humans. *Journal Of International Medical Research*, Sep-Oct, 2001; 29 (5): 392-396.
52. Smedman A, Vessby B. Conjugated linoleic acid supplementation in humans -metabolic effects. *Lipids*, Aug. 2001; 36 (8): 773-781.
53. Riserus U, et al. Conjugated linoleic acid (CLA) reduced abdominal adipose tissue in obese middle-aged men with signs of the metabolic syndrome: a randomised controlled trial. *International Journal Of Obesity & Related Metabolic Disorders*, Aug, 2001; 25 (8): 1129-35.
54. Blankson H, et al. Conjugated linoleic acid reduces body fat mass in overweight and obese humans. *Journal of Nutrition,* Dec, 2000; 130 (12): 2943-2948.
55. Noone EJ, et al. The effect of dietary supplementation using isomeric blends of conjugated linoleic acid on lipid metabolism in healthy human subjects. *British Journal of Nutrition,* Sept, 2002; 88 (3): 243-251.
56. Malpuech-Brugère CB, et al. Effects of Two Conjugated Linoleic Acid Isomers on Body Fat Mass in Overweight Humans. *Obesity Research,* Apr, 2004; 12: 591-598.
57. Kreider RB, et al. Effects of conjugated linoleic acid supplementation during resistance training on body composition, bone density, strength, and selected hematological markers. *Journal Of Strength And Conditioning Research,* Aug, 2002; 16 (3): 325-34.
58. Zambell KL, et al. Conjugated linoleic acid supplementation in humans: effects on body composition and energy expenditure. *Lipids,* Jul, 2000; 35 (7): 777-782.
59. Mozaffarian D, et al. Dietary fats, carbohydrate, and progression of coronary atherosclerosis in postmenopausal women. *American Journal of Clinical Nutrition*, 2004; 80: 1175-1184.
60. Dhiman TR, et al. Conjugated linoleic acid content of milk from cows fed different diets. *Journal of Dairy Science*, Oct, 1999; 82 (10): 2146-2156.
61. French P, et al. Fatty acid composition, including conjugated linoleic acid, of intramuscular fat from steers offered grazed grass, grass silage, or concentrate-based diets. *Journal of Animal Science*, Nov, 2000; 78 (11): 2849-2855.
62. O'Sullivan A, et al. Grass silage versus maize silage effects on retail packaged beef quality. *Journal of Animal Science,* 2002; 80: 1556–1563.
63. Hebeisen DF, et al. Increased concentrations of omega-3 fatty acids in milk and platelet rich plasma of grass-fed cows. *International Journal for Vitamin and Nutrition Research*, 1993; 63 (3): 229-233.
64. Simopoulos AP, Salem N Jr. Egg yolk as a source of long-chain polyunsaturated fatty acids in infant feeding. *American Journal of Clinical Nutrition*, Feb, 1992; 55 (2): 411-414.

Chapter 27

1. Smith R. The most important BMJ for 50 years? *British Medical Journal*, Jun, 2003; 326: 0-f.
2. Wald NJ, Law MR. A strategy to reduce cardiovascular disease by more than 80%. *British Medical Journal,* Jun 28, 2003; 326 (7404): 1419.
3. Regush NM. Shabby Medical Thinking. *British Medical Journal Rapid Responses*. Available online: http://bmj.bmjjournals.com/cgi/eletters/326/7404/1419#33770 (accessed Sept. 3, 2004).

4. Banerjee SK, Maulik SK. Effect of garlic on cardiovascular disorders: a review. *Nutrition Journal*, Nov 19, 2002; 1 (1): 4.
5. Campbell JH, et al. Molecular basis by which garlic suppresses atherosclerosis. *Journal of Nutrition*, Mar, 2001; 131 (3s): 1006S-1009S.
6. Efendy JL, et al. The effect of the aged garlic extract, 'Kyolic', on the development of experimental atherosclerosis. *Atherosclerosis*, Jul 11, 1997; 132 (1): 37-42.
7. Koscielny J, et al. The antiatherosclerotic effect of Allium sativum. *Atherosclerosis*, May 1999; 144 (1): 237-49.
8. Budoff MJ, et al. Inhibiting progression of coronary calcification using Aged Garlic Extract in patients receiving statin therapy: a preliminary study. *Preventive Medicine*, Nov, 2004; 39 (5): 985-991.
9. Kiesewetter H, et al. Effects of garlic coated tablets in peripheral arterial occlusive disease. *Clinical Investigator*, May 1993; 71 (5): 383-386.
10. Rose KD, et al. Spontaneous Spinal Epidural Hematoma with Associated Platelet Dysfunction from Excessive Garlic Ingestion: A case Report. *Neurosurgery*, 1990; 26: 880–882.
11. Sunter W. Warfarin and garlic. *Pharmacology*, 1991; 246: 722.
12. Burnham BE. Garlic as a possible risk for postoperative bleeding. *Plastic and Reconstructive Surgery*, 1995; 95: 213.
13. Fugh-Berman A. Herb-drug interactions. *Lancet*, 2000; 355: 134–138.
14. Petry JJ. Garlic and postoperative bleeding. *Plastic and Reconstructive Surgery*, 1995; 96: 483–484.
15. Gao CM, et al. Protective effect of allium vegetables against both esophageal and stomach cancer: a simultaneous case-referent study of a high-epidemic area in Jiangsu Province, China. *Japanese Journal of Cancer Research*, Jun, 1999; 90 (6): 614-621.
16. Hu J, et al. Diet and brain cancer in adults: a case-control study in northeast China. *International Journal of Cancer*, Mar, 1999; 31; 81 (1): 20-23.
17. Steinmetz KA, et al. Vegetables, fruit, and colon cancer in the Iowa Women's Health Study. *American Journal of Epidemiology*, 1994; 139: 1-15.
18. Hsing AW, et al. Allium vegetables and risk of prostate cancer: a population-based study. *Journal of the National Cancer Institute*, 2002 Nov 6; 94 (21): 1648-1651.
19. Hong JY, et al. Inhibitory effects of diallyl sulfide on the metabolism and tumorigenicity of tobacco-specific carcinogen 4-methylnitrosamino-1-3-pyridyl 1-butanone (NNK) in A/J mouse lung. *Carcinogenesis*, 1992; 13: 901-904.
20. Sparnins VL, et al. Effects of organosulfur compounds from garlic and onions on benzo[a]pyrene-induced neoplasia and glutathione S-transferase activity in the mouse. *Carcinogenesis*, Jan 1988; 9 (1): 131-134.
21. Wargovich MJ, et al. Chemoprevention of N-nitrosomethylbenzylamine-induced esophageal cancer in rats by the naturally occurring thioether, diallyl sulfide. *Cancer Research*, 1998; 48 (23): 6872-6875.
22. Nishino H, et al. Antitumor-promoting activity of garlic extracts. *Oncology*, 1989; 46: 277-280.
23. Schaffer EM, et al. Garlic and associated allylsulfur components inhibit N-methyl-N-nitrosourea induced rat mammary carcinogenesis. *Cancer Letters*, 1996; 102: 199-204.
24. Schaffer EM, et al. Garlic powder and allyl sulfur compounds enhance the ability of dietary selenite to inhibit 7,12-dimethylbenz(a)anthracene-induced mammary DNA adducts. *Nutrition and Cancer*, 1997; 27: 162-168.
25. Liu JZ, et al. Inhibition of 7,12-dimethylbenz(a)anthracene-induced mammary tumors and DNA adducts by garlic powder. *Carcinogenesis*, 1992; 13:1847-1851.
26. Nishiyama N, et al. Beneficial effects of aged garlic extract on learning and memory impairment in the senescence-accelerated mouse. *Experimental Gerontology*, 1997; 32: 149-160

27. Moriguchi T, et al. Anti-aging effect of aged garlic extract in the inbred brain atrophy mouse model. *Clinical and Experimental Pharmacology and Physiology*, 1997; 24: 235-242.
28. Hu JJ, et al. Protective effects of diallyl sulfide on acetaminophen-induced toxicities. *Food and Chemical Toxicology*, Oct, 1996; 34 (10): 963-969.
29. Josling P. Preventing the common cold with a garlic supplement: a double-blind, placebo-controlled survey. *Advances in Therapy*, Jul-Aug, 2001; 18 (4): 189-193.
30. Song K, Milner JA. The Influence of Heating on the Anticancer Properties of Garlic. *Journal of Nutrition*, Mar 1, 2001; 131 (3): 1054S-1057.
31. Yin MC, Cheng WS. Inhibition of Aspergillus niger and Aspergillus flavus by some herbs and spices. *Journal of Food Protection*, 1998; 61: 123-125.
32. Chen HC, et al. Antibacterial properties of some spice plants before and after heat treatment. *Zhonghua Min Guo Wei Sheng Wu Ji Mian Yi Xue Za Zhi*, Aug, 1985; 18 (3): 190-195.
33. Chen JH, et al. Chronic consumption of raw but not boiled Welsh onion juice inhibits rat platelet function. *Journal of Nutrition*, Jan 2000; 130 (1): 34-37.
34. Ali M, et al. Effect of raw versus boiled aqueous extract of garlic and onion on platelet aggregation. *Prostaglandins, Leukotrienes, and Essential Fatty Acids*, Jan, 1999; 60 (1): 43-47.
35. Fox C, et al. Magnesium: its proven and potential clinical significance. *Southern Medical Journal*, Dec, 2001; 94 (12): 1195-1201.
36. Shechter M, et al. Effects of oral magnesium therapy on exercise tolerance, exercise-induced chest pain, and quality of life in patients with coronary artery disease. *American Journal of Cardiology*, Mar 1, 2003; 91 (5): 517-521.
37. Shechter M, et al. Beneficial antithrombotic effects of the association of pharmacological oral magnesium therapy with aspirin in coronary heart disease patients. *Magnesium Research*, Dec, 2000; 13 (4): 275-284.
38. Shechter M, et al. Oral magnesium therapy improves endothelial function in patients with coronary artery disease. *Circulation*, Nov 7, 2000; 102 (19): 2353-2358.
39. Guerrero-Romero F, et al. Oral magnesium supplementation improves insulin sensitivity in non-diabetic subjects with insulin resistance. A double-blind placebo-controlled randomized trial. *Diabetes & Metabolism*, Jun, 2004; 30 (3): 253-258.
40. Rodriguez-Moran M, Guerrero-Romero F. Oral magnesium supplementation improves insulin sensitivity and metabolic control in type 2 diabetic subjects: a randomized double-blind controlled trial. *Diabetes Care*, Apr, 2003; 26 (4): 1147-1152.
41. Ford ES, Mokdad, AH. Dietary Magnesium Intake in a National Sample of U.S. Adults. *Journal of Nutrition*, 2003; 133: 2879-2882.
42. Fox CH, et al. Magnesium deficiency in African-Americans: does it contribute to increased cardiovascular risk factors? *Journal of the National Medical Association*, 2003 Apr; 95 (4): 257-62.
43. Massey LK, Whiting SJ. Caffeine, urinary calcium, calcium metabolism and bone. *Journal of Nutrition*, 1993; 123: 1611-1614.
44. Massey LK, Berg T. Effect of dietary caffeine on urinary excretion of calcium, magnesium, phosphorus, sodium, potassium, chloride and zinc in healthy males. *Nutrition Research*, 1985; 5:1281-1284.
45. Figures for Lipitor based on retail price for 90 x 10mg Lipitor tablets, obtained from Walgreen's web site on Sept. 29, 2006 (http://www.walgreens.com). Prices for all supplements except Life Extension Two-Per-Day obtained from Bodybuilding.com on Sept 29, 2006. Price for Life Extension Two-Per-Day obtained from www.lef.org on September 29, 2006.
46. No author listed. Vegetables Without Vitamins. *Life Extension Magazine*, Mar, 2001. Available online:

http://www.lef.org/magazine/mag2001/mar2001_report_vegetables.html (accessed
September 8, 2005).

Chapter 28
1. Pate RR, et al. Physical activity and public health. A recommendation from the Centers
    for Disease Control and Prevention and the American College of Sports Medicine,
    Journal of the American Medical Association, Feb, 1995; 273: 402 - 407.
2. No listed author. Prevalence of physical activity, including lifestyle activities among
    adults--United States, 2000-2001. *MMR Weekly*, Aug. 15, 2003; 52 (32); 764-769.
3. Lee IM, Skerrett PJ. Physical activity and all-cause mortality: what is the dose-response
    relation? *Medicine and Science in Sports and Exercise*, 2001; 33 (6 Suppl): S459-S471.
4. Lee I-M., et al. The "Weekend Warrior" and Risk of Mortality. *American Journal of
    Epidemiology*, Oct 1, 2004; 160 (7): 636-641.
5. Dupen F, et al. The source of risk factor information for general practitioners: is physical
    activity under-recognised? *Medical Journal of Australia*, Dec 6-20, 1999; 171 (11-12):
    601-603.
6. Pierson LM, et al. Effects of combined aerobic and resistance training versus aerobic
    training alone in cardiac rehabilitation. *Journal of Cardiopulmonary Rehabilitation*, Mar-
    Apr, 2001; 21 (2): 101-110.
7. Paffenbarger RS Jr, et al. Physical activity as an index of heart attack risk in college
    alumni. *American Journal of Epidemiology,* 1978; 108: 161–175.
8. Dorn J, et al. Results of a multicenter randomized clinical trial of exercise and long-term
    survival in myocardial infarction patients: The National Exercise and Heart Disease
    Project (NEHDP). *Circulation*, Oct, 1999; 100: 1764-1769.
9. Arbab-Zadeh A, et al. Effect of aging and physical activity on left ventricular
    compliance. *Circulation,* Sep, 2004; 110: 1799-1805.
10. No listed author. Lifelong exercise prevents heart disease. *Washington Times*, Sep. 14,
    2004. Available online: http://washingtontimes.com/upi-breaking/20040914-105102-
    2529r.htm (accessed September 8, 2005).
11. Tabata I, et al. Effects of moderate-intensity endurance and high-intensity intermittent
    training on anaerobic capacity and VO2max. *Medicine & Science in Sports & Exercise*,
    Oct, 1996; 28 (10): 1327-1330.
12. Laursen PB, Jenkins DG. The scientific basis for high-intensity interval training:
    optimising training programmes and maximising performance in highly trained
    endurance athletes. *Sports Medicine*, 2002; 32 (1): 53-73.
13. Warburton DER, et al. Effectiveness of High-Intensity Interval Training for the
    Rehabilitation of Patients With Coronary Artery Disease. *American Journal of
    Cardiology*, 2005; 95: 1080–1084.
14. Persinger R, et al. Consistency of the talk test for exercise prescription. *Medicine &
    Science in Sports & Exercise,* Sept, 2004; 36 (9): 1632-1636.

Chapter 29
1. Lee DR, McKenzie RB. *Getting Rich in America.* HarperPerennial, New York, NY,
    2000.
2. Berkman LF, Syme SL. Social networks, host resistance, and mortality: a nine-year
    follow-up study of Alameda County residents. *American Journal of Epidemiology,* Feb,
    1979; 109 (2): 186-204.
3. House JS, et al. The association of social relationships and activities with mortality:
    prospective evidence from the Tecumseh Community Health Study. *American Journal of
    Epidemiology,* Jul, 1982; 116 (1): 123-140.
4. Seeman TE. Health promoting effects of friends and family on health outcomes in older
    adults. *American Journal of Health Promotion,* Jul-Aug 2000; 14 (6): 362-370.

5. Cohen S, et al. Emotional Style and Susceptibility to the Common Cold. *Psychosomatic Medicine*, Jul-Aug, 2003; 65: 652-657.
6. Helgeson VS, Fritz HL. Cognitive Adaptation as a Predictor of New Coronary Events After Percutaneous Transluminal Coronary Angioplasty. *Psychosomatic Medicine*, 1999; 61: 488-495.
7. Butler G, Hope T. *Managing Your Mind: The Mental Fitness Guide*. Oxford University Press, 1996.
8. Thayer RE, et al. Self-regulation of mood: strategies for changing a bad mood, raising energy, and reducing tension. *Journal of Personality and Social Psychology*, Nov, 1994; 67 (5): 910-925.
9. Jin P. Efficacy of Tai Chi, brisk walking, meditation, and reading in reducing mental and emotional stress. *Journal of Psychosomatic Medicine*, May, 1992; 36 (4): 361-370.
10. Roth DL, Holmes DS. Influence of aerobic exercise training and relaxation training on physical and psychologic health following stressful life events. *Psychosomatic Medicine*, Jul-Aug, 1987; 49 (4): 355-65.
11. Blumenthal JA, et al. Effects of Exercise Training on Older Patients With Major Depression. *Archives of Internal Medicine*, 1999; 159: 2349-2356.
12. Babyak M, et al. Exercise treatment for major depression: maintenance of therapeutic benefit at 10 months. *Psychosomatic Medicine*, Sep-Oct, 2000; 62: 633–638.
13. Martinsen EW, et al. Comparing aerobic with nonaerobic forms of exercise in the treatment of clinical depression: a randomized trial. *Comprehensive Psychiatry*, Jul-Aug, 1989; 30 (4): 324-331.
14. Wells AS, et al. Alterations in mood after changing to a low-fat diet. *British Journal of Nutrition*, Jan, 1998; 79 (1): 23-30.
15. Kaplan JR, et al. The effects of fat and cholesterol on social behavior in monkeys. *Psychosomatic Medicine*, Nov-Dec, 1991; 53 (6): 634-642.
16. Hibbeln JR. Fish consumption and major depression. *Lancet*, 1998; 351: 1213.
17. Hibbeln JR. Seafood consumption and homicide mortality. A cross-national ecological analysis. *World Review of Nutrition and Dietetics*, 2001; 88: 41-46.
18. Tanskanen A, et al. Fish Consumption and Depressive Symptoms in the General Population in Finland. *Psychiatric Services*, Apr, 2001; 52: 529-531.
19. Magnusson A, et al. Lack of seasonal mood change in the Icelandic population: results of a cross-sectional study. *American Journal of Psychiatry*, 2000; 157: 234-238.
20. Cott J, Hibbeln JR. Lack of seasonal mood change in Icelanders. *American Journal of Psychiatry*, 2001; 158: 328.
21. Iribarren C, et al. Dietary intake of n-3, n-6 fatty acids and fish: Relationship with hostility in young adults--the CARDIA study. *European Journal of Clinical Nutrition*, Jan, 2004; 58: 24-31.
22. Peet M, Horrobin DF. A dose-ranging study of the effects of ethyl-eicosapentaenoate in patients with ongoing depression despite apparently adequate treatment with standard drugs. *Archives of General Psychiatry*, Oct, 2002; 59 (10): 913-919.
23. Stoll AL, et al. Omega 3 fatty acids in bipolar disorder: a preliminary double-blind, placebo-controlled trial. *Archives of General Psychiatry*, May, 1999; 56 (5): 407-412.
24. Peet M, et al. Two double-blind placebo-controlled pilot studies of eicosapentaenoic acid in the treatment of schizophrenia. *Schizophrenia Research*, 2001; 49 (3): 243-251.
25. Peet M, Horrobin DF. A dose-ranging exploratory study of the effects of ethyl-eicosapentaenoate in patients with persistent schizophrenic symptoms. *Journal of Psychiatric Research*, Jan-Feb, 2002; 36 (1): 7-18.
26. Hamazaki T, et al. The Effect of Docosahexaenoic Acid on Aggression in Young Adults. A Placebo-controlled Double-blind Study. *Journal of Clinical Investigation*, Feb, 1996; 97 (4): 1129-1134.

27. Sawazaki S, et al. The effect of docosahexaenoic acid on plasma catecholamine concentrations and glucose tolerance during long-lasting psychological stress: a double-blind placebo-controlled study. *Journal of Nutritional Science and Vitaminology*, Oct, 1999; 45 (5): 655-665.

28. Fontani G, et al. Cognitive and physiological effects of Omega-3 polyunsaturated fatty acid supplementation in healthy subjects. *European Journal of Clinical Investigation*, 2005; 35 (11): 691–699.

29. *Ninth Special Report to the U.S. Congress on Alcohol and Health*. National Institute on Alcohol Abuse and Alcoholism, National Institutes of Health, Bethesda, Maryland, 1987.

Chapter 30

1. Mokdad AH, et al. Actual Causes of Death in the United States, 2000. *Journal of the American Medical Association*, 2004; 291: 1238-1245.

2. *The Economic Costs of Alcohol and Drug Abuse in the United States, 1992*. Prepared by the Lewin Group for the National Institute on Drug Abuse and the National Institute on Alcohol Abuse and Alcoholism, May 1998.

3. Murray CJL, Lopez AD. *The Global Burden of Disease: a comprehensive assessment of mortality and disability from diseases, injuries and risk factors in 1990 and projected to 2020*. Cambridge, Mass: Harvard University Press on behalf of the World Health Organization and the World Bank, 1996.

4. Rehm J, Sempos CT. Alcohol consumption and all-cause mortality. *Addiction*, 1995; 90: 471-480.

5. White IR. The level of alcohol consumption at which all-cause mortality is least. *Journal of Clinical Epidemiology*, 1999; 52: 967-975.

6. Holman CDJ, et al. Meta-analysis of alcohol and all-cause mortality: a validation of NHMRC recommendations. *Medical Journal of Australia*, 1996; 164: 141-145.

7. Andreasson S, et al. Alcohol, social factors and mortality among young men. *British Journal of Addiction*, 1991; 86: 877-887.

8. National Highway Traffic Safety Administration. *Traffic safety facts 2001, alcohol*. Washington, D.C.: Department of Transportation, 2001.

9. Middleton K, et al. Moderate alcohol use and reduced mortality risk: Systematic error in prospective studies. *Addiction Research and Theory*, Apr 4, 2006. Available online: http://www.journalsonline.tandf.co.uk/media/e05d2179yndqwke0mtfg/contributions/m/3/5/0/m350jp7v218202g8.pdf (accessed April 10, 2006).

10. Trevisan MT, et al. Drinking Pattern and Mortality: The Italian Risk Factor and Life Expectancy Pooling Project. *Annals of Epidemiology*, Jul, 2001; 11 (5): 312-319.

11. McKee M, Britton A. The positive relation between alcohol and coronary heart disease in Eastern Europe: potential physiological mechanisms. *Journal of the Royal Society of Medicine*, 1998; 91: 402-407.

12. Puddey IB, et al. Influence of drinking on cardiovascular disease and cardiovascular risk factors--a review. *Addiction*, 1999; 94: 649-663.

13. Murray RP, et al. Alcohol volume, drinking pattern and cardiovascular disease morbidity and mortality: is there a U-shaped function? *American Journal of Epidemiology*, 2002; 155: 242-248.

14. Rehm J, et al. Average volume of alcohol consumption, patterns of drinking and risk of coronary heart disease - a review. *Journal of Cardiovascular Risk*, 2003; 10: 15-20.

15. Puddey IB, et al. Influence of pattern of drinking on cardiovascular disease and cardiovascular risk factors - a review. *Addiction*, May, 1999; 94 (5): 649-663.

16. Nissen MB, Lemberg L. The "holiday heart" syndrome. *Heart & Lung*, Jan, 1984; 13 (1): 89-92.

17. Panos RJ, et al. Sudden death associated with alcohol consumption. *Pacing and Clinical Electrophysiology*, Apr, 1988; 11 (4): 423-424.

18. Kupari M, Koskinen P. Alcohol, cardiac arrhythmias and sudden death. *Novartis Foundation Symposium*, 1998; 216: 68-79.
19. Klatsky AL. Alcohol, coronary disease, and hypertension. *Annual Review of Medicine*, 1996; 47: 149-160.
20. Henriksson KM, et al. Body composition, ethnicity and alcohol consumption as determinants for the development of blood pressure in a birth cohort of young middle-aged men. *European Journal of Epidemiology*, 2003; 18 (10): 955-963.
21. Potter JF, Beevers DG. Pressor effect of alcohol in hypertension. *Lancet*, Jan 21, 1984; 1 (8369): 119-122.
22. Rao MN, et al. Light, but not heavy alcohol drinking, stimulates paraoxonase by upregulating liver mRNA in rats and humans. *Metabolism*, 2003; 52 (10): 1287-1294.
23. Rimm EB, et al. Review of moderate alcohol consumption and reduced risk of coronary heart disease: is the effect due to beer, wine, or spirits? *British Medical Journal*, Mar, 1996; 312: 731-736.
24. Hendriks HF, et al. Effect of moderate dose of alcohol with evening meal on fibrinolytic factors. *British Medical Journal*, 1994; 308: 1003-1006.
25. Prickett CD, et al. Alcohol: Friend or foe? Alcoholic beverage hormesis for cataract and atherosclerosis is related to plasma antioxidant activity. *Nonlinearity in Biology, Toxicology, and Medicine*, Oct-Dec, 2004; 2: 353-370.
26. Zador P, et al. Alcohol-related relative risk of driving fatalities and driver impairment in fatal crashes in relation to driver age and gender: An update using 1996 data. *Journal of Studies on Alcohol*, 2000; 61: 387-395.
27. Moskowitz H, Fiorentino D. *A Review of the Literature on the Effects of Low Doses of Alcohol on Driving Related Skills. Pub. No. DOT HS-809-028.* Springfield, VA: U.S. Department of Transportation, National Highway Traffic Safety Administration, 2000.
28. Kesmodel U, et al. Moderate alcohol intake in pregnancy and the risk of spontaneous abortion. *Alcohol and Alcoholism*, Jan-Feb, 2002; 37 (1): 87-92.
29. Floyd RL, et al. Alcohol use prior to pregnancy recognition. *American Journal of Preventive Medicine*, Aug, 1999; 17 (2): 101-107.
30. Camargo CA Jr. Moderate alcohol consumption and stroke. The epidemiologic evidence. *Stroke*, Dec, 1989; 20 (12): 1611-1626.
31. Iso H, et al. Alcohol intake and the risk of cardiovascular disease in middle-aged Japanese men. *Stroke*, May, 1995; 26 (5): 767-773.
32. Tsugane S, et al. Alcohol consumption and all-cause and cancer mortality among middle-aged Japanese men: seven-year follow-up of the JPHC study Cohort I. Japan Public Health Center. *American Journal of Epidemiology*, Dec 1, 1999; 150 (11): 1201-1207.
33. Grant BF, Dawson DA. Age at onset of alcohol use and its association with DSM-IV alcohol abuse and dependence: results from the National Longitudinal Alcohol Epidemiologic Survey. *Journal of Substance Abuse*, 1997; 9: 103-110.
34. Toumbourou JW, et al. Adolescent alcohol-use trajectories in the transition from high school. *Drug and Alcohol Review*, Jun, 2003; 22 (2): 111-116.

Epilogue

1. Whyte WH, Nocera J. *The Organization Man.* Doubleday, New York, 1956.
2. Gold T. The effect of peer review on progress. Looking back on 50 years in science. *Journal of American Physicians and Surgeons,* 2003; 8 (3): 80-82.

Appendix A

1. Fraser GE. Associations between diet and cancer, ischemic heart disease, and all-cause mortality in non-Hispanic white California Seventh-day Adventists. *American Journal of Clinical Nutrition*, Sept. 1999; 70 (3): 532S-538S.

2. Phillips RL. Role of lifestyle and dietary habits in risk of cancer among Seventh-Day Adventists. *Cancer Research*, Nov. 1975; 35: 3513-3522.
3. Layman DK, et al. Dietary protein and exercise have additive effects on body composition during weight loss in adult women. *Journal of Nutrition*, Aug, 2005; 135:1903-1910.
4. Layman DK, et al. A reduced ratio of dietary carbohydrate to protein improves body composition and blood lipid profiles during weight loss in adult women. *Journal of Nutrition*, Feb, 2003.133: 411-417.
5. Hakala P, Karvetti RL. Weight reduction on lactovegetarian and mixed diets. Changes in weight, nutrient intake, skinfold thicknesses and blood pressure. *European Journal of Clinical Nutrition*, Jun. 1989; 43 (6): 421-430.
6. Key TJ, et al. Dietary habits and mortality in 11 000 vegetarians and health conscious people: results of a 17 year follow up. *British Medical Journal*, Sept 28, 1996; 313 (7060): 775-779.
7. Thorogood M, et al. Risk of death from cancer and ischaemic heart disease in meat and non-meat eaters. *British Medical Journal*, Jun, 1994; 308: 1667-1670.
8. Key TJ, et al. Mortality in vegetarians and non-vegetarians: detailed findings from a collaborative analysis of 5 prospective studies. *American Journal of Clinical Nutrition*, 1999; 70 (S): 516S-524S.
9. Key TJ, et al. Mortality in British vegetarians: review and preliminary results from EPIC-Oxford. *American Journal of Clinical Nutrition*, 2003; 78: 533S-538S.
10. Chang-Claude J, et al. Mortality pattern of German vegetarians after 11 years of follow-up. *Epidemiology*, Sep, 1992; 3 (5): 395-401.
11. Chang-Claude J, et al. Dietary and lifestyle determinants of mortality among German vegetarians. *International Journal of Epidemiology*, Apr, 1993; 22 (2): 228 236.
12. Enstrom JE. Health practices and cancer mortality among active California Mormons. *Journal of the National Cancer Institute*, Dec 6, 1989; 81 (23): 1807-1814.
13. Enstrom JE, et al. The relationship between vitamin C intake, general health practices, and mortality in Alameda County, California. *American Journal of Public Health*, Sep, 1986; 76 (9): 1124-1130.

Appendix B

1. Ornish D, et al. Can lifestyle changes reverse coronary heart disease? The Lifestyle Heart Trial. *Lancet*, Jul 21, 1990; 336 (8708): 129-133.
2. Vona M, et al. Impact of physical training and detraining on endothelium-dependent vasodilation in patients with recent acute myocardial infarction. *American Heart Journal*, Jun, 2004; 147 (6): 1039-1046.
3. Watts K, et al. Exercise training normalizes vascular dysfunction and improves central adiposity in obese adolescents. *Journal of the American College of Cardiology*, May 19, 2004; 43 (10): 1823-1827.
4. Karason K, et al. Weight loss and progression of early atherosclerosis in the carotid artery: a four-year controlled study of obese subjects. *International Journal of Obesity and Related Metabolic Disorders*, Sep, 1999; 23 (9): 948-956.
5. Raitakari M, et al. Weight reduction with very-low-caloric diet and endothelial function in overweight adults: role of plasma glucose. *Arteriosclerosis, Thrombosis, and Vascular Biology*, Jan, 2004; 24 (1): 124-128.
6. Maron DJ. Flavonoids for reduction of atherosclerotic risk. *Current Atherosclerosis Reports*, Jan, 2004; 6 (1): 73-78.
7. Ornish D, et al. Intensive lifestyle changes for reversal of coronary heart disease. *Journal of the American Medical Association*, Dec 16, 1998; 280 (23): 2001-2007.

8. Koertge J, et al. Improvement in medical risk factors and quality of life in women and men with coronary artery disease in the Multicenter Lifestyle Demonstration Project. *American Journal of Cardiology*, Jun 1, 2003; 91 (11): 1316-1322.

9. Ornish D. *Dr. Dean Ornish's Program for Reversing Heart Disease: The Only System Scientifically Proven to Reverse Heart Disease Without Drugs or Surgery*. Ivy Books, 1995.

10. De Lorgeril M, et al. Mediterranean alpha-linolenic acid-rich diet in secondary prevention of coronary heart disease. *Lancet*, 1994; 343: 1454-1459.

11. Warner M. Is a Trip to McDonald's Just What the Doctor Ordered? *New York Times*, May 2, 2005.

12. Gittleman AL, *Beyond Pritikin,* Bantam Books, 1996.

Appendix C

1. American Heart Association. Heart Disease and Stroke Statistics--2004 Update. AHA web site. Available online: http://www.americanheart.org/downloadable/heart/1079736729696HDSStats2004Update REV3-19-04.pdf (accessed September 8, 2005).

2. Murphy ML, et al. Treatment of chronic stable angina. A preliminary report of survival data of the randomized Veterans Administration cooperative study. *New England Journal of Medicine,* Sep 22, 1977; 297 (12): 621-627.

3. Peduzzi P, et al. Twenty-two-year follow-up in the VA Cooperative Study of Coronary Artery Bypass Surgery for Stable Angina. *American Journal of Cardiology*, Jun 15, 1998; 81(12):1393-1399.

4. CASS Principal Investigators and Associates. Myocardial infarction and mortality in the coronary artery surgery study (CASS) randomized trial. *New England Journal of Medicine*, Mar 22, 1984; 310: 750-758.

5. Alderman EL, et al. Ten-year follow-up of survival and myocardial infarction in the randomized Coronary Artery Surgery Study. *Circulation*, Nov, 1990; 82: 1629-1634.

6. European Coronary Surgery Study Group. Long-term results of prospective randomised study of coronary artery bypass surgery in stable angina pectoris. *Lancet*, Nov. 27, 1982; 2 (8309): 1173-1180.

7. Varnauskas E, for the European Coronary Surgery Study Group. Twelve-year follow up of survival in the randomized European Coronary Surgery Study. *New England Journal of Medicine*, 1998; 319: 332-337.

8. Hueb W, et al. The Medicine, Angioplasty, or Surgery Study (MASS-II): A Randomized, Controlled Clinical Trial of Three Therapeutic Strategies for Multivessel Coronary Artery Disease. One-Year Results. *Journal of the American College of Cardiology*, May 19, 2004: 43 (10): 1743–1751.

9. Hueb WA, et al. The medicine, angioplasty or surgery study (MASS): a prospective, randomized trial of medical therapy, balloon angioplasty or bypass surgery for single proximal left anterior descending artery stenoses. *Journal of the American College of Cardiology*, 1995; 26: 1600-1605.

10. Madsen JK, et al. Danish multicenter randomized study of invasive versus conservative treatment in patients with inducible ischemia after thrombolysis in acute myocardial infarction (DANAMI). Danish trial in acute myocardial infarction. *Circulation*, 1997; 96: 748-755.

11. Takaro T, et al. The VA cooperative randomized study of surgery for coronary arterial occlusive disease II. Subgroup with significant left main lesions. *Circulation*, Dec, 1976; 54 (6 Suppl): III107-117.

12. RITA-2 trial participants. Coronary angioplasty versus medical therapy for angina: the second randomised intervention treatment of angina (RITA-2) trial. *Lancet*, 1997; 350: 461-468.

13. Pitt B, et al. Aggressive lipid-lowering therapy compared with angioplasty in stable coronary artery disease. Atorvastatin versus revascularization treatment investigators. *New England Journal of Medicine*, 1999; 341: 70-76.
14. Sievers B, et al. Medical therapy versus PTCA: a prospective, randomized trial in patients with asymptomatic coronary single-vessel disease. *Circulation,* 1993; 88(I): 297.
15. Bucher HC, et al. Percutaneous transluminal coronary angioplasty versus medical treatment for non-acute coronary heart disease: meta-analysis of randomised controlled trials. *British Medical Journal*, Jul. 8, 2000; 321: 73-77.
16. Berger A, et al. Surgery for Coronary Artery Disease. Long-Term Patency of Internal Mammary Artery Bypass Grafts. Relationship With Preoperative Severity of the Native Coronary Artery Stenosis. *Circulation*, 2004; 110: II-36 – II-40.
17. Desai ND, et al. A randomized comparison of radial-artery and saphenous-vein coronary bypass grafts. *New England Journal of Medicine*, Nov 25, 2004; 351 (22): 2302-2309.
18. FitzGibbon GM, et al. Coronary bypass graft fate: long-term angiographic study. *Journal of the American College of Cardiology*, Apr, 1991; 17 (5): 1075-1080.
19. Andreasen JJ, et al. Emergency coronary artery bypass surgery after failed percutaneous transluminal coronary angioplasty. *Scandinavian Cardiovascular Journal,* Jun, 2000; 34 (3): 242-246.
20. Schiele TM, et al. Vascular restenosis--striving for therapy. *Expert Opinion on Pharmacotherapy,* 2004; 5 (11): 2221-2232.
21. Hambrecht R, et al. Percutaneous Coronary Angioplasty Compared With Exercise Training in Patients With Stable Coronary Artery Disease: A Randomized Trial. *Circulation*, Mar, 2004; 109: 1371-1378.
22. Winslow CM, et al. The appropriateness of performing coronary artery bypass surgery. *Journal of the American Medical Association,* 1988; 260 (4): 505-509.

Appendix D
1. Khaw KT, et al. Association of hemoglobin A1c with cardiovascular disease and mortality in adults: The European Prospective Investigation into Cancer in Norfolk. *Annals of Internal Medicine*, 2004; 141:413-420.
2. Benjamin SM, et al. Estimated number of adults with prediabetes in the US in 2000: opportunities for prevention. *Diabetes Care*, Mar, 2003; 26 (3): 645-649.
3. Ridker PM, Cook N. Clinical usefulness of very high and very low levels of C-reactive protein across the full range of Framingham Risk Scores. *Circulation*, 2004; 109: 1955-1959.
4. Madjid M, et al. Leukocyte count and coronary heart disease: implications for risk assessment. *Journal of the American College of Cardiology*, Nov 16, 2004; 44 (10): 1945-1956.
5. Ernst E, et al. Leukocytes and the risk of ischemic diseases. *Journal of the American Medical Association,* May 1, 1987; 257 (17): 2318-2324.

Appendix E
1. Stacey M. Foreword to: McCully K, McCully M. *The Heart Revolution*. Harper Collins, New York, NY, 1999.
2. Domagala TB, et al. Hyperhomocysteinemia following oral methionine load is associated with increased lipid peroxidation. *Thrombosis Research*, Aug 15, 1997; 87 (4): 411-416.
3. Lawrence de Koning AB, et al. Hyperhomocysteinemia and its role in the development of atherosclerosis. *Clinical Biochemistry*, Sep. 2003; 36 (6): 431-441
4. Welch GN, Loscalzo J. Mechanisms of Disease: Homocysteine and Atherothrombosis. *New England Journal of Medicine*, Apr 9, 1998; 338: 1042-1050.

5. Robinson K, et al. Hyperhomocysteinemia and Low Pyridoxal Phosphate: Common and Independent Reversible Risk Factors for Coronary Artery Disease. *Circulation*, Nov, 1995; 92: 2825-2830.

6. Quinlivan EP, et al. Importance of both folic acid and vitamin B12 in reduction of risk of vascular disease. *Lancet*, 2002; 359 (9302): 227-228.

7. den Heijer M, et al. Vitamin supplementation reduces blood homocysteine levels: a controlled trial in patients with venous thrombosis and healthy volunteers. *Arteriosclerosis Thrombosis and Vascular Biology*, Mar, 1998; 18 (3): 356-361.

8. Stampfer MJ, et al. A prospective study of plasma homocyst(e)ine and risk of myocardial infarction in US physicians. *Journal of the American Medical Association*, Aug 1992; 268: 877-881.

9. Zylberstein DE, et al. Serum homocysteine in relation to mortality and morbidity from coronary heart disease: a 24-year follow-up of the population study of women in Gothenburg. *Circulation*, Feb 10, 2004; 109 (5): 601-606.

10. Liem AH, et al. Efficacy of folic acid when added to statin therapy in patients with hypercholesterolemia following acute myocardial infarction: a randomised pilot trial. *International Journal of Cardiology*, Feb, 2004; 93 (2-3): 175-179.

11. Toole JF, et al. Lowering homocysteine in patients with ischemic stroke to prevent recurrent stroke, myocardial infarction, and death: the Vitamin Intervention for Stroke Prevention (VISP) randomized controlled trial. *Journal of the American Medical Association*, 2004; 291 (5): 565-575.

12. Righetti M, et al. Effects of folic acid treatment on homocysteine levels and vascular disease in hemodialysis patients. *Medical Sciences Monitor*, Apr, 2003; 9 (4): PI19-24.

13. Schnyder G, et al. Effect of homocysteine-lowering therapy with folic acid, vitamin B12, and vitamin B6 on clinical outcome after percutaneous coronary intervention: the Swiss Heart study: a randomized controlled trial. *Journal of the American Medical Association*, 2002; 288 (8): 973-979.

14. Wood S. NORVIT: B6 and folic acid combination may increase stroke, MI risk. *HeartWire*, TheHeart.org, Sep 5, 2005.

15. Toole JF, et al. Lowering plasma total homocysteine to prevent recurrent stroke, myocardial infarction, and death in ischemic stroke patients: results of the Vitamin Intervention for Stroke Prevention (VISP) Randomized Trial. *Journal of the American Medical Association,* 2004; 291: 565–575.

16. Spence DJ, et al. Vitamin Intervention for Stroke Prevention Trial: An Efficacy Analysis. *Stroke*, Nov, 2005; 36 (11): 2404-2409.

17. Zhou J, et al. Dietary Supplementation With Methionine and Homocysteine Promotes Early Atherosclerosis but Not Plaque Rupture in ApoE-Deficient Mice. *Arteriosclerosis Thrombosis and Vascular Biology*, 2001; 21: 1470-1476.

18. Wang H, et al. Hyperhomocysteinemia accelerates atherosclerosis in cystathionine beta - synthase and apolipoprotein E double knock-out mice with and without dietary perturbation. *Blood*, 2003; 101 (10): 3901-3907.

19. den Heijer M, et al. Vitamin supplementation reduces blood homocysteine levels: a controlled trial in patients with venous thrombosis and healthy volunteers. *Arteriosclerosis Thrombosis and Vascular Biology*, Mar, 1998; 18 (3): 356-361.

20. Dinckal MH, et al. Effect of homocysteine-lowering therapy on vascular endothelial function and exercise performance in coronary patients with hyperhomocysteinaemia. *Acta Cardiologica*, Oct, 2003; 58 (5): 389-396.

21. Ueland P, Refsum H. Plasma homocysteine, a risk factor for vascular disease: plasma levels in health, disease, and drug therapy. *Journal of Laboratory and Clinical Medicine*, 1989; 114: 473-501.

22. Haulrik N, et al. Effect of protein and methionine intakes on plasma homocysteine concentrations: a 6-mo randomized controlled trial in overweight subjects. *American Journal of Clinical Nutrition*, Dec, 2002; 76 (6): 1202-1206.
23. Mann NJ, et al. The effect of diet on plasma homocysteine concentrations in healthy male subjects. *European Journal of Clinical Nutrition*, Nov, 1999; 53 (11): 895-899.
24. Herrmann W, et al. Total homocysteine, vitamin B(12), and total antioxidant status in vegetarians. *Clinical Chemistry*, Jun, 2001; 47 (6): 1094-1101.
25. Obeid R, et al. The impact of vegetarianism on some haematological parameters. *European Journal of Haematology*, Nov-Dec, 2002; 69 (5-6): 275-279.
26. Appel LJ, et al. Effect of Dietary Patterns on Serum Homocysteine: Results of a Randomized, Controlled Feeding Study. *Circulation*, 2000; 102: 852-857.
27. Samman S, et al. A mixed fruit and vegetable concentrate increases plasma antioxidant vitamins and folate and lowers plasma homocysteine in men. *Journal of Nutrition*, Jul, 2003; 133 (7): 2188-2193.
28. Broekmans WM, et al. Fruits and vegetables increase plasma carotenoids and vitamins and decrease homocysteine in humans. *Journal of Nutrition*, Jun, 2000; 130 (6): 1578-1583.
29. Schoene NW, et al. Effect of oral vitamin B6 supplementation on in vitro platelet aggregation. *American Journal of Clinical Nutrition*, May 1986; 43: 825-830.
30. Levene CI, Murray JC. The aetiological role of maternal vitamin-B6 deficiency in the development of atherosclerosis. *Lancet*, Mar 19, 1977; 1 (8012): 628-630.
31. Friso S, et al. Low plasma vitamin B-6 concentrations and modulation of coronary artery disease risk. *American Journal of Clinical Nutrition*, Jun, 2004; 79: 992-998.
32. Friso S, et al. Low Circulating Vitamin B6 Is Associated With Elevation of the Inflammation Marker C-Reactive Protein Independently of Plasma Homocysteine Levels. *Circulation*, Jun, 2001; 103: 2788-2791.

Appendix F

1. Ervin RB, et al. Dietary intakes of selected minerals for the United States population: 1999-2000. *Advance Data*, Apr 27, 2004; 341: 1-5.
2. Saari JT. Copper deficiency and cardiovascular disease: role of peroxidation, glycation, and nitration. *Canadian Journal of Physiology and Pharmacology,* 2000; 78 (10): 848-855.
3. Klevay LM. Dietary copper and risk of coronary heart disease. *American Journal of Clinical Nutrition*, May 1, 2000; 71(5): 1213-1214.
4. Klevay LM, et al. Cardiovascular Disease from Copper Deficiency--A History. *Journal of Nutrition*, 2000; 130: 489S-492S.
5. Klevay LM, Viestenz KE. Abnormal electrocardiograms in rats deficient in copper. *American Journal of Physiology*, 1981; 240: H185-H189.
6. Elsherif L, et al. Congestive heart failure in copper-deficient mice. *Experimental Biology and Medicine*, Jul, 2003; 228 (7): 811-817.
7. Elsherif L, et al. Regression of dietary copper restriction-induced cardiomyopathy by copper repletion in mice. *Journal of Nutrition*, Apr, 2004; 134 (4): 855-860.
8. Coulson WF, Carnes WH. Cardiovascular studies on copper-deficient swine V. The histogenesis of the coronary artery lesions. *American Journal of Pathology*, 1963; 43: 945-954.
9. Hamilton IM, et al. Marginal copper deficiency and atherosclerosis. *Biological Trace Element Research*, 2000; 78 (1-3): 179-189.
10. Reiser S, et al. Indices of copper status in humans consuming a typical American diet containing either fructose or starch. *American Journal of Clinical Nutrition*, 1985; 42: 242-251.

11. Spencer JC, et al. Direct relationship between the body's copper/zinc ratio, ventricular premature beats, and sudden coronary death. *American Journal of Clinical Nutrition*, Jun, 1979; 32: 1184-1185.
12. Lukaski HC, et al. Effects of dietary copper on human autonomic cardiovascular function. *European Journal of Applied Physiology*, 1988; 58: 74–80.
13. Milne DB, et al. Low dietary zinc alters indices of copper function and status in postmenopausal women. *Nutrition*, Sep, 2001; 17 (9): 701-708.
14. Klevay LM, et al. Increased cholesterol in plasma in a young man during experimental copper depletion. *Metabolism*, 1984; 33: 1112-1118.
15. Fields M, et al. The influence of gender on developing copper deficiency and on free radical generation of rats fed a fructose diet. *Metabolism*, Sep, 1992; 41 (9): 989-994.
16. Fields M, et al. Sexual differences in the expression of copper deficiency in rats. *Proceedings of the Society for Experimental Biology and Medicine*, Nov, 1987; 186 (2): 183-187.
17. Klevay LM, Halas ES. The effects of dietary copper deficiency and psychological stress on blood pressure in rats. *Physiology & Behavior*, Feb, 1991; 49 (2): 309-314.
18. Turnlund JR, et al. Long-term high copper intake: effects on indexes of copper status, antioxidant status, and immune function in young men. *American Journal of Clinical Nutrition*, Jun 2004; 79: 1037-1044.

Appendix G

1. Stephens NG, et al. Randomised controlled trial of vitamin E in patients with coronary disease: Cambridge Heart Antioxidant Study (CHAOS). *Lancet*, Mar 23, 1996; 347 (9004): 781-786.
2. Bowry VW, Stocker R. Tocopherol-mediated peroxidation. The prooxidant effect of vitamin E on the radical-initiated oxidation of human low-density lipoprotein. *Journal of the American Chemical Society*, 1993;115: 6029-6044.
3. Abudu N, et al. Vitamins in human arteriosclerosis with emphasis on vitamin C and vitamin E. *Clinica Chimica Acta*, 2004; 339: 11-25.
4. Huang HY, Appel LJ. Supplementation of diets with alpha-tocopherol reduces serum concentrations of gamma- and delta-tocopherol in humans. *Journal of Nutrition*, 2003; 133: 3137-3140.
5. van Haaften RI, et al. Inhibition of various glutathione S-transferase isoenzymes by RRR-alpha-tocopherol. *Toxicology In Vitro*, 2003; 17: 245-251.
6. GISSI-Prevenzione Investigators. Dietary supplementation with n-3 polyunsaturated fatty acids and vitamin E after myocardial infarction: results of the GISSI-Prevenzione trial. *Lancet*, Aug 7, 1999; 354 (9177): 447-455.
7. Lee IM, et al. Vitamin E in the primary prevention of cardiovascular disease and cancer: the Women's Health Study: a randomized controlled trial. *Journal of the American Medical Association*, 2005; 294 (1): 56-65.
8. Vivekananthan DP, et al. Use of antioxidant vitamins for the prevention of cardiovascular disease: meta-analysis of randomised trials. *Lancet*, Jun 14, 2003; 361 (9374): 2017-2023.
9. Jiang Q, et al. Gamma-tocopherol, but not alpha-tocopherol, decreases proinflammatory eicosanoids and inflammation damage in rats. *FASEB Journal*, May, 2003; 17 (8): 816-822.
10. Saldeen T, et al. Differential effects of alpha- and gamma-tocopherol on low-density lipoprotein oxidation, superoxide activity, platelet aggregation and arterial thrombogenesis. *Journal of the American College of Cardiology*, Oct, 1999; 34 (4): 1208-1215.

11. Liu M, et al. Mixed tocopherols have a stronger inhibitory effect on lipid peroxidation than alpha-tocopherol alone. *Journal of Cardiovascular Pharmacology,* May, 2002; 39 (5): 714-721.

12. Ohrvall M, et al. Gamma, but not alpha, tocopherol levels in serum are reduced in coronary heart disease patients. *Journal of Internal Medicine,* Feb, 1996; 239 (2): 111-117.

13. Kontush A, et al. Lipophilic antioxidants in blood plasma as markers of atherosclerosis: the role of alpha-carotene and gamma-tocopherol. *Atherosclerosis,* May, 1999; 144 (1): 117-122.

14. Kushi L, et al. Dietary Antioxidant Vitamins and Death from Coronary Heart Disease in Postmenopausal Women. *New England Journal of Medicine,* 1996; 334, 1156-1162.

15. Liu M, et al. Mixed tocopherols inhibit platelet aggregation in humans: potential mechanisms. *American Journal of Clinical Nutrition,* Mar, 2003; 77 (3): 700-706.

16. Himmelfarb J, et al. Alpha and gamma tocopherol metabolism in healthy subjects and patients with end-stage renal disease. *Kidney International,* 2003; 64 (3): 978-991.

17. Huang HY, et al. Supplementation of diets with alpha-tocopherol reduces serum concentrations of gamma- and delta-tocopherol in humans. *Journal of Nutrition,* Oct, 2003; 133 (10): 3137-3140.

18. Olmedilla B, et al. A European multicentre, placebo-controlled supplementation study with alpha-tocopherol, carotene-rich palm oil, lutein or lycopene: analysis of serum responses. *Clinical Science,* Apr, 2002; 102 (4): 447-456.

19. Morinobu T, et al. Measurement of vitamin E metabolites by high-performance liquid chromatography during high-dose administration of alpha-tocopherol. *European Journal of Clinical Nutrition,* Mar, 2003; 57 (3): 410-414.

20. Mahabir S, et al. Randomized, placebo-controlled trial of dietary supplementation of alpha-tocopherol on mutagen sensitivity levels in melanoma patients: a pilot trial. *Melanoma Research,* 2002; 12 (1): 83-90.

21. Smith KS, et al. Vitamin E supplementation increases circulating vitamin E metabolites tenfold in end-stage renal disease patients. *Lipids,* Aug, 2003; 38 (8): 813-819.

22. Cooney RV, et al. Effects of dietary sesame seeds on plasma tocopherol levels. *Nutrition and Cancer,* 2001; 39 (1): 66-71.

23. Ikeda S, et al. Dietary sesame seeds elevate alpha- and gamma-tocotrienol concentrations in skin and adipose tissue of rats fed the tocotrienol-rich fraction extracted from palm oil. *Journal of Nutrition,* Nov, 2001; 131 (11): 2892-2897.

24. Umeda-Sawada R, et al. The Metabolism and n-6/n-3 Ratio of Essential Fatty Acids in Rats: Effect of Dietary Arachidonic Acid and a Mixture of Sesame Lignans (sesamin and episesamin). *Lipids,* 1998; 33: 567-572.

Appendix H

1. Scientific Steering Committee on behalf of the Simon Broome Register Group. Risk of fatal coronary heart disease in familial hypercholesterolaemia. *British Medical Journal,* 1991; 303: 893-896.

2. Sijbrands EJG, et al. Mortality over two centuries in large pedigree with familial hypercholesterolaemia: family tree mortality study. *British Medical Journal,* Apr, 2001; 322: 1019-1023.

3. Williams RR, et al. Evidence that men with familial hypercholesterolemia can avoid early coronary death. An analysis of 77 gene carriers in four Utah pedigrees. *Journal of the American Medical Association,* 1986; 255: 219-224.

4. Vuorio AF, et al. Familial hypercholesterolemia in the Finnish North Karelia. A molecular, clinical, and genealogical study. *Arteriosclerosis, Thrombosis, and Vascular Biology*, 1997; 17: 3127-3138.
5. Alonso R, et al. Benefits and risks assessment of simvastatin in familial hypercholesterolaemia. *Expert Opinion on Drug Safety*, Mar, 2005; 4 (2): 171-181.
6. Goldman L, et al. Cost-effectiveness considerations in the treatment of heterozygous familial hypercholesterolemia with medications. *American Journal of Cardiology*, Sep 30, 1993; 72 (10): 75D-79D.
7. Sinzinger H, O'Grady J. Professional athletes suffering from familial hypercholesterolaemia rarely tolerate statin treatment because of muscular problems. *British Journal of Clinical Pharmacology*, Apr, 2004; 57 (4): 525-528.
8. Cooper F. *Cholesterol and the French Paradox.* Zeus Publications, Queensland, Australia, 2006.

Made in the USA
Lexington, KY
26 July 2010